T0136486

CLINICAL SKILLS, DIAGNOSTICS AND REASONING

EUREKA

CLINICAL SKILLS, DIAGNOSTICS AND REASONING

Ben Lovell MBBS MRCP FHEA MSc FAcadMEd DRCOG
Associate Professor of Medical Education
Consultant Physician in Acute Medicine,
University College London Hospitals NHS Foundation Trust

Mark Lander BSc MBBS MRCP
Specialist Registrar in Acute Medicine,
University College London Hospitals NHS Foundation Trust

Nick Murch MBBCh PG Cert Med. Ed. FRCP
Acute Medicine Clinical Lead,
Royal Free London NHS Foundation Trust
Honorary Clinical Associate Professor,
University College London Medical School

© **Scion Publishing Ltd, 2020**

ISBN 9781911510505

First published 2020

All rights reserved. No part of this book may be reproduced or transmitted, in any form or by any means, without permission.

A CIP catalogue record for this book is available from the British Library.

Scion Publishing Limited

The Old Hayloft, Vantage Business Park, Bloxham Road, Banbury OX16 9UX, UK

www.scionpublishing.com

Important Note from the Publisher

The information contained within this book was obtained by Scion Publishing Ltd from sources believed by us to be reliable. However, while every effort has been made to ensure its accuracy, no responsibility for loss or injury whatsoever occasioned to any person acting or refraining from action as a result of information contained herein can be accepted by the authors or publishers.

Readers are reminded that medicine is a constantly evolving science and while the authors and publishers have ensured that all dosages, applications and practices are based on current indications, there may be specific practices which differ between communities. You should always follow the guidelines laid down by the manufacturers of specific products and the relevant authorities in the country in which you are practising.

Although every effort has been made to ensure that all owners of copyright material have been acknowledged in this publication, we would be pleased to acknowledge in subsequent reprints or editions any omissions brought to our attention.

Registered names, trademarks, etc. used in this book, even when not marked as such, are not to be considered unprotected by law.

Clinical photography ©Sam Scott-Hunter (www.samscotthunter.co.uk)
    except where indicated in the Appendix

Cartoons by James Pollitt (www.jamespollitt-graphicnarratives.co.uk)

Other line artwork by Matthew McClements at Blink Studio Ltd (www.blink.biz)

Cover design by Andrew Magee Design Ltd

Typeset by Evolution Design and Digital, Kent, UK

Printed in the UK

Last digit is the print number: 10 9 8 7 6 5

Contents

Preface   vii

Acknowledgements   viii

Abbreviations   ix

1   Consultation and communication skills   1

2   Clinical reasoning   19

3   The general examination   35

4   Cardiovascular system   61

5   Respiratory system   99

6   Gastrointestinal system   127

7   Genitourinary system   159

8   Female reproductive system   181

9   Nervous system   213

10 Cranial nerves and ophthalmology   249

11 Musculoskeletal system   275

12 Psychiatry   301

13 Endocrine system   327

14 Paediatrics   353

15 Critically ill patients   377

16 Special circumstances   395

Appendix: Figure acknowledgements   411

Index   413

Preface

Healthcare students are very good at remembering things. Years of interviews, revision and examinations have trained you how to place limitless complex information into your head and retrieve it when required. Traditional medical textbooks focus on this process: teaching students to *know* what a healthcare professional *knows*.

This book takes a different approach. We want to teach you to *think* like a healthcare professional *thinks*. Possessing the knowledge is only part of the equation. Using this knowledge to make a reasoned diagnosis, and then develop a management plan for individual patients: this is the very soul and centre of clinical medicine. In our case studies, we lay out the thought processes and logical steps required when a healthcare professional meets a new patient. We show how some conditions can be ruled out or ruled in, and why diagnosis A is more likely than diagnosis B or C. Our ambition is to demystify the diagnostic process, and show you that clinical reasoning can be learned and developed, just like anything else.

The cases presented in this textbook bring the patient stories to life. There are two purposes to this. First, it is much easier to recall things that are cognitively linked to a specific person or context. Secondly, examining the patient version of the clinical case humanises the case. We show the patient's story because, in one sense, this is the only story. Patients bring their stories to doctors, and ask us to help them make sense of them, to influence them, to change them for the better. The illustrated cases help reinforce this message: it is never a case of *"how do you treat pneumonia?"*, but *"how do you treat this patient who has pneumonia?"*.

Finally, we hope you enjoy reading this book. Have fun with your learning if you can.

Ben Lovell
Mark Lander
Nick Murch

Acknowledgements

We would like to thank Sam Scott-Hunter for his excellent clinical photographs, as well as our models Marcus and Jessica who appear in them.

We would also like to thank James Pollitt for his cartoons, and Matthew McClements, who provided the other illustrations.

Abbreviations

ABPI	ankle brachial pressure index		**COPD**	chronic obstructive pulmonary disease
ACE	angiotensin-converting enzyme		**CPR**	cardiopulmonary resuscitation
ACh	acetylcholine		**CREST**	Calcinosis, Raynaud's syndrome, oEsophageal dysmotility, Sclerodactyly, Telangiectasia
ACS	acute coronary syndrome			
ACTH	adrenocorticotrophic hormone			
ADH	antidiuretic hormone		**CSF**	cerebrospinal fluid
AED	anti-epileptic drug		**CT**	computed tomography
AF	atrial fibrillation		**CXR**	chest radiograph
AKI	acute kidney injury		**DKA**	diabetic ketoacidosis
ARB	angiotensin receptor blocker		**DMARD**	disease-modifying antirheumatic drug
ATP	adenosine triphosphate			
AV	atrioventricular		**DNACPR**	do not attempt CPR
BAD	bipolar affective disorder		**DNAR**	do not attempt resuscitation
BMI	body mass index		**DoLS**	Deprivation of Liberty Safeguard
BP	blood pressure		**DRE**	digital rectal examination
bpm	beats per minute		**DVLA**	Driver and Vehicle Licensing Agency
CBT	cognitive behavioural therapy		**DVT**	deep vein thrombosis
CCB	calcium channel blocker		**ECG**	electrocardiogram
CCF	congestive cardiac failure		**EEG**	electroencephalogram
CHD	coronary heart disease		**EMG**	electromyography
CKD	chronic kidney disease		**ENT**	ear, nose and throat
CN	cranial nerve		**ESR**	erythrocyte sedimentation rate
CNS	central nervous system		**FAST**	focused assessment with sonography for trauma
CO	cardiac output			

FSH	follicle-stimulating hormone		**LSD**	lysergic acid diethylamide
GABA	gamma-aminobutyric acid		**LUTS**	lower urinary tract symptoms
GALS	gait, arms, legs and spine		**MCP**	metacarpophalangeal
GCS	Glasgow Coma Scale		**MCV**	mean cell volume
GH	growth hormone		**MDMA**	3,4-methylenedioxy-methamphetamine
GHB	gamma-hydroxybutyric acid		**MDT**	multidisciplinary team
GI	gastrointestinal		**ME**	myalgic encephalomyelitis
GMC	General Medical Council		**MI**	myocardial infarction
GnRH	gonadotrophin-releasing hormone		**MMSE**	Mini-Mental State Examination
GORD	gastro-oesophageal reflux disease		**MRC**	Medical Research Council
GP	general practitioner		**MRI**	magnetic resonance imaging
GTN	glyceryl trinitrate		**MRSA**	methicillin-resistant *Staphylococcus aureus*
GU	genitourinary			
HHS	hyperosmolar hyperglycaemic state		**MS**	multiple sclerosis
HIV	human immunodeficiency virus		**MSE**	mental state examination
HPV	human papillomavirus		**MSK**	musculoskeletal
HR	heart rate		**NA**	noradrenaline
HRT	hormone replacement therapy		**NAFLD**	non-alcoholic fatty liver disease
IBD	inflammatory bowel disease		**NASH**	non-alcoholic steatohepatitis
IBS	irritable bowel syndrome		**NCS**	nerve conduction studies
IGF	insulin-like growth factor		**NEAD**	non-epileptic attack disorder
IIH	idiopathic intracranial hypertension		**NMDA**	*N*-methyl-D-aspartate
IUCD	intrauterine contraceptive device		**NMJ**	neuromuscular junction
IUGR	intrauterine growth restriction		**NSAID**	non-steroidal anti-inflammatory drug
IV	intravenous			
JVP	jugular venous pressure		**NSTEACS**	non-ST elevation ACS
KUB	kidneys, ureter, bladder		**NSTEMI**	non-ST elevation MI
LGA	large for gestational age		**OA**	occipitoanterior
LH	luteinising hormone		**OCD**	obsessive–compulsive disorder
LMN	lower motor neuron		**OCP**	oral contraceptive pill
LOS	lower oesophageal sphincter		**OGD**	oesophagogastroduodenoscopy
LP	lumbar puncture		**OGTT**	oral glucose tolerance test

OP	occipitoposterior		SIADH	syndrome of inappropriate ADH
OT	occipitotransverse		SLE	systemic lupus erythematosus
OTC	over the counter		SNRI	serotonin–noradrenaline reuptake inhibitor
PCOS	polycystic ovarian syndrome			
PE	pulmonary embolism		SNS	sympathetic nervous system
PEFR	peak expiratory flow rate		SOL	space-occupying lesion
PET	positron emission tomography		SSRI	selective serotonin reuptake inhibitor
PID	pelvic inflammatory disease			
PIH	pregnancy-induced hypertension		STEMI	ST elevation MI
PMB	post-menopausal bleeding		STI	sexually transmitted infection
PND	paroxysmal nocturnal dyspnoea		SV	stroke volume
PNS	peripheral nervous system		SVC	superior vena cava
PPE	personal protective equipment		TB	tuberculosis
PPI	proton pump inhibitor		TCA	tricyclic antidepressant
PR	per rectum		TIA	transient ischaemic attack
PSIS	posterior superior iliac spines		TPN	total parenteral nutrition
PTH	parathyroid hormone		TPR	total peripheral resistance
PTSD	post-traumatic stress disorder		TSH	thyroid-stimulating hormone
PUD	peptic ulcer disease		UC	ulcerative colitis
PVD	peripheral vascular disease		UMN	upper motor neuron
REM	rapid eye movement		US	ultrasound
RIF	right iliac fossa		UTI	urinary tract infection
SA	sinoatrial		VRE	vancomycin-resistant enterococci
SFH	symphyseal fundal height		VSD	ventricular septal defect
SGA	small for gestational age		VTE	venous thromboembolism
			WCC	white cell count

Chapter 1
Consultation and
communication skills

Starter questions

1. Why might you put some of the *past medical history* or *drug history* in the *history of presenting complaint* section?
2. Why is it important to look at patients moving around the ward or when they are coming into the clinic room?
3. When might it be necessary to use closed rather than open questions?
4. Should you make notes during a consultation?

Answers to questions are to be found in *Section 1.9*.

1.1 Introduction

When you first start in clinical areas you might feel that you have some of the medical knowledge but without much chance to interact with patients, relatives or other healthcare staff. If you feel nervous, remember that patients are also often apprehensive about speaking to someone about their health, especially if they are worried they may get bad news. A daily occurrence for you might be a once in a lifetime occurrence to them. They may not remember what you say or do, but will always remember how you made them feel. Being asked personal questions and being examined can be embarrassing, even distressing for some people, so keep this in mind and thank them for their time and cooperation.

Developing your 'presence' (a combination of appearance including body language, communication skills, confidence, knowledge and personality) will help you to appear confident and give you a sense of authority, but be careful to not appear overconfident or arrogant. Show an interest in the patient, and ask them about themselves as a person, not just a patient. Enquire about occupations and pets, for example; you'll hear some fascinating stories.

1.2 The consultation

The consultation is the interaction between the clinician and the patient or the patient's relatives. There are numerous reasons why patients seek healthcare advice (**Table 1.1**); do not assume you know why they are there, as they may have a different agenda to you.

Table 1.1 *Some common reasons why patients seek healthcare advice*

Reason	Reasoning	Example
To register with a practice / healthcare professional	This is an opportunity to meet your new patient and get a benchmark set of tests	Registering with a new healthcare professional often requires a medication review, check on height and weight (for body mass index), blood pressure and urine dipstick check
To establish relationship with the healthcare professional	Some patients like to see if they get on with their healthcare practitioner, or if they trust them	Personal or mental health problem, to see what relationship is like with the practitioner
To establish a health risk	Do their family or friends have a history of significant disease?	Heart disease, cancer, diabetes, blood pressure, cholesterol
To monitor trends	Many patients need regular check-ups and monitor risks that trend over time without being noticed	Weight, body mass index, blood pressure
To check up on physical and mental health	Patients often have stresses in life that may lead to deteriorations in physical and mental health and require review	During pregnancy After childbirth After surgery After bereavement
To aid wellbeing	Patients occasionally have things in their life that are impacting on physical and mental health	Diets Sleep disturbances Weight Exercise
For regular recommended check-ups	Regular milestones to have check-ups at	Regular check-ups for babies and children to assess growth and development All adults should consider a check-up every 3 years; every year if aged >75
For regular follow-up of abnormal results	Review of previous abnormalities	Bone density scans Abnormal radiology Abnormal blood tests
For screening	Regular screening is advised for certain genders at certain ages	Breast cancer, prostate, colonic and cervical cancers
For vaccinations	To promote herd immunity in the general population or for those travelling abroad	Measles, mumps, rubella, tetanus, polio, diphtheria, pertussis, BCG, human papillomavirus (HPV), influenza vaccine (seasonal), pneumococcal and meningococcal vaccinations if at risk (e.g. hyposplenism) Hepatitis and influenza vaccine (seasonal) for healthcare workers or those in at-risk groups

Reason	Reasoning	Example
Medication reviews	Repeat prescriptions need periodic review	Asthma medication, antihypertensives, antidepressants, analgesics and many others
Travel advice	When going away on holiday or business it may be prudent to have travel advice	Water drinking advice Vaccination advice Prophylaxis advice (e.g. malaria, mosquito nets)
Administrative support	To provide or sign documentation	Signing passport documents or photos Letter for social services or JobCentre Sick or 'fit to work' notes Referrals for private healthcare Medical certificates for adventure sports, e.g. endurance sports such as Channel swimming
Family planning advice or genitourinary (GU) health screening	Advice on safe sex, contraception, and screening for sexually transmitted infections (STIs)	Oral contraceptive pill, coils, caps, condoms, implants, sterilisation Screening for and treating STIs
Concern about others	When concerned about relatives, neighbours, friends	e.g. when concerned for child or elder abuse, undiagnosed mental health issues or self-neglect
To get a particular problem reviewed	Review of a problem; note there may be a hidden agenda!	Lumps, bumps, discharges, concerns, who knows what will present next time?

The medical consultation is the basic tool for making an accurate diagnosis or management plan. The accurate medical history lays the foundations for further specific questioning, concise and appropriate physical examinations, and investigations. The examination and investigations are there to confirm or refute the potential diagnoses (differential diagnoses) raised from the history. Good communication skills are essential in order to ensure accurate information is obtained from the patient or carer, to guide the management plans. Communication skills also improve the quality and comprehensibility of the information received by the patient; in addition they enhance your rapport and ultimately, your relationship with the patient.

The history guides the examination and then any appropriate investigations, and as such you may be the first person to see them and start them on their path. An incorrect or inadequate history may lead to an incorrect patient journey, including unnecessary investigations. It is imperative to listen to the patient and gather information from other sources including relatives, witnesses, hospital records and radiology or pathology results already on electronic systems.

Try to gather as much information as possible in advance but be prepared to have an open mind and avoid cognitive bias (see *Chapter 2*). Always question previous diagnoses if there is a lack of supporting evidence, as they may have been attributed to the patient in error in the past. Some previous diagnoses are hinted at by the medications taken, but be aware some drugs have dual uses (e.g. alpha blockers for hypertension and prostate disease).

A full consultation takes as long as it requires. At the beginning of your career, it can easily take an hour to take a full history, carry out an examination and document findings. This will reduce with practice and experience.

1.2.1 First impressions

The first impression of a patient is full of useful clues about their physical and psychological state. For example, does their behaviour change when you enter the room or when their family or friends are present? Sometimes there is a 'gut feeling' when seeing patients. If your gut feeling is telling you that there is something wrong with a patient that you cannot name, this is your accrued experiential wisdom recognising that someone does not quite fit the illness script or exemplar in your mind (see *Section 2.2.2*). This sometimes leads to the healthcare professional getting a 'sense' that a patient is not well. If another healthcare professional says they are worried or that a patient is sick but cannot articulate why, then they may well be correct.

1.2.2 Appearance

Students and those in training often spend time worrying about what to wear when in clinical areas. You should feel comfortable, able to perform your job and instil confidence in patients and the general public.

The general advice is to dress respectfully and to appear clean. Despite limited evidence, patients often perceive that uniforms worn outside of the clinical setting pose an infection control risk. Patients and relatives often judge the professionalism of the person looking after them based on their appearance. Dressing professionally instils confidence in patients, and therefore trust; patients sometimes feel that a healthcare worker dressed too casually (or revealing a lot of their body) may not take their job, or their patient, as seriously as a smartly dressed professional, which leads to anxiety (**Figure 1.1**). How you dress therefore plays a role in developing a rapport between you and the patient. You should:

- wear clear identifiers (name badge and identification), so patients and other staff know who you are and that you have a right to be there
- avoid excessive cleavage, leg or chest exposure
- wear comfortable soft-soled, closed-toe shoes; you will be in them for many hours, standing or walking (and even running) in them
- consider covering tattoos if potentially offensive.

Patients, particularly in hospitals, often have lowered immunity and therefore are more vulnerable to infection, especially the more serious infections found in clinical areas. In order to minimise the transmission of infection between yourself and patients (and vice versa), you should:

- wear short-sleeved shirts, or shirts with sleeves folded to the elbow when providing patient care; there is limited evidence that being 'bare below the elbows' reduces the risk of passing infection between patients, but this policy has been taken up by most clinical institutions
- change into and out of uniforms, including scrubs, at work; this prevents infections from being brought into hospital
- change your clothes at the earliest opportunity if they are soiled (e.g. with blood) as they are unhygienic and look unprofessional to patients
- tie long hair back
- keep fingernails short and clean
- avoid false nails, hand or wrist jewellery (except perhaps a wedding band)
- regularly wash uniforms and work clothes at the highest temperature possible
- avoid excessive badges, lanyards, folders, dirty pens or equipment that could cause cross-contamination; consider cleaning your equipment with antibacterial or antifungal wipes when appropriate
- avoid free-flowing scarves and ties.

'Infection control' is the process of preventing the transmission of healthcare-acquired infections amongst patients, staff and visitors.

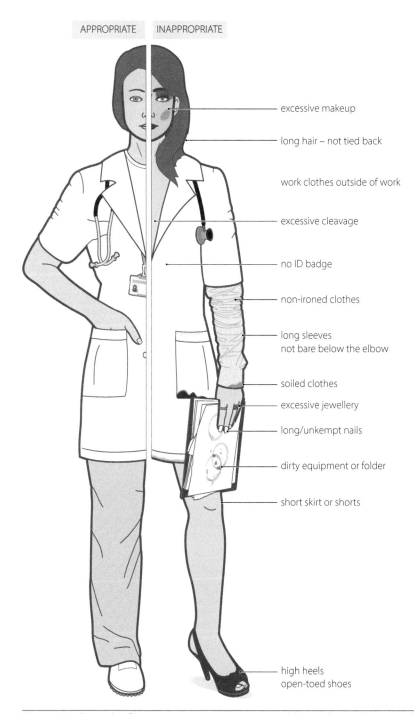

APPROPRIATE   INAPPROPRIATE

excessive makeup

long hair – not tied back

work clothes outside of work

excessive cleavage

no ID badge

non-ironed clothes

long sleeves
not bare below the elbow

soiled clothes

excessive jewellery

long/unkempt nails

dirty equipment or folder

short skirt or shorts

high heels
open-toed shoes

Figure 1.1 Example of inappropriate appearance at work (many, but perhaps not all, of these issues apply equally to men).

Medical uniforms

Historically, medical professionals have worn white coats or scrubs. White coats are much less common in the UK now due to infection control, but they may still be seen in some institutions. Some specialties often use scrubs, particularly surgical, anaesthetic and emergency specialties. Scrubs are thought to reduce the risk of infection, as they are washed after every use. However, there is some evidence that patients prefer their doctors to be in smarter attire, such as shirts, especially in outpatient departments.

1.2.3 Environment

The way a clinical area is set up helps to promote (or reduce) the opportunity for positive body language. Always assess first for one's own safety when in a clinical area, so you should perform a brief risk assessment before entering any area. In order to ensure that you are not left open to risk of violence or litigation (both very rare, but unfortunately they do occasionally occur), ensure a chaperone is available if appropriate, and be aware of the exits in case of emergency (**Figure 1.2**).

Ask yourself whether the setting is appropriate or not. Is it suitably private? What is the temperature of the room? Is there a gown or sheets present if an examination is required? Is it possible to get to the level of patient, either by sitting or crouching or elevating the bed during an examination? Patients feel a little intimidated if they feel their doctor or nurse is standing over them when talking to them. Therefore make sure there are chairs available that put you at face level with the patient during conversations, whether they are sitting in a chair or lying on a couch or a bed.

1.2.4 Communication skills

These are the skills needed to enable conveying information to or from another individual or group in an effective way. Communication can be verbal (words), non-verbal (body language), written or pictorial. A large proportion of our communication is non-verbal; how it is said is often more important than the content.

Open and closed questions

Open and closed questions are ways of asking for information, and should be used in combination as required. Certain situations may lend themselves more to one style than the other, but generally you should start with open questions then hone in with closed ones if required.

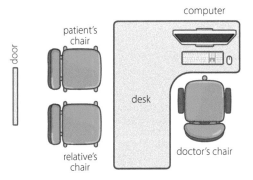

EXAMPLES OF POOR PRACTICE

- desk is perceived barrier
- attention on computer screen
- doctor cannot easily see patient enter and may be trapped

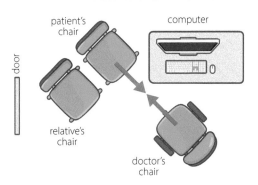

EXAMPLES OF BETTER PRACTICE

- less of a perceived barrier
- easier to flip attention from patient to screen and vice versa
- doctor can see patient enter, and less difficult to leave in an emergency

Figure 1.2 How to set up a clinical room.

Closed questions

Closed questions (e.g. *How old are you? Do you feel hot?*) have very short concise answers. They give you facts, are quick and easy and leave the questioner in control of the conversation. However, they do not allow the patient to provide rich, complex information about their health or illness. Using closed questions allows you to lead the conversation, and may therefore address your agenda but not necessarily that of the patient. Therefore closed questions are not appropriate for gathering information at the outset of the consultation, but are useful for clarifying, checking and quantifying the symptoms the patient wants to discuss.

Open questions

Open questions are broader questions that invite the patient to give a descriptive, detailed answer, e.g. *How do you feel?* They have a tendency to lead to long answers that require follow-up with other open, or even closed, questions for clarification. They allow the person answering to think and reflect, offering opinions and feelings, and it may be perceived that you hand the control of the conversation over to the respondent. With practice you will learn to guide the conversation without leading it with closed questions.

Body language

More than 50 percent of communication is non-verbal. The appropriate use of receptive body language and correct tone of voice are critical for healthcare professionals. Generally an open posture is preferred when trying to communicate with patients, relatives or other healthcare professionals. Crossed legs or arms suggest an unwillingness to interact. You should face the person with whom you are interacting, whilst maintaining an appropriate level of eye contact (**Table 1.2**).

Presence

The clinical presence is the person and atmosphere you choose to project during your consultations. Tips to optimise your presence as a healthcare professional include:

- Dress appropriately and comfortably
- Have an open body posture, and carry yourself with positive posture, displaying confidence
- Smile when introducing yourself and your role

Table 1.2 *Non-verbal communication and how to optimise it*

Non-verbal communication	Potential problems	Possible solutions to consider
Posture	Slumped in chair or looking out of the window indicates a lack of interest	The body should ideally be positioned facing the other people in the room Sit up straight when possible
Limb positioning	'Arms crossed' or rising shoulders seem threatening or hostile	Relaxed and open position of arms is a positive, receptive signal
Eye contact	Studying the floor, looking away when responding, or failing to make eye contact, likely signal nervousness or lack of trust	Maintaining eye contact communicates your attention, interest and focus on the other person
Facial expressions	Be aware that others usually pick up subconscious grimaces or smiles – the mouth and face need to be conveying the same message	A simple smile (with eye contact) conveys a message of a positive and helpful attitude as well as confidence Nods signal agreement
Tone of voice	Using jargon, speaking too quietly or quickly or mumbling	Clearly spoken words, delivered at an unhurried pace and a moderate tone of voice

- Remember, patients and relatives are usually more scared or worried than you, but you must also accept they may be experts in their conditions
- Speak clearly and concisely
- Practise active listening
- Show 'in the moment humility'; if you are unsure about something, say so; don't make things up but say that you'll find out from someone who will know or that you are prepared to look it up
- Show an interest in what's going on and don't be afraid to ask questions if you're unsure what is happening.

Active listening

Active listening means taking part in the conversation and working on the rapport between the parties involved. Some tips:

- Maintain an appropriate level of eye contact throughout
- Keep open, relaxed, yet professional body language (uncrossed legs and arms, leaning slightly forward in chair if seated)
- Ask open questions then try to funnel the answer by asking more closed ones if appropriate
- Nod to show you acknowledge what the patient says
- Find shared common ground – e.g. enquire about pets, ask where they are from, ask about employment. Shared experiences mean they are much more likely to build a rapport with you, communicate effectively and have a positive experience at what can be a scary time
- Avoid interrupting

- Summarise and negotiate a list of their concerns, agreeing which are the most urgent / worrying.

Suggested active listening techniques:
- **Mimicry** – repeat the last thing they said as well as using the same body language
- **Rephrasing** – reiterate their comments in a new sentence to show understanding
- **Reflecting** – put their feelings into words for them in an empathetic manner – legitimising their emotions ('it's OK to feel like that').

Some particular groups (such as those with sensory or learning difficulties) provide more challenges in trying to establish a rapport or gain a history or consent. **Table 1.3** has some suggested techniques for these groups.

Cultural awareness

Cultural awareness is of paramount importance and includes the need to be aware of and accept differences in gender, sexual orientation, socioeconomic status, disability, age, ethnicity and language. Certain groups often have particular expectations from healthcare professionals; some patients still dress in their best clothes to see you! You should have an understanding of the potential variation in approach needed to these different individuals and should react to cues appropriately. Some patients request to be seen by someone of a particular gender; this should be accommodated if you can, but is not always possible. Personal feelings should not affect the behaviour of healthcare professionals towards patients or relatives.

1.3 Initiating the consultation

The consultation begins before the first direct interaction with the patient from the moment they arrive, the way they have accessed seeing you, for example via ambulance or patient transport and how they enter the room, or you enter theirs. Some patients may have been in hospital for a period of time, so be aware

you may be entering their personal space. The introduction sets the environment for the whole future relationship. During the introduction it can be possible to assess the patient's gait and mobility, and upper limb strength and coordination, as well as their hearing and speech.

Table 1.3 *Some common difficulties when communicating with patients and relatives / carers and how to address them*

Patient group	Potential problems	Possible solutions to consider
Learning difficulties	Not enough time for consultation	Book an enhanced slot, particularly for the first appointment
		Talk directly to the patient, bringing the carer into the conversation with the patient's permission
	Difficult for them to understand you	Make eye contact, try to build rapport and establish trust
		Make all reasonable adjustments possible
	Unable to gain information from patient	A 'health passport' contains important information about the patient and is owned by the patient; it lists the patient's likes and dislikes, sleeping and behaviour patterns, preferred communication methods as well as clinical information; an example is the 'red bag' scheme
	Gaining trust and consent for examination	Tell the patient and carer what is going to happen in the consultation; demonstrate any examinations or procedures before performing and consider sedation in rare cases.
	Information inaccessible to patient	Visual aids: picture mats, photos, videos, face pain scale, emojis
		Check understanding
Visual impairment	Unable to read the medical information and literature provided	Encourage people to bring their usual aids including guide dogs
		Show the person where the bathroom and call button, etc. are, rather than giving directions
		Make handwriting more legible by choosing a dark felt tip pen and write neatly using thicker strokes. Ensure letters are in large font or Braille if possible and required.
Hearing impairment	Lip reading difficulty	Face the person so they can see your lips
		Make sure you are well lit so the person can see both your body and face clearly
		Speak clearly and at a normal pace – do not shout
		Use gestures to help explain what you are saying
		Use whole sentences rather than one-word replies – lip reading is often pattern recognition
		Be patient – if you are asked to repeat something, vary it slightly
		Write or draw what you mean
		Check, if appropriate, whether they have their hearing aid with them and if working
	Hearing aid problems	Use the stethoscope in reverse for problems with the ear itself (conductive hearing loss). Speak into it as a mouthpiece and place the tips in the patient's ears

Table 1.3 *(cont'd)*

Patient group	Potential problems	Possible solutions to consider
	Sign language difficulties	Try to arrange someone who can sign if possible – note there are different types of sign language even in English
Speech impairment or muteness	Unable to understand patient	Allow them time to write down things when needed
Child patients	Parents interrupting	Speak to the patient where possible; they need to be heard; consider other adjustments as above
Patient unhappy with waiting	Angry patient	Don't accept blame unless it is your fault *'Hello Miss France, my name is Kevin Jennings, one of the doctors. Thank you for waiting.'* *'I understand that it can be frustrating'* Say *'thank you for waiting'* as opposed to *'sorry about the wait.'* Of course, remember your safety first. If the patient is aggressive or abusive, you must leave to maintain your safety

Tips for introducing yourself to patients include:
- Assess the most appropriate method for introduction each time
- In a clinic hold the door open for the patient
- Ask permission to enter a patient's room, or to open curtains around their bed
- Smile when introducing yourself and your role
- Establish what the patient wants to be called, and try to remember their name for future meetings.

Some patients prefer to be titled, e.g. Mr. Lowe or Dr Roberts; some will want to be called by their first name. This preference may guide what to call yourself. If they want to be called by a title you may want to call yourself by your title, e.g. Dr Khan or Professor Summerskill, or your full name and position. If they prefer first names, consider using yours.

Establish why the patient thinks they are there and what the purpose of the interaction is.

Try not to project stress, time constraints, personal views or biases on the patient or relatives. Also avoid being dismissive of a patient's frustrations or concerns, particularly if they have waited a long time to be seen.

1.3.1 Developing rapport

Rapport is a state of harmony that allows more effective communication between those involved. It puts both parties at ease, increasing the amount of important and potentially sensitive information shared.

Empathy plays a role in the establishment and maintenance of a good rapport. Patients are more likely to be honest and forthcoming to a doctor exhibiting empathy and compassion. This can be demonstrated by showing respect for a patient's beliefs and practices and supporting them in their own decision-making. If patients have capacity then they are allowed to make what may be seen as 'unwise' decisions, and they should have your support if appropriate.

You must gain consent to speak to, and then examine the patient. First establish the reason for the consultation so that both parties are clear as to the expected outcomes. Ask the patient early on about any concerns or expectations, as they may not be able to focus on the rest of the consultation until these are addressed.

1.4 Gathering information

Communication can be verbal or non-verbal. If a patient is avoiding eye contact or has a closed body posture then something might be making them feel uncomfortable. Generally, use open questions where possible and follow up with closed questions if appropriate. Find out what is their first language; it is much easier for both you and the patient to use an appropriate interpreter or a translation service, instead of being unclear with each other due to linguistic limitations.

There is often a complex interplay between acute and chronic health issues, the patient's lifestyle, their social set-up and their relationships with family and friends. Be wary of using relatives (especially children) as interpreters, especially if conveying potentially sensitive information.

Always introduce yourself, and any others present, and check the identity of the patient and their preferred name. Also check the identity of any others present as their relationship may not be immediately obvious; don't assume the relationship! Direct the conversation to the patient themself where possible, rather than towards a relative or friend. Check if the patient wants others to stay during the consultation (where possible), and ensure a chaperone is present (and name documented) for any examination that requires one. Try to avoid situations with the possibility of exposing either yourself or the patient to potential risk including violence, spurious accusations or potential cross-infection.

1.4.1 Taking the history

Do not fall into the trap of interrupting patients during their opening statements. This interruption gives the patient the impression that they are being hurried or that you are not listening. Most patients will 'run out of steam' within 30 seconds but this brief period allows the patient or relative to feel heard.

Allow the patient to finish speaking then follow up with appropriate questions – try not to interrupt and allow silence if appropriate, as the patient will often offer information when there is an obvious opportunity.

Helping to build rapport
- Ask how they are; offer them a seat / glass of water
- Empathise with any emotion they display / verbalise and acknowledge the difficulty / stress of situations they could be experiencing (watch them carefully)
- Listen and respond to the things they say.

Keeping the pace of the conversation steady, and the language suitable for the individual (usually plain layman's terms unless medical or scientific), helps with the overall experience.

Some tips for effective communication include using only one or two information words in a sentence. Don't overburden the patient with questions. Use layman's terms rather than medical terms when possible, whilst speaking at a steady pace, giving the person plenty of time to respond to what you've said. Check that they have understood what you have said by asking them to tell you what they think you said; this can be very enlightening. Don't be afraid to use pictures or symbols to reinforce ideas, as appropriate.

1.5 The medical history

The consultation, and thus the documentation of the history, should have a familiar appearance. This structure should be clear in your mind before seeing the patient and has a relatively standardised format:
- Presenting complaint (PC)
- History of presenting complaint (HPC)
- Past medical history (PMH)
- Medication / drug history (DH)
- Family history (FH)
- Social history (SH)
- Systems review

1.5.1 Presenting complaint (PC)

This is one word or phrase in the patient's own words. A good question to gain the presenting complaint is 'Why am I seeing you today?' Record the answer in the notes, e.g. "shortness of breath" or "vomiting".

1.5.2 History of presenting complaint (HPC)

This is an elaboration on the presenting complaint; it should explore important facets of the chief complaint and will help to guide towards a differential diagnosis. Common questions might include:
- When did the PC first start? How did it start?
- What other symptoms are associated with the PC?
- Has the patient ever had this before?
- Is the PC a constant phenomenon or does it come and go? If it is intermittent, what brings it on? How regularly does it occur?
- What treatments has the patient tried for this problem, if any? Did they work?

1.5.3 Past medical history (PMH)

This is a representation of important medical and surgical conditions that can be listed in chronological order, order of relative importance or in the order recounted. Ask about previous operations, when they were, if they have had previous hospital admissions, whether they see a specialist for any conditions, or if they attend the GP regularly. Would they describe themselves as usually fit and well?

Use the acronym **MJ THREADS** to remember the important previous co-morbidities in older patients:
- **M**I (myocardial infarction; heart attack)
- **J**aundice
- **T**uberculosis (TB)
- **H**ypertension
- **R**heumatic fever (rare in the UK now)
- **E**pilepsy
- **A**sthma/COPD
- **D**iabetes
- **S**troke

Many older patients struggle to remember the details and dates of all of their past medical history, particularly for illnesses in the distant past. Using their medical records is a useful way of filling in the blanks, assuming the records are correct and you have access to them. If a patient can't remember the exact date of a procedure or a diagnosis, ask them if they remember whether it was in their 20s, 30s, 40s, etc. This is usually sufficient.

1.5.4 Medication / drug history (DH)

This includes medications that are currently being taken or that have been used in the preceding weeks and months. Also ask specifically about over-the-counter (OTC) medications, dietary supplements and herbal remedies. These substances are often forgotten by patients or considered irrelevant as they were not prescribed, and they can, rarely, lead to side-effects or affect how well their other medications work. An allergy history should be elicited, along with the reaction caused.

Ask specifically if patients take medications including OTC drugs such as antacids, analgesics (painkillers) or sedatives. Patches (nicotine, painkillers, etc.) may not be seen as medication by the patient. Oxygen is also a prescribed drug.

1.5.5 Family history (FH)

This section highlights any potential genetic illnesses in the family. Common inherited illnesses that should be elicited in the family history include:
- sudden unexplained or cardiac death
- some cancers, such as colon, breast and ovarian
- heart attacks or strokes under the age of 50
- rare neurological illnesses
- autoimmune diseases
- kidney disease.

1.5.6 Social history (SH)

The social history gives you the opportunity to learn about your patient as a person. What is their day-to-day life like? What do they do for work and in their free time? The purpose of the social history is to generate a clear idea of how the patient lives their life, how they manage, and what their priorities are. This helps you to 'humanise' the patient (instead of considering them as a clinical puzzle to be solved) and facilitates your decision-making process when creating a holistic management plan. It also allows you to comprehend how their daily life impacts upon their health, and how their health (or illnesses) impact upon their lives.

Subsections of the social history include employment, functionality, and use of illicit or non-prescribed drugs and alcohol.

Employment history

Asking about employment (past and present) provides information regarding exposure to potential precipitants of disease, e.g. tobacco smoke, asbestos, alcohol, sun or potential allergens. People who spent all of their working lives in pubs have often been exposed to tobacco smoke during that time. Factory workers, farmers, carpenters, and many others in manual professions are exposed to irritants and chemicals that cause or exacerbate respiratory diseases; these conditions may improve if they go on holiday, for example.

Functional history

'Functional' in this context means how the patient interacts with and copes within their usual environment. It is particularly relevant in older patients or those with disabilities. Elements of the functional history include:

- How do they manage to walk (often called 'mobilise')?
- Are they independently mobile or do they use walking aids, such as sticks, a walking frame or wheelchair?
- Are they able to leave their home? If so, is that alone, or with assistance?
- If they are unable to leave their home, can they walk around the house, or are they bed-bound or chair-bound? Has this led to pressure ulcers?
- Do they live in their own home, or in a facility such as a residential or nursing home?
- Do they have any carers? If so, how many times

a day or week do they visit and what sort of activities do they help with?
- If there are no carers, does the patient need family members or friends and neighbours to visit them regularly to help?

If you are assessing a patient during an acute illness, then you should ask about their functionality when they were last well; this is called their 'premorbid state', or their 'functional baseline'. You can use this information to help qualify how their acute illness has affected their functional status, and use it as a target for potential rehabilitation after the acute illness is over.

Drugs, alcohol and smoking

These substances have a profound impact on patients' physical and psychosocial health. Ask patients politely about their recreational habits, and without judgement. Patients sometimes lie, particularly about their smoking and alcohol consumption, if they sense a judgemental attitude, usually out of embarrassment.

Smoking

Ask about their smoking history, including when they started and whether they still smoke. Some will say they have given up, meaning that morning! You can record the smoking history as number of cigarettes per day, or as 'pack years' if they are long-term smokers.

> **'Pack years' is a useful way of quantifying a patient's long-term smoking habits**. One pack year is 20 cigarettes/day for one year. Therefore:
> - Someone who smoked 20 cigarettes/day for 40 years has 40 pack years
> - Someone who smoked 40 cigarettes/day for 40 years has 80 pack years
> - Someone who smoked 10 cigarettes/day for 40 years has 20 pack years
> - Someone who smoked 60 cigarettes/day for 60 years has 180 pack years

If someone does smoke, ask what it is they smoke; do not assume they mean tobacco. Do they use shisha? Do they smoke marijuana? Both substances are associated with more severe lung damage in comparison to cigarettes. If they roll their own cigarettes, ask how long a pack of tobacco lasts (often they will not use filters so the effects may be even more deleterious). Also ask about e-cigarettes and vaping, although the long-term effects of these substances on health are currently unknown.

Alcohol

Ask about alcohol consumption, and ask about what type of alcohol, e.g. strong beer or spirits. 'Occasionally' or 'socially' is not particularly meaningful. If someone is uncertain about how many units of alcohol they drink, try rephrasing the question; for example, ask how long a bottle of vodka (for example) usually lasts.

> **It is not recommended to exceed 14 units of alcohol per week**. As a rough guide, one unit of alcohol is:
> - one 25 ml measure of spirits, e.g. vodka
> - one small glass of wine (125 ml)
> - half a pint of medium strength beer/cider (4% alcohol by volume)
>
> Note, stronger beers (5–6% ABV) have 2.5–3 units in a pint, rather than 2.

Other drugs

Asking about recreational drug use should be considered in every history, especially in higher risk patients, such as those with heavy alcohol intake, chaotic social situations, or with mental health disorders.

Common drugs of abuse are cannabis, cocaine, amphetamines, and oral or injectable opiates.

So-called 'legal highs' and synthetic cannabinoids are becoming more common recreational drugs. A good way of covering all forms of drugs of abuse is to ask if they've ever smoked, swallowed, snorted or injected any drugs, including body-building or performance-enhancing medications.

1.5.7 Systems review

This is an overview of all the major body systems, i.e. respiratory, gastroenterological, cardiovascular, neurological, psychiatric, musculoskeletal and dermatological. It acts as a screen for potential problems.

This section sounds lengthy, but it usually involves asking general screening questions, such as:
- Any problems with the bowels or waterworks?
- Any headaches, seizures, numbness or weakness?
- Any breathing difficulties?
- Any heart problems?
- Any aches, pains or swelling in your joints or muscles?
- Any rashes?
- How is your mood?

1.6 Explanation and planning

Once the relevant information has been gathered, potential differential diagnoses should be presented back to the patient or their representative in small bite-sized portions, without jargon. It is sometimes useful to draw simple diagrams or offer patients the opportunity to see their radiology (X-rays or scans) or blood result trend on the computer. Patients and relatives will often look things up themselves so be prepared for them to have some understanding and questions regarding the potential diagnoses. If they ask a question

that cannot be answered immediately then let them know you will check this for them or ask someone else who is better placed to make that assessment.

Try to avoid false reassurance, and explain the relative likelihood of the various differential diagnoses. The potential risks and benefits of both investigations and potential therapies should be explained in as simple terms as is appropriate. There should be an agreed management plan including both the immediate management of the current medical condition as well as the further investigation of the differential diagnoses. The location for management and time of review are needed, as well as considering potential plans for discharge if appropriate. Treatment escalation plans should be considered, discussed and documented (see *Section 2.7.2*).

1.6.1 Finishing off

At the end of the consultation thank the patient for their time and summarise the main outcomes for them. You should, where possible, follow up the patient, to assess your own decision-making and for self-appraisal of the differential diagnoses suggested.

1.7 Breaking bad news

Telling people bad news is a very sensitive issue. A common scenario is having to tell a patient an unwelcome diagnosis. If it is potentially a difficult conversation, then consider the SPIKES model (**Table 1.4**) as an aide memoire.

1.8 Ethico-legal considerations

Consent should be obtained from the patient (or their designated deputy, if the patient lacks capacity) before looking at their notes or results, and before speaking to or examining the patient. This is often assumed but should be clarified when required.

Health records must be clear, accurate, factual and legible and should be contemporaneous. They must include all relevant clinical findings, the decisions made, information given to patients, and drugs or treatment prescribed. Personal views about the patient's behaviour or temperament should not be included unless they have a potential bearing on treatment, or it is deemed necessary for the protection of staff or other patients.

Documentation in the notes or on prescriptions should be made legibly in black ink, with capital letters for drug names. All entries should be dated and timed, with a legible signature, grade and contact details documented. Each leaf paper of the clinical notes should have at least three patient identifiers on them (preferably on both sides in case of photocopying / scanning.

Health records should not be altered or tampered with, other than to correct inaccurate or misleading information. Any such amendments must be made in a way that makes it clear what has been altered, who made the alteration and when. Healthcare professionals should ensure that their manner of keeping records facilitates access by patients if requested. It is helpful to order, flag or highlight records so that when access is given, any information which should not be disclosed (such as that which identifies third parties) is readily identifiable.

Patient-identifiable information should not be removed from the clinical area, and information should only be shared with the minimum number of people necessary to care for the patient. Patients and their results should not be discussed in public areas including canteens, lifts, etc. Social media sites should be treated the same as any other public area. Breaches of patient confidentiality will lead to disciplinary action including large financial penalties.

Data protection must be maintained for both written and electronic records. Destroying patient-identifiable data requires paper pulping or shredding, and encryption and destruction software for electronic data. All data must only be kept for the minimum time needed for use, then destroyed appropriately.

Table 1.4 *Using SPIKES as a tool to help communicate, including breaking bad news*

Part of conversation	Potential problems	Possible solutions	Phrases to consider
Setting	Where to break bad news	A comfortable, quiet and private area, preferably with somewhere to sit. Have tissues and water available where possible. Arrange chairs so they all face each other without physical barriers, e.g. a desk. Ensure unlikely to be interrupted by telephone, bleep, people wanting to access room.	*'Would you like to discuss this somewhere a little more private?'*
		Other healthcare workers who know the patient or can provide support in breaking the diagnosis, e.g. nurse specialists or their own nurse.	
	Who to have with you or them	Ask the patient if they want anyone to be with them. If there is someone else there already, check to see if your patient would prefer them to stay or leave, after checking the relationship.	*'Would you prefer to have a family member or friend here?'*
Perception	What they already understand	Discuss any symptoms the patient has been experiencing up to this point. Discuss the events leading up to now: scans, blood results, biopsies, etc.	*'Could you tell me what's happened up to this point?'*
		Establish what the patient already knows or is expecting. Establish the patient's current emotional state and if there is anything particular on the patient's mind (any ideas, concerns or expectations the patient might have).	*'The reason we did the tests was so we could find out why you have been experiencing these symptoms.'*
		The patient may not be aware of the possible diagnoses but often fears the worst.	*'What did you think these tests were looking for, or might show?'*
Invitation	Check if the patient wants to receive all the information today	Some patients, who recognise that the news isn't what they hoped for, may want to put it off until family are present, or after a holiday or family occasion, etc.	*'I have the result here, how much would you like to know today?'*

Part of conversation	Potential problems	Possible solutions	Phrases to consider
Knowledge	Check what you and they know about the subject matter	Ensure you deliver the information in manageable chunks, and regularly check for understanding.	*'As you know, we performed a test and the results were not as we hoped.'*
		Make sure your tone is respectful, at a slow pace and clear. Allow pauses.	
		Some patients do not hear or remember anything after a word such as 'cancer'. After giving the diagnosis, it's wise to wait for the patient to re-initiate the conversation.	*'I'm sorry to tell you this… but the results show you have cancer.'*
		Give the patient time and space to have an emotional reaction. They often go quiet, ask questions, go into denial, start crying, or become hysterical or angry.	*'I'm so sorry I had to break this news to you.'*
Empathy		Recognise and respond to emotions with acceptance, empathy and concern.	*'I can see that this is not the news that you expected, I'm so sorry.'*
		Acknowledge and reflect their emotions and body language.	
		Give the patient time to have their emotional reaction. People often find it very uncomfortable watching patients like this, but give the patient space to just react.	
		If they are asking questions like *'What will happen next?'* then they are ready to receive answers to their questions.	
Summary / strategy		Check understanding.	*'Can I check what you think is going on?'*
		Summarise important points – those with an emotional response will not take in much information.	
		Make a plan to meet again / plan the next steps.	
		Ensure you answer any questions or concerns.	
		Offer ongoing assistance to the patient, such as giving them details of a clinical nurse specialist or specialty team, if appropriate.	*'I'm so sorry, but at this stage, I don't have enough information to answer that.'*
		Highlight other sources of information / support (groups, websites, charities) as well as written material to take away.	

1.9 Answers to starter questions

1. It is useful to have information about chronic disorders, relevant family history or medications in the *history of presenting complaint* (HPC) section, especially if they impact upon the PC. For example, in a case of pneumonia, the patient's smoking status provides important information about their acute illness. If someone with chronic lung disease has previous admissions to the intensive care unit, this suggests that their disease is severe.

2. It is useful to look at patients moving around the ward or coming into the clinic room, even when not formally assessing them, to see how they move when not obviously observed. Assessing gait is a useful test of multiple functions, and some patients change their behaviour when they feel observed.

3. It might it be necessary to use closed rather than open questions in a few situations. An obvious example is when refining your questioning after an open question. Other less obvious uses include when there are only a few choices possible – such as asking the specific frequency or dose of a drug if the patient cannot remember the name. It might also be necessary to ask very specific questions, such as 'do you take ibuprofen or paracetamol?' Many patients do not appreciate that OTC medications are drugs too.

4. Note-taking during a consultation may be seen as rude or intrusive by patients, but it is necessary if remembering important details is difficult. Many professionals make notes during a consultation early in their career, but the need to do this should diminish with time. You should make any notes as soon as possible after the consultation.

Chapter 2
Clinical reasoning

Starter questions

1. Can medical histories be taken by computer programs?
2. How many diagnoses are patients allowed to have?
3. Is it possible to teach doctors how to think?

Answers to questions are to be found in *Section 2.8*.

2.1 Introduction

Clinical reasoning is the process of thinking critically, analysing information pertaining to a patient and their illness, using clinical judgement and problem-solving to generate and test hypotheses to reach a diagnosis, and instigating and evaluating investigations.

It is involved in:

- diagnostic reasoning
- prioritising patients
- creating summaries and formulations of a patient's illness
- planning and interpreting investigations
- making management plans.

Clinical reasoning is not solely for making diagnoses. It is a skill required for every interaction with patients in order to guide their healthcare. It is used to recognise sick or deteriorating patients, identify errors, and when discussing treatment options with the multidisciplinary team. It guides every decision we make with patients.

2.2 Diagnostic reasoning

Diagnostic reasoning is the translation of medical information (i.e. a patient's symptoms, signs, examination results and investigation results) into a rational diagnosis, using your medical knowledge and experience. There are different methods of reasoning; in practice an experienced clinician would be able to use more than one, employing the most useful in any given situation. These methods include:

- hypothetico-deductive reasoning
- pattern recognition, e.g. illness scripts
- heuristics
- dual process theory
- metacognition
- recognition of reg flags.

19

Understanding why errors are made during diagnostic reasoning, and reflecting on the process of reaching a decision, will help to improve your reasoning and decision-making.

2.2.1 Hypothetico-deductive reasoning

The hypothetico-deductive approach is a method of analytical reasoning and it forms the basis of the scientific method. As the medical history is taken and the patient examined, a working list of diagnoses is developed; these are called the 'differential diagnoses' (**Figure 2.1**). These differential diagnoses are the 'hypotheses' of hypothetico-deductive reasoning. Further history, examination and clinical investigations are then chosen in order to corroborate or refute these diagnoses until the one 'true' diagnosis remains.

For example, consider a patient presenting with the following problems:

- Polyuria and polydipsia (excessive thirst and urination)
- Weight loss
- Chronic cough
- Strong smoking history
- Constipation
- Depression.

In the case above, potential causes of excessive thirst include hyperglycaemia, hypercalcaemia, diabetes insipidus and diuretic medication overuse. Each of the other symptoms has a similar list of potential causes and associations. You must direct the history to explore any connections between these causes. For example, a differential diagnosis for chronic cough is asthma, so the doctor asks about the other features of asthma (wheezing and breathlessness) to support or refute asthma as a differential. As each symptom is explored, the associated features are linked together until a unifying diagnosis is achieved (**Figure 2.2**).

This analytical approach is particularly useful for medical students and junior doctors, who may not have enough clinical experience to use pattern recognition (see *Section 2.2.2*).

2.2.2 Pattern recognition

Experienced physicians will develop mental 'illness scripts' or 'illness exemplars'; these are cognitive frameworks that incorporate the relevant information about a specific illness. These are remembered and compared with a newly-presenting patient; if the presentation matches an illness script this provides a quick diagnosis. A common illness script used by experienced physicians is the patient 'archetype'. This is a hypothetical patient with all of the characteristics of a particular disease. For example, the archetype in **Figure 2.3** is of a 'Cushingoid' patient; a patient with hypercortisolism.

Another example is if a patient presented with a cough, breathlessness and a fever; this compares with the classic exemplar of a chest infection. The doctor is therefore able to generate a rapid diagnosis and initiate treatment with antibiotics. It negates the requirement to build up a list of differential diagnoses via the hypothetico-deductive approach.

2.2.3 Dual process theory

This is the theory that human reasoning and decision-making incorporates two systems:

- System 1 is automatic, implicit, rapid and experiential
- System 2 is purposeful, explicit, slow and analytical.

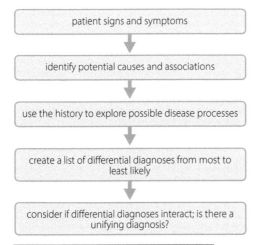

Figure 2.1 A template of the hypothetico-deductive approach.

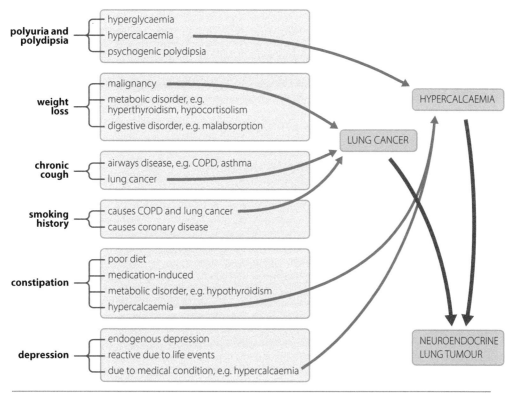

Figure 2.2 The hypothetico-deductive approach to diagnosis, using the example of a neuroendocrine lung tumour.

Both systems are present within the realm of clinical reasoning. When collating and amalgamating data from the patient history and examination, system 1 offers up 'immediate' differential diagnoses, often based on pattern recognition. Therefore, system 1 thinking is more closely related to professional experience and illness scripts. System 1 thinking is useful for reaching rapid diagnoses, but is vulnerable to 'knee-jerk' reaction to the information: jumping to a foregone diagnostic conclusion without a considered approach.

System 2 thinking is more closely bound to the hypothetico-deductive approach to clinical reasoning, and is therefore more commonly employed by less experienced clinicians.

Dual process theory recognises that both systems play a part in clinical reasoning. An experienced doctor quickly generates one or several differential diagnoses for a patient (system 1), and then uses a considered and analytical

approach to verify, justify or refute them (system 2). A less experienced clinician also uses both systems, but their system 1 thinking is more prone to error, due to a lack of illness scripts to guide them. An example is shown in **Figure 2.4**.

2.2.4 Heuristics

Heuristics are embedded mental 'rules of thumb' or cognitive shortcuts that facilitate rapid analysis and reasoning when solving a problem. They're commonly expressed in terms of 'common sense' approaches, or useful maxims to help make general inroads into a clinical reasoning process.

A commonly cited heuristic in medicine is 'if you hear hoof beats, they are more likely to be caused by a horse than a zebra'. In other words, look for the simplest, most common explanation to a problem first. This is often shortened to the warning 'don't think zebras': don't diagnose the least likely or rarest diagnosis when a more likely or common one will fit.

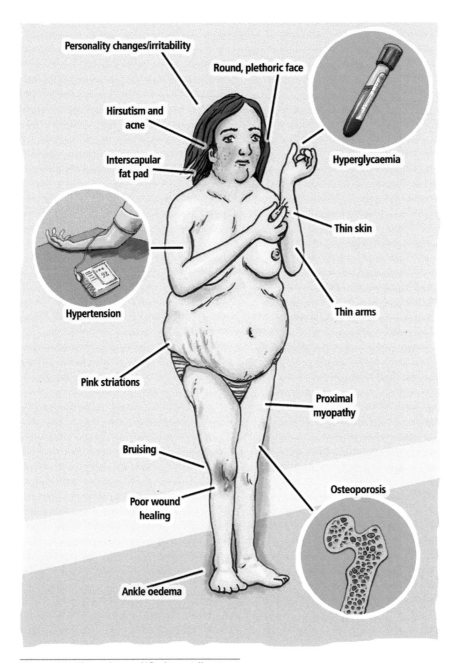

Figure 2.3 The archetypal 'Cushingoid' patient.

Other common medical heuristics are listed in **Table 2.1**.

Heuristics are a way of simplifying difficult decisions. Doctors use heuristics both consciously and unconsciously on a daily basis. They are invaluable tools when working in fast-paced environments, such as the emergency department. However, they hold the potential for introducing cognitive errors.

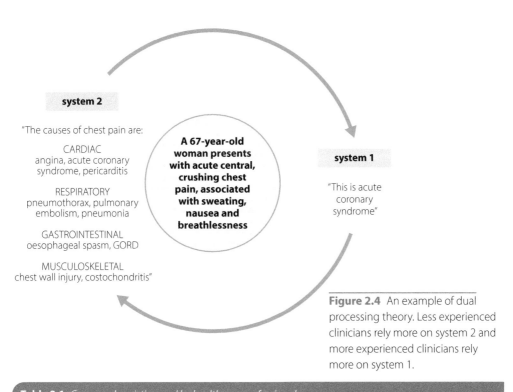

"The causes of chest pain are:

system 2

CARDIAC
angina, acute coronary
syndrome, pericarditis

RESPIRATORY
pneumothorax, pulmonary
embolism, pneumonia

GASTROINTESTINAL
oesophageal spasm, GORD

MUSCULOSKELETAL
chest wall injury, costochondritis"

A 67-year-old woman presents with acute central, crushing chest pain, associated with sweating, nausea and breathlessness

system 1

"This is acute coronary syndrome"

Figure 2.4 An example of dual processing theory. Less experienced clinicians rely more on system 2 and more experienced clinicians rely more on system 1.

Table 2.1 *Common heuristics used by healthcare professionals*

Heuristic	Meaning	Example
First do no harm ('If in doubt, do nowt')	In clinical uncertainty, no treatment is the least injurious option for the patient	A surgeon is uncertain whether an operation will improve a patient's condition or not. The potential risks of the operation may outweigh the risks of leaving the condition untreated, but it is impossible to be certain. The surgeon elects not to perform the surgery.
Recognition heuristic	Using a single feature or a few features of a history to reach a rapid diagnosis based on pattern recognition	Rapidly diagnosing a pulmonary embolism (PE) in a patient with acute pleuritic pain and breathlessness following an operation, as the patient has the 'classic' features of a PE
Treat the patient, not the numbers	Make management plans based on the patient's whole clinical status and wishes, rather than on test results or quantitative measurements	A patient is incidentally found to have a slow heart rate of 40 beats per minute at a check-up (normal is 60–100). However, the patient feels completely well, so the doctor decides not to implant a pacemaker.
Rapid screening tools	These are quick decision aids to identify or rule out serious medical conditions based on simple criteria.	The FAST criteria: if a patient has one of the following features they may be having a stroke and an ambulance should be called: **F**ace drooping **A**rm weakness **S**peech disturbance **T**ime to call ambulance

2.3 Errors and bias

Errors in diagnostic reasoning rarely come from incompetence or poor knowledge; rather from imperfect thinking processes. These types of mistakes are called 'human factors', as they relate to the fact that healthcare professionals are human beings who are prone to mental slips, lapses in judgement and misperception of clinical information; particularly when tired, very busy or under pressure.

Errors and biases result in patient harm, and reducing their prevalence and impact is of crucial importance.

2.3.1 Cognitive errors

Whilst heuristics play an important role in making rapid decisions, they have the potential to induce cognitive errors. Cognitive errors are 'thinking mistakes'. Even though a doctor has all the necessary information to make a reasoned decision or diagnosis, a cognitive error leads them down the wrong mental pathway. Cognitive errors are responsible for the vast majority of medical errors and clinical mistakes. They usually occur when system 1 thinking completely replaces or overpowers system 2 thinking.

Common cognitive errors are explored in **Table 2.2**.

Table 2.2 *Common cognitive errors encountered in clinical reasoning*

Cognitive error	Meaning	Example
The anchoring heuristic	Remaining bound to one's initial diagnosis, and interpreting information in a way that supports this 'anchoring diagnosis'	A doctor diagnoses a patient with pleuritic pain due to a chest infection. He attributes the elevated D-dimer (a blood chemical that is classically elevated in blood clots) level to the infective inflammatory process. An eventual CT scan reveals a pulmonary embolism.
The representative heuristic	Arriving at a rare diagnosis due to the 'textbook' nature of the clinical scenario	A doctor treats a woman with recurrent abdominal pains, hypertension and a psychiatric history, and diagnoses acute intermittent porphyria – a rare metabolic disorder – due to the classical features of the disease. The patient in fact has the much more common diagnoses of hypertension and irritable bowel syndrome.
Premature closure	Settling on a hypothetical diagnosis without accruing enough data to verify or refute it	A busy emergency department doctor encounters a young female patient with severe lower abdominal left-sided pain. She recognises the classic signs of appendicitis and refers her to the surgeons without doing a pregnancy test. Further investigation reveals an ectopic pregnancy.
The availability heuristic	The thinker has a tendency to diagnose conditions that they find easier to recall and describe	A patient with severe nausea and vomiting is found to have pancreatitis. His doctor remembers that the commonest causes of pancreatitis are gallstones and alcohol, so recommends abstinence from alcohol and requests ultrasound scans of the biliary system. However, the patient actually has autoimmune pancreatitis (rare).

Although over-reliance on system 1 thinking is the root cause of most cognitive errors, system 1 thinking is not a bad thing. It helps senior clinicians make rapid and safe decisions based on minimal data and their professional experience. However, it must be balanced out by parallel system 2 thinking.

2.3.2 Cognitive bias

A bias is an inclination to a particular decision, outcome or way of thinking. Most cognitive biases are unconscious, so doctors are unaware if they are affecting their clinical reading, and to what extent. Some biases can be thought of as personality traits, such as:

- **risk aversion**: choosing safe options for the patient at all times, even if this results in suboptimal outcomes

- **tolerance to risk**: choosing potentially more risky options for the patient if the outcomes could be good
- **overconfidence**: unwillingness to reflect upon one's own thinking or make any changes
- **sensitivity to hierarchy**: inability or strong aversion to challenging more senior doctors' clinical reasoning
- **blind obedience**: unthinking acceptance of another (usually senior) doctor's assessment.

Other biases are related to how a patient or a clinical problem is perceived on a case-by-case basis (**Table 2.3**).

2.3.3 External pressures

Doctors are more prone to making cognitive errors when under external pressures, such as:

- **time constraints**: trying to finish the work before the end of the shift

Table 2.3 *Common cognitive biases that affect clinical reasoning*

Cognitive error	Meaning	Example
Illusory correlation	Perceiving a relationship between two phenomena that isn't actually there	A doctor prescribes antibiotics to all patients with a fever, and sees that resolution of the fever as confirmation that antibiotics 'cure' all fevers, whereas the majority of the patients had a viral infection that simply ran its course and the antibiotics did nothing
The framing effect	The manner in which a disease or treatment is presented to a doctor affects their opinion of it	A doctor is much less likely to choose a treatment option if they hear that it has a 25% mortality rate than if it is presented as having a 75% survival rate
Ascertainment bias	Seeing what you expect to see, or using stereotyping or profiling in clinical reasoning	A homeless alcoholic man presents to the emergency department complaining of a headache and asking for sedatives. The attending doctor decides that the patient is drug-seeking, and discharges him from the department. The patient has a generalised seizure outside the hospital.
Recent case bias	After encountering a rare case, repeatedly suspecting it in consequent cases	A doctor misses a diagnosis of a rare sarcoma in a patient presenting with shoulder pain. She then screens all new patients with shoulder pain for sarcoma for fear of missing another case.

- **senior pressure**: being given large amounts of work by a senior colleague
- **split focus**: trying to stay on top of many different tasks at the same time.

These external pressures are not exclusive to doctors. They affect all people working in healthcare, and therefore all have the potential to cause patient harm.

2.3.4 Internal pressures

Internal pressures refer to the biopsychosocial factors within the doctor that influence their thinking processes and induce biases and cognitive errors. The commonest internal factors that significantly affect clinical reasoning are the HALT factors:

- **H**ungry
- **A**ngry (or experiencing another emotion that destabilises thinking, such as sadness)
- **L**ate for work
- **T**ired

These factors are transient phenomena that have profound influences on doctors' behaviour and thought processes.

2.3.5 Getting the diagnosis wrong

Diagnostic accuracy is hard to measure, but diagnostic mistakes are made by all doctors at all levels of experience and seniority. Some mistakes have no effect on the patient, whilst some cause serious harm. It is therefore expected that diagnostic errors will happen, and the task of a healthcare system and the individual doctor is to reduce the volume and the impact of these errors to an absolute minimum.

Doctors are encouraged to report their own errors without fear of judgement or penalty, as part of a no-blame culture. This recognises that doctors do not make mistakes out of negligence, malignity or incompetence. Once a mistake is reported, the details are analysed by an investigator, who determines the individual

factors that led to its occurrence. The doctor in question is included in this investigation, and is invited to reflect on the entire case in order to facilitate their own learning and perhaps recognise and address the cognitive errors and biases that caused it.

2.3.6 Metacognition

Metacognition is a way of avoiding unconscious biases and errors, or noticing them in your own thinking before they can cause patient harm. It is the process of 'thinking about thinking' or 'mindful thinking'.

Metacognition can be a parallel process to usual thinking, and generally focuses on asking oneself questions such as:

- 'Is there anything else that this could be?'
- 'Is this the most likely diagnosis or do I want it to be the diagnosis?'
- 'How much is my decision being influenced by the fact that I am hungry / angry / late / tired?'

Metacognition can also be a reflective process, after the fact. Reflective practice is a common aspect of the postgraduate curriculum in most healthcare systems. It encourages doctors to critique and analyse their own actions and mental processes, and helps them bring previously unacknowledged cognitive biases to light. This therefore helps the doctor recognise if they are, for example, risk averse, risk tolerant, or perhaps overconfident in their clinical reasoning. Metacognition is therefore a skill that can be learned and practised.

> **The enormous role cognitive error plays in everyday medicine has only been recognised in recent years.** Postgraduate teaching and training has undergone a substantive evolution to incorporate metacognitive thinking, reflective practice and self-identification of 'thinking mistakes'.

2.4 Prioritising patients

Rapid prioritisation of patients is a crucial skill for healthcare workers, requiring good history-taking skills and recognition of red flag features. In the emergency department, the sickest patients must be identified and seen first. In the GP surgery, prioritising helps decide whether a patient needs to be seen the same day, as a routine appointment within a week, or referred to the emergency services.

2.4.1 How to prioritise patients

Prioritisation is a challenging skill to learn. As a doctor, there are multiple competing demands for your attention and time, and the people you interact with often have different priorities to your own. Assessing and treating patients in a safe and efficient manner depends on your ability to recognise emergencies, scan histories and clinical examinations for red flags, and differentiate between illness and disease.

Recognising emergencies

Acute derangement of the basic physiological parameters is a common feature of most medical emergencies (**Figure 2.5**). These parameters are the 'vital signs', and they serve as the primary red flags for any disease process:

- Blood pressure
- Heart rate
- Respiratory rate
- Oxygen saturations
- Core temperature.

Many hospitals use an Early Warning Score (EWS) for inpatients to help doctors and nurses prioritise the more unwell patients. The EWS is generated from a scoring sheet that assigns points to different vital signs. A patient with completely normal vital signs has an EWS of 0, which allows the doctor to safely move them down their list of priorities. An extremely unwell patient with very abnormal vital signs receives a higher EWS, such as 8–10, and must therefore be seen very urgently.

Red flags

A red flag symptom is a clinical feature that raises the seriousness or urgency of the potential diagnosis. Whilst many red flag symptoms eventually prove to be innocuous, they should act as a cognitive trigger, and prompt a refocus of the patient examination to exclude serious illness.

Common red flags are detailed in **Table 2.4**.

Disease versus illness

When prioritising patients, it is important to detect whether the patient is at their usual health baseline, or whether there is an acute deterioration in their health status. A patient may have multiple diseases but not be necessarily ill. Many patients are able to lead normal lives whilst suffering from a chronic condition, such as diabetes, and do not consider themselves 'ill' for most of the time.

2.4.2 Triage

Triage is the system of classifying the severity and urgency of an illness to ensure that patients are seen in a safe and timely manner. This prioritisation necessitates a rapid evaluation of the patient's presenting symptoms.

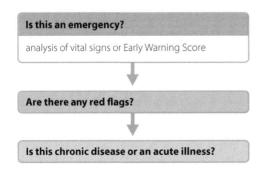

Figure 2.5 The process of prioritising patients.

In emergency departments, the first healthcare professional a patient encounters **is the triage nurse**, who takes a quick history, records their vital signs, and assigns them a triage category, often based on a traffic light system:

- Red = emergency: patient must be seen by a doctor immediately
- Yellow = urgent: patient must be seen within the hour
- Green = non-urgent: patient can wait in a queue to see the doctor

| Table 2.4 | | | Common 'red flags' that should alert the history-taker / examiner to the possibility of a serious or dangerous diagnosis requiring urgent treatment |

Presenting symptom	Red flag	Explanation
Back pain	Neurological impairment	Whilst musculoskeletal back pain is one of the commonest presenting complaints to primary care, the presence of sensory or motor impairment implies that the spinal cord has been damaged – this requires emergency evaluation to prevent permanent disability
Headache	Thunderclap onset	This is the hallmark of a subarachnoid haemorrhage, a potentially fatal condition
Syncope / collapse	Self-injury	This implies that the patient has no warning (or presyncope) that they are going to collapse, and is associated with epileptogenic or arrhythmogenic causes
Cough	Haemoptysis	This can herald lung cancer or tuberculosis
Gastro-oesophageal reflux disease (GORD)	Iron-deficiency anaemia	This can be found in gastric or oesophageal bleeding, due to severe inflammation or peptic ulceration
Head injury	Loss of consciousness	This implies significant concussion, or an intracranial haemorrhage
Loss of appetite	Significant unintentional weight loss	This is a constitutional feature of malignancy of any part of the body

2.5 Summarising and formulation

Summarising is the process of encapsulating and reiterating the key points of a clinical story into a brief paragraph. This is done to help the listener comprehend what you think are the key features of the patient's story. Formulation is the process of conceptualising the clinical case by articulating potential diagnoses, and exploring the causes and outlining a management plan.

2.5.1 Summarising the history

A clinical summary is three or four sentences of information that effectively highlight the issues identified in the history and examination. As a general rule, a good case summary should include:

- **important positive findings**, e.g. 'the patient has experienced recurrent central chest pain'
- **salient negative findings**, e.g. 'there are no ECG findings in keeping with coronary ischaemia'.

A case summary should not include unimportant negative findings, i.e. negative findings not related to the case. For example, there is no need to mention that the patient does not have nail clubbing, when summarising a case of heavy periods (menorrhagia).

If there are numerous positive or negative findings, group them into one broad category. For example, instead of stating: 'There is no sign of clubbing, palmar erythema, Dupuytren's contractures, leukonychia or asterixis', state simply: 'There are no peripheral signs of chronic liver disease'.

Template for summary

A useful template for an effective clinical summary is:

- **Sentence 1**: The name, age and presenting complaint of the patient
- **Sentence 2**: Important features of the history of presenting complaint
- **Sentence 3**: Past medical history and drug history relevant to the current presentation
- **Sentence 4**: Important psychosocial factors that influence the current presentation.

2.5.2 Summarising the examination

When presenting the examination findings, use the chronological order of the examination itself as a template. This means beginning the presentation with:

- the general impression of the patient
- peripheral findings in the hands
- signs detected in the face, eyes, mouth and neck
- signs detected in the chest or abdomen, as appropriate.

Again, it is not necessary to list all negative findings, only those pertinent to the positive findings.

2.5.3 Formulation

The clinical formulation begins with a concise summary, but then synthesises the clinical history and examination findings to form a provisional diagnosis. In addition, the formulation should:

- outline any differential diagnoses
- suggest potential investigations to confirm or refute the diagnosis
- discuss the biological, psychological and social factors that have predisposed, precipitated and perpetuated the current clinical condition
- outline a holistic treatment plan that addresses the likely prognosis.

Differential diagnosis

It is rare to immediately arrive at one single diagnosis in a clinical case. Instead, doctors state the single most likely (primary) diagnosis, followed by a list of differential diagnoses, which are the possible alternatives if the primary diagnosis proves to be false. The primary diagnosis is influenced by the patient's signs and symptoms, epidemiological factors, and the doctor's clinical knowledge and ability.

For example, if a patient presents with a chronic bilateral headache which has been slowly worsening over a period of weeks, the doctor may make a primary diagnosis of tension-type headache, and a differential diagnosis of an intracranial tumour. Their case formulation would mention the clinical features that strengthen or weaken the case for their diagnoses, and propose their investigations, such as a CT scan of the head.

Case 2.1: Worsening breathlessness and cough

The following case illustrates a biopsychosocial approach to the management of a 64-year-old man with a new diagnosis of chronic obstructive pulmonary disease (COPD).

History summary

Mr Townsend is a 64-year-old retired gardener who presents with worsening breathlessness and cough. His symptoms have been gradually worsening over a 6-month period, and are associated with production of small amounts of clear sputum but no haemoptysis. He has no previous respiratory diagnosis, but is a lifelong smoker of tobacco, and currently smokes 30 cigarettes a day. He is worried that his symptoms are deteriorating and is frightened that he might have lung cancer.

Examination summary

Mr Townsend is comfortable at rest, but notably breathless on walking. His respiratory rate is 20 breaths per minute, his heart rate is 84 beats per minute, and his blood pressure is 134/67 mmHg. His oxygen saturations are 97% on room air. There is no nail clubbing. Auscultation and percussion of the chest are normal.

Case 2.1 *continued*

Formulation

Mr Townsend is experiencing worsening respiratory symptoms, which are chiefly cough, breathlessness on exertion and mild sputum production. Considering his smoking history, the most likely diagnosis is COPD. A differential diagnosis would be an interstitial lung disease such as fibrosis, but the absence of nail clubbing and crackles make this less likely. A second differential diagnosis would be lung cancer, although he has not experienced any red flag symptoms such as weight loss, anorexia or haemoptysis.

2.5.4 Medical records

Legality

Medical notes are legal documents. Keeping clear and contemporaneous notes is a key obligation in the General Medical Council's *Good Medical Practice* guide for UK doctors. Such notes are a record of the doctor's findings, thinking processes and reasoning, formulations and management plans. All interactions with a patient must be documented in their medical notes. This ensures that:

- future healthcare professionals are able to gain a clear insight into the clinical case from reading your notes
- you are able to recall important features of the case when you reread your notes at a later date
- in the rare cases of medico-legal investigations and complaints, there is a comprehensive record of what occurred; this is crucial if the patient or another party is making allegations about you or the hospital.

For these reasons it is commonly stated that 'if it isn't documented in the notes, then it didn't happen'.

Medical records must fulfil certain criteria:

- They must be legible.
- They must be comprehensible.
- Only common abbreviations that are generally understood should be used, e.g. ECG for electrocardiogram.
- Each entry must have the date and time it was written clearly documented alongside.
- Each entry must be completed with the writer's name, job title, contact number and signature.
- They must be contemporaneous – written at the time of the events being recorded or as soon after as possible.

Pejorative, sarcastic or facetious entries in patient notes are unprofessional. Be mindful that patients have a legal right to see their own notes; don't write anything down that you would not say directly to the patient.

Confidentiality

Medical notes are bound by doctor–patient confidentiality. Paper notes must be kept in the clinical areas, and never removed from the hospital unless accompanying the patient to another medical institution. Electronic notes should be password protected.

Identifiable patient details must be sent by encrypted email only – a facility that is provided by most hospitals and surgeries. Texting patient details is considered an insecure method of communication, due to concerns about confidentiality. Any documentation with patient identification details must be destroyed, rather than simply thrown away.

Data protection is an important responsibility for healthcare professionals, and breaches often have serious repercussions. Patients must be able to trust doctors to keep their stories and lives private and secure.

2.5.5 Presenting patients

Communication of clinical information is ubiquitous in healthcare. Presenting patients is the process of transmitting a patient's story and your analysis from one healthcare professional to another. This happens at the beginning and end of every shift, when patients move from one department to another, or when referring patients from your care to another doctor or to a specialist. This process must be precise and efficient in order to avoid the 'Chinese whisper' effect, especially when the patient's information is passed from doctor to doctor to doctor.

> **Errors in communication are a contributing factor in 30% of medical malpractice cases**. Presenting clinical cases to colleagues therefore demands careful attention to detail, and efficient organisation of clinical information into comprehensible and logical data sets. Medical students spend much time learning how to present patients to their tutors, in order not only to assess their history-taking ability, but also to refine their communication skills.

Medical students usually find that each doctor has their own preferred style for presenting patients. However, a good presentation should be:

- **concise**: extraneous information is distracting and sometimes confusing for the listener – only include information that is relevant to the clinical case
- **organised**: each section of the medical history (see *Section 1.5*) should be clearly defined by the presenter
- **coherent**: each section of the history should be presented in a bullet point style, rather than in continuous prose, as bullet points are easier for the listener to follow
- **complete**: the presentation should be concluded with a summary and, if appropriate, a formulation of the case.

2.6 Investigations

The selection of investigation follows on immediately from the case formulation, and establishes how you will confirm or refute your primary diagnosis, or ascertain which of your differential diagnoses is the correct one.

Choosing clinical investigations in order to confirm or discount a provisional diagnosis requires careful consideration of the following factors:

2.6.1 Accuracy

There are two metrics used to classify the accuracy of a clinical test.

Sensitivity

This is the ability of a test to correctly detect patients who have the illness. A test with a high sensitivity (>95%) yields very low numbers of false negative results, so it is useful for ruling out a potential diagnosis. In other words, a negative test result is very likely to be a true negative.

A high sensitivity test may still have a high level of false positives, i.e. a low specificity.

An example of a high sensitivity test is a computed tomography (CT) scan to detect lung cancer.

Specificity

This is the ability of a test to correctly detect patients who do not have the illness. A test with a high specificity yields very low numbers of false positive results, so it is useful for confirming a diagnosis. In other words, a positive result is very likely to be a true positive.

A high specificity test may still have a high level of false negatives, i.e. a low sensitivity.

An example of a high specificity test is lumbar puncture to detect subarachnoid haemorrhage.

2.6.2 Availability

More complex investigations are not available at every institution, and doctors must use the resources at their disposal. The 'gold standard' investigation for a pulmonary embolism is a CT pulmonary angiogram, an image modality that may not be available in smaller hospitals, so doctors there may opt for the slightly less sensitive ventilation / perfusion scan instead.

2.6.3 Discomfort or harm to patient

Whilst some investigations are non-invasive, such as an electrocardiogram, others may cause pain or carry a risk of complications. In these cases, the risks and benefits of the test must be discussed with the patient. For example, a coronary angiogram carries a very small risk of MI, but has an extremely high sensitivity and specificity for diagnosis of coronary artery disease. Therefore the doctor may elect to perform CT coronary angiography, which is less accurate but non-invasive and therefore carries a low risk of harm.

2.6.4 Prevalence of the potential diagnosis

Following the heuristic that hoofbeats usually mean horses, not zebras, it is good practice to investigate for the common causes of a patient's symptoms first. For example, a patient with a new diagnosis of hypertension is much more likely to have essential hypertension, rather than a phaeochromocytoma (a rare catecholamine-secreting tumour), so imaging of the adrenals and measuring catecholamine levels are not considered 'first-line' investigations.

2.6.5 Financial considerations

Some tests are considerably more expensive than others. Doctors have a responsibility to ensure that their institution has the appropriate funds to provide equitable healthcare for all patients. For this reason, inexpensive investigations are common, even if the accuracy is imperfect. For example, nearly all patients presenting to hospital undergo blood tests. Blood results often do not clinch the ultimate diagnosis in the way an expensive full body magnetic resonance imaging

(MRI) scan would, but they provide the doctors with more medical data in order to reach a diagnosis.

2.6.6 Benefits of a diagnosis

Not all symptoms require investigation. If a clinical diagnosis is apparent, then a treatment plan is possible without tests. An example would be a patient presenting to the GP with a cough and green sputum production. The GP will prescribe a short course of oral antibiotics for a chest infection without performing blood testing or a chest X-ray. A patient presenting with viral symptoms would not need investigation, as there is no treatment for common colds, other than simple home remedies.

In palliative care, doctors make decisions about investigating symptoms in accordance with the patient's prognosis and quality of life. For example, if an elderly patient with terminal cancer developed heartburn, her palliative care doctor may suggest treating the symptoms with antacid therapy, rather than performing an endoscopic examination of the stomach and oesophagus, as there would be no possible finding on endoscopy that would alter the patient's treatment or prognosis.

2.6.7 Example investigations

Mr Townsend (*Case 2.1*) requires investigations to support or rule out the differential diagnoses of COPD and possible lung cancer. Lung function testing is a non-invasive and accurate method of diagnosing small airway obstruction (see *Section 5.7.3*), with a sensitivity and specificity of around 90%. Both chest X-ray and a chest CT detect lung lesions in keeping with cancer, but a chest X-ray is a better test as it is accurate, non-invasive, involves much lower doses of radiation than a CT scan, and is much less expensive to perform.

2.7 Problem-based management plans

The management plan details how to treat the patient after making a diagnosis. In some environments, such as the GP surgery, there is no

access to the tests you need to narrow down your list of differential diagnoses to a single diagnosis, such as X-rays, CT scan and lung function tests.

Therefore GPs often include the investigations they would like to do in their management plans. However, most management plans are made after the diagnosis has been ascertained.

Problem-based management plans should use a biopsychosocial approach to treating the whole patient, rather than focusing on treating just the disease. Patients should be involved in the formation of management plans. This requires taking time to explain the different options to patients, as well as the risks and benefits of the different treatments available.

> **The acronym PARQ is a useful way of discussing each treatment option with patients**:
> - **P**lan: this encompasses the details of the doctor's proposed management plan
> - **A**lternatives: this explores other potential approaches to treatment
> - **R**isks: this details the potential risks of the plan
> - **Q**uestions: this encourages the patient to ask any questions about the proposed treatment

2.7.1 Example management plan

Consider *Case 2.1*. Mr Townsend's lung function tests reveal an obstructive lung defect in keeping with COPD. His chest X-ray does not show any lung tumour. He requires treatment to improve his symptoms.

Biological

Mr Townsend requires inhalers to maintain bronchodilation and improve his symptoms of breathlessness. He must stop smoking to prevent deterioration of his condition.

Psychological

Mr Townsend is likely to need help to stop smoking. Nicotine replacement therapy and smoking cessation nurses may be useful in supporting him through this lifestyle change, which many people find challenging.

Social

Mr Townsend has found it difficult to go to his social club due to his breathlessness, which has

been making him feel isolated and miserable. Reclaiming his independence and social life is an important motivator for him to stay abstinent from tobacco and control his symptoms.

2.7.2 Treatment escalation planning

Not every treatment is appropriate for every patient. For example, transferring a patient who is dying of an advanced, incurable and end-stage disease to the intensive care unit for intubation, ventilation or renal replacement therapy is often not appropriate. The patient is likely to die irrespective of these interventions, and will likely suffer harm and distress through the move.

Treatment escalation plans describe the decisions made about what would be appropriate treatment to offer a patient, should they deteriorate at some point in the near future. This is relevant not only to hospital inpatients but also to patients who are at home or in care homes. Sometimes, not returning to hospital and being allowed to die naturally at home (with the appropriate support) if community-based treatments fail, is the right decision for a patient.

Treatment escalation planning balances the likelihood of a given treatment being beneficial to a patient, i.e. helping them to recover or stabilise, against the side-effects, invasiveness and potential suffering caused by that treatment. Be mindful that the decisions made are individualised to the patient in front of you rather than the diseases or co-morbidities that they have. Whilst in the UK it remains that a clinician decides what treatments are and are not offered to patients, all treatment escalation plans must be discussed with and explained to patients and those important to them. This conversation must be clearly recorded in their medical record so that other healthcare professionals can access it when needed.

Treatment escalation plans are intentionally made in advance. They often require actions to be carried out to ensure that appropriate care is possible, particularly when setting up support for a person to die at home. Delaying decisions to the point at which there is no more time often leads to rash decisions that are not appropriate to the patient they affect, resulting in harm and suffering.

The decisions cover all treatments including intravenous (IV) medications, clinically assisted nutrition and hydration, non-invasive ventilation, invasive organ support and cardiopulmonary resuscitation (CPR). If it is decided that CPR is not appropriate then a "Do Not Attempt Cardiopulmonary Resuscitation" (DNACPR or DNAR) order must be completed.

2.8 Answers to starter questions

1. The history taker must be responsive to the information that they uncover, analysing and creating meaning from what the patient is and is not saying, and adapt the ongoing history to gain insight into the biopsychosocial causes and effects of their symptoms. This requires a human ability to make intuitive and analytical connections between data.

2. As medical science advances, more patients are living longer and with more co-morbidities. Whilst it is possible for a healthy young patient to present to a doctor with a single diagnosis, such as a urinary tract infection, older patients commonly experience acute worsening of their chronic conditions during times of intercurrent illness. Therefore a clinical formation for an older patient usually comprises a list of diagnoses, which may be a domino effect: one health problem exacerbating or triggering other acute problems.

3. Medical education has historically focused on the transmission, retention and recall of information. Clinical reasoning and critical thinking were tacit abilities that doctors developed 'on the job' as they accrued experience. It is now apparent that the ability to reflect on one's own thinking processes, use a blend of knowledge and experience to make analytical and intuitive insights into a clinical case, and weigh up different approaches in patient management, can be explicitly taught to learners. Medical teachers are increasingly using reflective practice and metacognitive techniques to enhance their students' reasoning skills.

Chapter 3
The general examination

Starter questions

1. Why is examination performed after the history has been taken?
2. Why is it necessary to examine patients when medical tests and imaging are so advanced?
3. Why might a patient refuse to be examined?
4. Is it possible to determine the blood pressure without using any equipment?
5. If oxygen saturation can be detected using a simple finger probe, why are arterial blood gas measurements needed?

Answers to questions are to be found in *Section 3.14.*

3.1 Introduction

Examination of the patient is at the heart of the physician's craft. Detecting clinical signs of disease, however subtle, and threading them together to form a rich understanding of the patient's physical health is a skill that must be practised and refined over time. It would take too long to examine every part of the body for every patient. Instead, a physician uses the information from the history and pieces together the pattern of symptoms to guide the appropriate body systems to examine. This chapter describes the structure followed when examining any body system. The details of individual body system examinations are described in later chapters; the parts of the body that are not covered, but are no less important, are described here. Usually, one begins with the peripheral examination before homing in on the particular organ system. This allows you to look for signs outside of the particular body system (such as in the fingernails or around the hair or eyes) before focusing on the organ's anatomical area. These peripheral signs give you a clear indication of how well the person is.

3.2 Approach and preparation

Throughout this book, we use the acronym 'ID CHECK' to signal the mandatory actions you must take before examining a patient.

These actions are described below.

- **ID**entify the patient and yourself
- **C**onsent
- **H**and washing
- **E**xposure
- **C**omfort maintained
- **K**indly proceed.

3.2.1 Identify the patient and yourself

Check the patient's identity to ensure you have not approached the wrong patient. This may seem obvious in the GP or clinic setting, after a consultation. However, in a busy hospital ward, you may well be asked to examine a patient without taking a history or establishing a relationship with them, and mistaken identities do happen.

Identify yourself; all healthcare workers should introduce themselves when they first meet a patient, regardless of why they are interacting with them. Develop the habit of saying "Hello, my name is ..." as the very first thing you say to a new patient. Introducing yourself politely and professionally is the first step in establishing a rapport and relationship of trust between a patient and healthcare professional. Remember that most patients meet many different people on their journey through ill health, which is bewildering and often frightening, especially when they feel unwell and vulnerable.

3.2.2 Consent

Always ask the patient's permission before undertaking any examination. This is firstly a courtesy; you are often asking the patient to at least partially undress, which can feel awkward and embarrassing for them. Secondly, examining a patient without consent, especially more intimate examinations involving the breasts, abdomen or genitalia, could be construed as assault. The patient answering "yes" or nodding their head in response to the simple question "Do you mind if I examine your chest now?" is sufficient consent.

3.2.3 Hand washing

Hospital-acquired infection is an infection obtained whilst being in hospital that would

not have been picked up outside of that environment. Common examples include MRSA (methicillin-resistant *Staphylococcus aureus*), C. diff. (*Clostridium difficile*) and VRE (vancomycin-resistant enterococci). These infections cause significant illness and even death. They are often difficult to treat and are easily spread from person to person through skin contact. The biggest cause of spread within hospitals is through poor hand hygiene. Always wash your hands, either with soap and water or alcohol hand gel, using the seven-stage hand washing technique (**Figure 3.1**), both before and after you examine a patient, even if it is just to take their pulse.

Some scenarios require you to wear gloves, aprons or face masks (collectively known as personal protective equipment or PPE). Gloves are worn when performing any internal (i.e. rectal or vaginal) examination, when touching any open wounds or sores, when performing procedures (such as venepuncture) or handling bodily fluids.

> **When washing your hands, the general rule is: alcohol gel if not contaminated, soap and water if contaminated**. Hands are considered as being contaminated if you have used gloves, come into contact with bodily fluids or been inside a room with infection control protocol.

Some patients with transmissible diseases are nursed in side rooms. This is to reduce the risk of spreading infections to other patients within the hospital. Wearing gloves and aprons (and face masks for infections such as TB or influenza) prevents microbes landing on your hands and clothing. By removing these inside the room and washing your hands with soap and water before leaving the room, you help to prevent spread when visiting other patients.

3.2.4 Exposure

It is difficult to palpate an abdomen or auscultate the lungs through the patient's clothes or hospital gown; too many clinical signs will be missed. This means the patient should be exposed. Privacy and dignity are paramount, so only expose the area

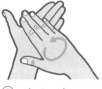

palm to palm

right palm over left dorsum and left palm over right dorsum

palm to palm, fingers interlaced

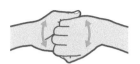

backs of fingers to opposing palms with fingers interlocked

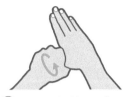

rotational rubbing of right thumb clasped in left palm, and vice versa

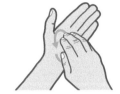

rotational rubbing, backwards and forwards with clasped fingers of right hand in left palm, and vice versa

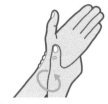

rotational rubbing of left wrist with right palm, and vice versa

Figure 3.1 Seven-stage hand washing technique.

necessary for examination. For ease, each area is described in the relevant systems examination in each chapter.

If, by exposing one area of their body, a patient must also expose another (for example, a person wearing a dress exposing their abdomen will also expose their groin and legs), ensure that sheets or drapes are available so that only the necessary area is exposed.

3.2.5 Comfort maintained

When asking a patient to undress and be examined, ensure that total privacy is maintained. Most clinic rooms have a screen or a curtain that conceals the examination couch, just in case someone walks into the room. Intimate examinations often involve briefly locking the examination room door to reassure the patient that no one can inadvertently enter – however, locking doors is acceptable only if the patient is aware and agrees.

If you are examining a patient on a hospital ward, ensure the curtains around the bed are completely closed. Leaving a gap of even an inch or two risks the patient feeling exposed and embarrassed.

Always provide a chaperone for an intimate examination of a patient of either gender. This is reassuring for the patient and protects the clinician from any spurious claims of molestation. In particular, for intimate examinations of female patients, provision of a female chaperone should be routine when the doctor is male.

Always ensure the patient is not in pain before starting the examination, and that they are able to remain in the same position throughout. Patients in severe pain will likely require analgesia before you commence.

> **Remember that some patients are comfortable sitting in a chair in front of you, but struggle to maintain the position necessary for the exam.** For example, patients with pulmonary oedema and orthopnoea become too breathless to lie at 45 degrees.

3.2.6 Kindly proceed

Once the above measures have been taken, you may begin the examination.

3.3 The 'endobedogram'

Every examination begins with looking at the patient. In a hospital setting this is from the end of the bed so in this book, we refer to this observation as the 'endobedogram' – but the same is needed when examining a patient in any clinical setting. It gives you the opportunity to get an impression of the patient's general state, and provides clues that are explored in the later examination.

Start by looking at the patient. Ask yourself:
- Does the patient look well?
- If not, what is it that makes them look unwell? Are they pale, in discomfort or breathless?
- Do they have any signs of medical therapy, e.g. intravenous infusions, oxygen therapy or bruises from recent blood tests?
- What is their body habitus (physical state)? Are they overweight or obese? Are they underweight?
- Do they appear appropriately dressed and are they clean and kempt?

> **Being unkempt tells you a lot about a person.** It may be that they are unable to maintain personal care due to financial, emotional, cognitive or functional reasons. Be sensitive when asking about this as there is often some embarrassment.

Next, look at what the patient has brought with them and at the area around them for clues pointing towards ill health:
- Are there any medications visible? If so, what is the drug and how is it taken (tablet, liquid or inhaled)? Remember that herbal remedies are often used by patients.
- Are there any mobility aids such as walking stick, Zimmer frame or wheelchair?
- If on the ward, are there any signs around the bed such as a "nil by mouth"?
- Is there any paraphernalia of smoking or recreational drug taking? These are sometimes seen in hospital as well as at the patient's home!

3.4 Vital signs

Vital signs are a collection of the basic physiological parameters, often called 'observations' or 'obs'. They are routine assessments, quick to carry out during a consultation and performed several times per day by nurses for hospital inpatients. They provide a sensitive measurement of severity of illness. They include:
- heart rate
- blood pressure
- respiratory rate
- oxygen saturation
- core temperature.

Additionally, urine output is recorded as a vital sign when necessary.

3.4.1 Heart rate

A normal heart rate is between 60 and 100 beats per minute (bpm). The causes of a fast or slow heart rate are detailed in *Section 4.5.4*.

To take the heart rate, locate the radial pulse (**Figure 3.2**). Either count the beats over a whole minute, or count the number of beats in 15 seconds then multiply by 4.

3.4.2 Blood pressure

Two measurements of blood pressure (BP) are taken: systolic, which is the arterial blood pressure during the heartbeat, and diastolic, which is the arterial blood pressure between heartbeats. Normal BP is 110–130mmHg (millimetres of mercury) systolic and 70–90mmHg diastolic.

Normal BP is required to perfuse the organs of the body. Low BP (hypotension) results in poor tissue perfusion which, if uncorrected, leads to multi-organ failure. Clinical signs of hypotension are listed in **Table 3.1**. High BP (hypertension) causes microvascular damage to organs, and if uncorrected, causes irreversible organ dysfunction (**Table 3.2**).

BP is measured over the brachial artery. A BP cuff (sphygmomanometer) is inflated to

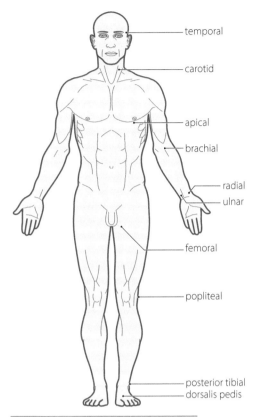

Figure 3.2 Location of palpable pulses.

temporal
carotid
apical
brachial
radial
ulnar
femoral
popliteal
posterior tibial
dorsalis pedis

Table 3.1 *Clinical signs of hypotension*

Organ system	Signs
Cardiovascular	Chest pain
	Hypothermia
Respiratory	Breathlessness
Abdominal	Abdominal pain
Neurological	Dizziness
	Collapse
	Drowsiness
	Loss of consciousness
Genitourinary	Low urine output

Table 3.2 *Long-term effects of untreated hypertension*

Organ system	Effects of hypertension
Cardiovascular	Heart failure
	Peripheral vascular disease
	Arterial aneurysm
	Arterial dissection
Respiratory	Pulmonary hypertension
Neurological	Stroke
	Intracerebral haemorrhage
Ophthalmological	Retinopathy
Genitourinary	Nephropathy

determine the systolic and diastolic pressure; the process is as follows:
- Ensure the patient is sitting comfortably in a chair or lying at 45 degrees in bed.
- Wash your hands.
- Ask the patient if they have had a BP reading performed before. If not, advise them that it is mildly uncomfortable, but not painful, and only requires a couple of minutes.
- Place the sphygmomanometer around their upper arm, and locate the radial pulse with your right hand. Use your left hand to slowly pump the sphygmomanometer pressure up. When the radial pulse disappears, then the sphygmomanometer pressure has overcome the systolic pressure (**Figure 3.3**). Note the sphygmomanometer pressure when this occurs – this is your estimate of the systolic pressure.
- Release the sphygmomanometer pressure.

Place your stethoscope over the brachial artery in the antecubital fossa (the 'crook' of the elbow). You will not hear any sounds, as there will be normal blood flow through the brachial artery.
- Gradually inflate the sphygmomanometer. When you reach the diastolic pressure, the brachial arterial pulse (**Figure 3.4**) will suddenly become audible. It sounds like a knocking or tapping.
- Continue to inflate the sphygmomanometer until the tapping sound disappears again – this is the systolic pressure. It should roughly

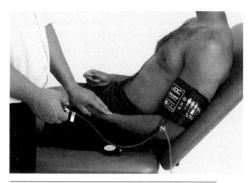

Figure 3.3 Estimate the systolic pressure by noting the pressure at which the radial pulse disappears.

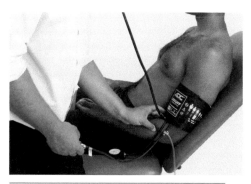

Figure 3.4 Auscultate over the brachial artery to determine the pressure when tapping appears and disappears, to determine the diastolic and systolic pressure, respectively.

equate to your initial estimate of systolic pressure.
- Deflate the sphygmomanometer and record the BP in the patient notes.
- Wash your hands.

3.4.3 Respiratory rate

This is the number of breaths per minute. Normal values are between 10 and 20 breaths. When a patient becomes unwell, an increased respiratory rate is often the first detectable abnormality in their vital signs, which probably represents an underlying sympathetic nervous response.

To take the respiratory rate, watch the rise and fall of the patient's chest and count the breaths over 20 seconds, then multiply the number by 3. It is best to measure the respiratory rate immediately after measuring the heart rate, without telling the patient what you are doing; informing someone that you are assessing their breathing often makes them subconsciously alter their respiratory rate.

3.4.4 Oxygen saturation

This is an estimate of the percentage of red blood cells that are oxygenated. Normal values are between 94% and 98% in healthy individuals. Patients with chronic respiratory diseases may have much lower O_2 saturations, at levels which are considered 'normal' for them, for example in the range of 88–92%. Therefore measurement of O_2 saturation in isolation is not helpful – a little background information about the patient is required.

Oxygen saturation is measured using a fingertip infrared device called a pulse oximeter. The device measures peripheral O_2 saturation by comparing the changes in different wavelengths of light as it passes through the finger. The result is not identical to arterial O_2 saturation but sufficiently similar for general clinical use.

3.4.5 Temperature

Temperature is measured with a digital thermometer under the tongue, or in the axilla or ear, depending on the circumstances. There is a different type of thermometer for each site; for example, the ear thermometer records the temperature from the tympanic membrane and is designed in a way that means it cannot touch and damage the membrane. Normal body temperature is between 35.5 and 37.5°C. Sometimes, if a patient is very unwell, it is necessary to measure their temperature rectally (a "core temperature"); however, this is not routine.

3.4.6 Urine output

Urine output is a vital sign but is only measured when strictly necessary because it usually requires insertion of a urinary catheter, which is unpleasant for the patient and carries an infection risk. However, in areas such as intensive care units it is recorded as a vital sign.

Decreased urine production is a clear sign of deteriorating kidney function. Normal urine output is over 0.5ml of urine per kilogram of body weight per hour, e.g. a healthy 80kg patient should pass a minimum of 40ml of urine per hour.

3.5 The peripheral examination

Examination of a body system starts with a look for signs of disease around the body before continuing to examine the function of the particular organs involved in that system. Usually, this starts with the hands and follows up the arms to the head and then continues down through the body until the area for organ examination is reached (such as the chest for the cardiovascular and respiratory systems, or the abdomen for the gastrointestinal (GI) system). The examination then continues down the body to finish at the legs and feet. Examination of the areas outside the particular area for an organ system is called the peripheral examination.

3.6 Hands

Take the patient's hand and feel the temperature using the back of your hand. Is it warm or cool? If cool, how far does this extend, i.e. does the patient have cool fingers or are they cool to the wrists or even elbows?

Look at the fingers for signs of clubbing (**Figure 3.5**):

■ Fluctuance (a softness or bogginess) of the nail beds (**Figure 3.6a**)

■ Loss of the normal nail bed angle

■ Increased nail bed convexity

■ 'Drumstick' appearance of the distal fingers.

Ask the patient to align the distal phalanges of both index fingers together (**Figure 3.6b**). Normally, there should be a diamond-shaped 'window' seen between the nails. When there is finger clubbing, this window is lost. This is known as the Schamroth sign. Causes of clubbing are listed in **Table 3.3**.

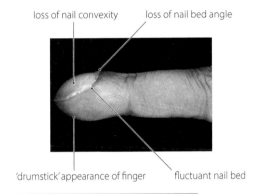

loss of nail convexity   loss of nail bed angle

'drumstick' appearance of finger   fluctuant nail bed

Figure 3.5 Features of finger clubbing.

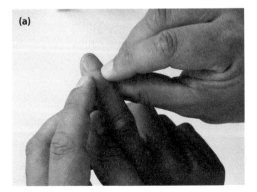

(a)

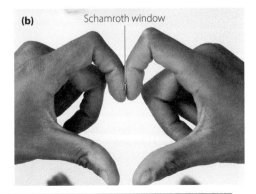

(b)   Schamroth window

Figure 3.6 Examination of clubbing: (a) feeling for nail bed fluctuance; (b) assessing for the Schamroth sign.

Look at the nails for changes indicating underlying disease (**Table 3.4**). Then look at the palms and backs of both hands. Observe the skin colour and the presence of any signs of chronic disease (**Table 3.5**).

3.6.1 Radial pulse

Palpate the radial pulse (**Figure 3.7**) and note:

■ Rate – the number of beats in 15 seconds, used to calculate heart rate in beats per minute
■ Rhythm – whether the pulse is regular or irregular. If irregular, is this a regularly irregular pulse (a regularly repeating irregular pattern) or irregularly irregular (a random and non-repeating pattern)?

Table 3.3 *Causes of clubbing*

Organ system	Causes of clubbing
Cardiovascular	Benign cardiac tumours
	Subacute bacterial endocarditis
	Congenital cyanotic heart disease
Respiratory	Lung cancer
	Bronchiectasis
	Cystic fibrosis
	Interstitial lung disease
GI	Cirrhotic liver disease
	Inflammatory bowel disease
Endocrinological	Graves' disease (called 'thyroid acropachy')
Non-pathological	Familial (called 'pseudoclubbing')

Table 3.5 *Hand changes associated with chronic disease*

Sign	Associated disease
Joint deformity	Musculoskeletal disease (rheumatoid or psoriatic arthritis, osteoarthritis, gout, etc.)
Muscle wasting	Arthritis
	Motor nerve injury or entrapment
Tar staining	Tobacco / cannabis smoking
Palmar erythema	Chronic liver disease
	Pregnancy
Janeway lesions and Osler's nodes	Subacute bacterial endocarditis

Table 3.4 *Nail changes associated with chronic disease*

Appearance	Medical term	Associated disease
Blue discolouration	Cyanosis	Low blood oxygen level
Spooning and upward growth	Koilonychia	Iron and B12 deficiency
White discolouration	Leukonychia	Low albumin levels
Raised nails separated from the nail bed	Onycholysis	Psoriasis (nails can also be pitted, ridged and discoloured)
Thickened nails	–	Peripheral vascular disease
		Nail bed trauma
		Fungal nail infections
Splinter haemorrhages	Splinter haemorrhages	Subacute bacterial endocarditis
		Systemic lupus erythematosus (SLE)

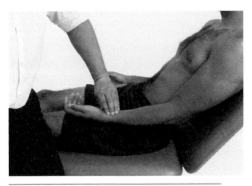

Figure 3.7 Palpate the radial pulse with your fingers.

- Volume – whether the vessel feels well filled or underfilled (indicating a low circulating blood volume)
- Character – the pattern of how the pulse reaches full volume and recedes. Appreciating varying pulse character takes practice.

3.7 Neck

The neck comprises multiple structures: bones, muscles, blood and lymphatic vessels, organs of speech, airways and the proximal oesophagus. Many signs of disease are found here.

3.7.1 Jugular venous pressure

The jugular venous pressure (JVP) is the movement seen when blood rises and falls within the jugular veins and is a representation of the pressure within the venous system as a whole. With the patient reclined at 45°, ask them to turn their head away from you, and look for the JVP (**Figure 3.8a**). Note that the position of the JVP changes depending on how flat the patient is. It appears falsely high if the patient is flatter than 45°

and falsely low if the patient is more upright. If the JVP is not visible, gently press in and upwards in the patient's right upper quadrant. This presses on the liver and increases the volume within the vena cava, thus causing the JVP to rise. Once pressure is removed, the JVP will drop again. This is called the hepatojugular reflex (**Figure 3.8b**).

The JVP is seen rather than felt. During diastole, the atria contract to push blood into the ventricles. As there is no valve separating the vena cava and right atrium, atrial contraction also causes a degree of back flow into the vena cava and thus the jugular vein. This is seen as an impulse spreading up the neck along the vein, which is sometimes difficult if the patient has

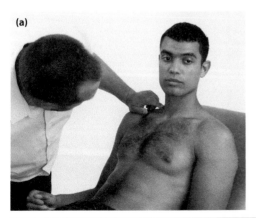

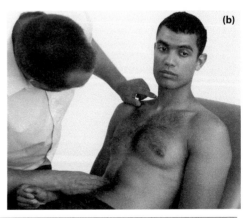

Figure 3.8 (a) Correct position for assessing the JVP; (b) using the hepatojugular reflex to accentuate the JVP.

much adipose tissue in the neck. Two aspects of the JVP are noted – the waveform and height.

JVP waveform

The JVP has a biphasic waveform (**Figure 3.9**). The periods of increase and decrease in venous pressure along the waveform are distinct and correspond to a part of the cardiac cycle (**Table 3.6**).

JVP height

The JVP height is the highest distance the impulse reaches above the sternal angle. A normal JVP height is 2cm. The JVP is reduced or not seen in low volume states such as severe dehydration or after heavy bleeding. There are many causes for a raised JVP which are distinguished according to the waveform, as listed in **Table 3.7**. The JVP will

rise with expiration and fall with inspiration due to changes in intrathoracic pressure. If this pattern is reversed then the JVP is said to be 'paradoxical'.

3.7.2 Carotid pulse

The carotid pulse is the pulsation felt over the carotid arteries. Palpate it gently (**Figure 3.10**) and note the character and volume (see *Section 4.5.7*). Only palpate one carotid artery at a time – if you press too hard on both at once this can impair blood flow to the brain. Listen over each

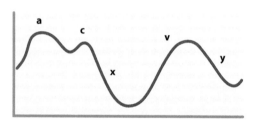

Figure 3.9 The JVP waveform.

Table 3.6 *Physiology of the JVP waveform*	
Waveform	**Physiology**
'a' wave	Atrial contraction
	Peak of a wave occurs at the end of atrial systole
'c' wave	Right ventricular contraction closing the tricuspid valve and causing it to bulge into the right atrium
'x' descent	Ventricular systole pulling tricuspid valve downwards
	Atrial relaxation and refilling due to low pressure
'v' wave	Venous filling from venous return against a closed tricuspid valve
'y' descent	Rapid atrial emptying following tricuspid valve opening

Table 3.7 *Causes of a raised JVP according to changes in waveform*	
Waveform	**Physiology**
Normal waveform	Bradycardia
	Fluid overload
	Heart failure
Absent pulsation	Superior vena cava (SVC) obstruction
Large 'a' wave	Tricuspid stenosis
	Right heart failure
	Pulmonary hypertension
Cannon 'a' wave	Atrial flutter
	Third-degree heart block
	Ventricular ectopic beats
	Ventricular tachycardia
Absent 'a' wave	Atrial fibrillation
Large 'v' wave	Tricuspid regurgitation
Absent 'x' descent	Tricuspid regurgitation
Prominent 'x' descent	Constrictive pericarditis
Slow 'y' descent	Tricuspid stenosis
	Cardiac tamponade
Prominent / deep 'y' descent	Constrictive pericarditis
Paradoxical JVP	Pericardial effusion
	Pericardial tamponade
	Constrictive pericarditis

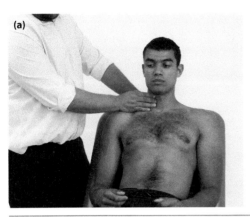
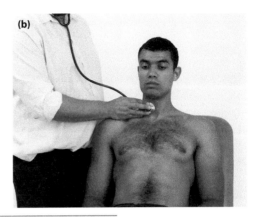

Figure 3.10 (a) Palpating the carotid pulse; (b) auscultating for carotid bruits.

carotid artery for evidence of a carotid bruit (see *Section 4.5.12*).

3.7.3 Neck masses

Stand behind the patient and, with the fingers of both hands, gently palpate the neck for any masses. The most common neck masses are listed in **Table 3.8**. Describe the mass in as much detail as possible:

- Site: where is the mass and how does its position relate to surrounding structures (**Figure 3.11**)?
- Size: how big is the mass?

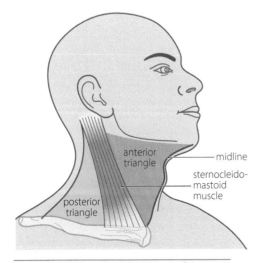

Figure 3.11 Anatomical divisions of the neck.

anterior triangle — midline — sternocleido-mastoid muscle — posterior triangle

Table 3.8 *Differential diagnosis for neck masses. The sternocleidomastoid marks the border between the anterior and posterior triangles of the neck. Note that some signs are found throughout the neck*

Location	Differential diagnosis
Midline	Lymph node
	Lipoma
	Sebaceous cyst
	Thyroid gland
	Thyroid nodule
	Thyroglossal cyst
Anterior triangle	Lymph node
	Lipoma
	Sebaceous cyst
	Salivary gland swelling
	Branchial cyst
	Carotid aneurysm
	Carotid body tumour
Posterior triangle	Lymph node
	Lipoma
	Sebaceous cyst
	Subclavian artery aneurysm
	Pharyngeal pouch
	Cystic hygroma

- Surface: what does the mass look like? Is it discoloured? Is there any discharge? Is it even visible at all?
- Shape: is the mass round, oval-shaped or irregular?
- Edge: is the mass smooth or irregular around its outside?
- Consistency: is the mass firm or soft? Can a fluctuance (suggesting it is fluid-filled) be felt?
- Pulsatility: is there a pulsation within the mass? Does this correspond with an arterial pulse? This would suggest the mass is vascular.
- Mobility: is the mass easy to move or is it tethered (attached) to a nearby structure?
- Tenderness: is the mass painful to touch?

Lymphadenopathy

Lymphadenopathy (enlarged lymph nodes) is the commonest cause of a neck mass. It is caused by infection or malignancy within a lymph node. 'Reactive lymphadenopathy' refers to lymph node enlargement in response to inflammation elsewhere in the body rather than the enlarged node itself. Lymphadenopathy is most easily felt in the neck, axillae and groins (**Figure 3.12**). It is usually local to, but can also be distant from a disease process.

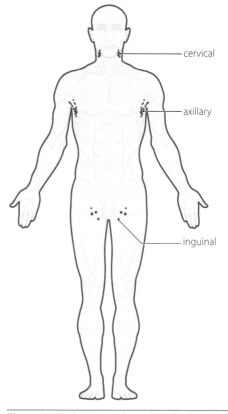

Figure 3.12 Areas to palpate lymphadenopathy.

3.8 Face

3.8.1 Face

Look at the patient's face. Do they have a particular 'facies' – a characteristic facial appearance associated with a certain condition? The commonest facies are given in **Table 3.9**.

3.8.2 Eyes

Gently pull down one of the lower eyelids and ask the patient to look up so that the conjunctiva is clearly seen (**Figure 3.13**). A pale conjunctiva (conjunctival pallor) is indicative of underlying anaemia. Then pull up one of the upper eyelids, ask the patient to look down and note the colour of the sclera (**Figure 3.14**). Jaundice causes a yellow discolouration of the sclera, called icterus.

3.9 Ear, nose and throat

The ear, nose and throat (ENT) are a complex set of organs with multiple functions. The ears are used in hearing and balance, the nose in smell and breathing and the throat (including the mouth) in tasting, breathing, talking and swallowing. Due to this they are partly examined in multiple systems examinations but their overall function is not part of any distinct body system.

Table 3.9	Stereotypical facial appearances (facies) and their disorders
Disorder	**Facial appearance**
Acromegaly	Coarse, enlarged facial features
Cushing's disease	'Moon face', oedematous skin, 'buffalo hump' over lower neck
Hyperthyroidism	Lid retraction with staring eyes
Hypothyroidism	Malar flush, loss of outer third of the eyebrows
Myasthenia gravis	Blank expression, bilateral ptosis
Myotonic dystrophy	Frontal balding, bilateral ptosis
SLE	'Butterfly rash' over nose and cheeks
Systemic sclerosis	Waxy skin, small mouth, 'beaked' nose

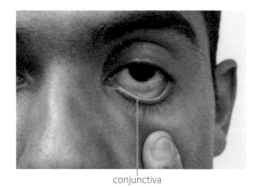

conjunctiva

Figure 3.13 Checking for conjunctival pallor; none seen.

sclera

Figure 3.14 Checking for discolouration of the sclera; none seen.

Diseases of the ear, nose or throat can be difficult to spot and often present through seemingly unrelated symptoms, so they should be thought of early and the organs examined closely.

3.9.1 The ENT history

Ear

Hearing loss

This is the commonest symptom of ear disease. It is unilateral or bilateral and may be to particular frequencies of sound. Ask when the hearing loss started and whether there is a family history of deafness which could imply a genetic cause. Ask about employment and exposure to loud noises (such as music concerts or working with loud machinery) which might cause hearing loss.

Dizziness

The feeling of being unbalanced is common and has many causes. Diseases of the inner ear cause vertigo which is the sensation of everything spinning. It is usually sudden and severe and is often accompanied by nausea and vomiting. Dizziness is described in many ways and causes include stroke, dehydration, low blood pressure or visual problems. A clear description is key in identifying the type of dizziness and its cause.

Other symptoms

Pain in and discharge from the ear (otalgia and otorrhoea, respectively) are often accompanied by itching. Ask about what the discharge consists of (wax, blood, pus or a mixture). Causes of this include infection, trauma and tumours. Pain may also be referred from elsewhere in the head and neck due to shared innervation, so the primary problem may be elsewhere (such as the teeth, throat or spine).

Tinnitus is a continuous ringing sound in the ears and is also associated with damage from sustained loud noise. Pulsatile tinnitus describes noises that come in waves or bursts. This is related to vascular malformations and tumours and should raise concern for careful investigation. 'Popping' noises and a feeling of increased pressure within the ear are associated with Eustachian tube pathologies.

Nose

Nasal obstruction is the commonest symptom of nasal diseases. Like hearing loss, it is unilateral or bilateral. Accompanying features such as sneezing, hay fever, or excessive secretions (with 'rhinorrhoea' describing excessive nasal secretions and 'postnasal drip' describing excessive secretions in the throat) suggest the cause may be due to irritation and inflammation of the mucosa. Sinusitis (inflammation of the sinuses) usually includes pain and headaches as well.

Nasal bleeding (epistaxis) is caused by trauma, mucosal damage or tumours. Always ask whether the patient takes blood-thinning medications (such as antiplatelets and anticoagulants) as these can make relatively minor bleeds heavy and difficult to stop.

Throat

Vocal changes such as a hoarse voice are caused by local inflammation and damage in the throat. Inflammation is caused by infections, overuse of the vocal cords (through prolonged singing or shouting) or chemical damage from chronic gastro-oesophageal reflux.

The vocal cords are innervated by the recurrent laryngeal nerves which are particularly susceptible to compression and damage from bronchial tumours. Ask about current or previous smoking and any constitutional symptoms suggestive of lung cancer (such as weight loss).

Ask the patient if they have any difficulty swallowing or if they cough after eating and/or drinking. If they do, establish the consistency of intake they cough after (i.e. thin liquids such as water, thick liquids such as custard or yoghurt, or solid food). For those with swallowing difficulties, this often presents with recurrent chest infections due to abnormal muscle control during swallowing.

3.9.2 Ear examination

Hearing assessment

Mask the ear not being tested by rubbing the tragus with one hand. At the same time, whisper a word or number from 60cm away from the ear being tested and ask the patient to repeat it back to you. If they cannot, repeat the process but whisper from 15cm away. Again, if the patient cannot repeat the word or number use a conversational voice from 15cm away.

Rinne's and Weber's tests

If the hearing is impaired this is either due to a conductive (how the sound travels to the tympanic membrane and is conveyed to the inner ear) or sensorineural (how the sound is received and processed by the nervous system) problem. Rinne's and Weber's tests are used to delineate these. They are explained in *Section 10.6.8*.

Otoscopy

This is the examination of the outer ear from pinna to tympanic membrane (**Figure 3.15**). Start by looking at the pinnae – the external ears:

- Are they symmetrical?
- Are there any deformities or scars?
- Are there any signs of infection (such as around recent piercings)?

Look behind the ear for any scars from previous surgery or swelling and/or redness indicating underlying infection. Then look in front of the ear for any sinuses or fistulae formed from chronic underlying infections.

Next examine the auditory canal and tympanic membrane. Turn the light of the otoscope on and place a speculum (disposable plastic) over the metal part. Gently pull the pinna upwards and backwards. Holding the otoscope like a pen and resting your hand lightly on the side of the patient's head, insert it into the external auditory meatus (the opening to the external auditory canal) and look through. Whilst slowly advancing the otoscope examine the auditory canal, noting the presence of:

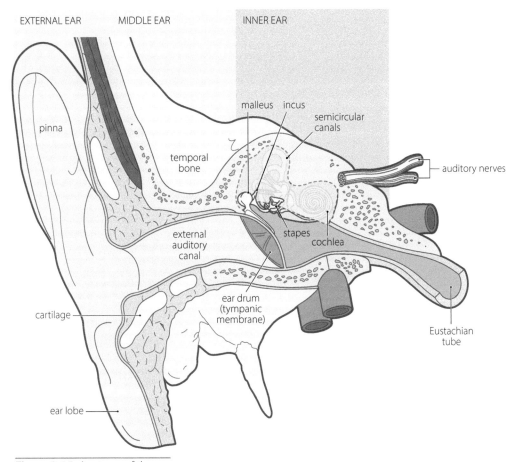

EXTERNAL EAR   MIDDLE EAR   INNER EAR

pinna

malleus   incus

semicircular
canals

temporal
bone

auditory nerves

external
auditory
canal

stapes

cochlea

cartilage

ear drum
(tympanic
membrane)

Eustachian
tube

ear lobe

Figure 3.15 Anatomy of the ear.

- excessive wax: a thick yellow/brown substance secreted by cells of the canal that traps bacteria, insects, water and dirt
- erythema: redness of the canal, suggesting infection, inflammation or irritation
- pus: highly suggestive of infection
- foreign bodies
- swellings: these could be within the canal and visible or seen to be bulging in from outside the canal.

Then examine the tympanic membrane. A normal membrane is pearly coloured and translucent. In a healthy membrane the light of the otoscope should reflect back (the light reflex). Other findings on the tympanic membrane are abnormal (**Table 3.10**).

3.9.3 Nose examination

Inspection

Begin by inspecting the nose for any deformity from the side and front. With the patient facing you, ask them to lean their head back slightly, and look to see if the cartilage is deviated or central. Deviation of the nasal cartilage obstructs smooth airflow during breathing. It is either congenital (from abnormal foetal development) or acquired (such as following a nasal injury).

With their head in a neutral position, gently press up the tip of their nose to elevate it so that the nasal cavity becomes visible. Shine a pen torch or otoscope light from outside to see more clearly. Look at the mucosa and note if it is inflamed or whether there is an excessive

Table 3.10 *Findings on the tympanic membranes*

Finding	Description
Normal	Pearly-grey colour
	Translucent
	Flat
	Light reflex present
Otitis media	Erythematous
	Bulging
	Fluid level may be visible behind
	Light reflex absent
Perforated tympanic membrane	Visible tear or hole within the membrane
	Blood or pus within the ear canal
Cholesteatoma	Hard, white, irregular mass on the membrane (usually in the superior portion)

amount of mucus, suggesting inflammation. Note also the presence of any masses or foreign bodies.

An ENT specialist may examine further by using Thudicum's speculum to widen the nasal passages to allow for better examination. This should only be performed by an experienced operator as improper use causes damage.

Palpation

Feel over the nasal bones at the top of the nose to assess their alignment and whether there is any deviation or pain. Continue down towards the tip of the nose, feeling for alignment and pain over the nasal cartilage.

Next assess nasal airflow by holding a cold metallic object under the nostrils and asking the patient to breathe slowly in and out through their nose. Watch the object for misting and note whether this occurs equally under both nostrils. Less misting under one suggests reduced airflow on that side.

3.9.4 Throat examination

The oropharynx

Ask the patient to open their mouth. Warn them beforehand, and then press down on the tongue using a tongue depressor. The aim is to see as much of the oropharynx as possible (**Figure 3.16**) but be careful not to touch the very back of the tongue or pharynx as this will cause gagging. Asking the patient to say 'ahh' will raise the palate and uvula to allow for a better view.

Pay attention to the following:

■ Dentition (the presence of teeth) and oral hygiene. Poor dentition is associated with nutritional deficiencies or repeated use of some types of antibiotics (especially tetracyclines) during childhood.

■ Colour and size of the tongue (relative to the size of the mouth). For example, a large

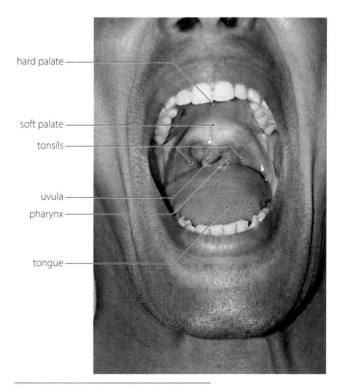

Figure 3.16 Anatomy of the oropharynx.

red tongue ('beef-red tongue') is caused by vitamin B12 deficiency.

■ Presence of central cyanosis, which is seen as a blue discolouration of the lips and under the tongue and suggests low circulating oxygen concentrations. Anyone with cyanosis should undergo detailed respiratory and cardiovascular system examinations.

■ Colour of the oropharyngeal mucosa. Redness is indicative of inflammation. Pus or a white coating suggests active bacterial and/or fungal infection.

■ Size and colour of the tonsils. Large, swollen and tender tonsils are diagnostic of tonsillitis. Sometimes small stones (tonsilloliths) are visible within the crevices. These are hard build-ups of bacteria and cellular debris and cause halitosis (bad breath).

Speech and swallowing

Note the patient's speech. Are they able to respond normally and make their speech audible and understandable?

■ Dysphonia describes abnormally quiet speech that the patient struggles to make louder.

■ Dysphasia describes difficulty in understanding and generating speech. It can be receptive, expressive or mixed:
  □ receptive dysphasia is the difficulty receiving and understanding information given to oneself
  □ expressive dysphasia is an inability to form and express speech, but knowing what one wants to say

■ Dysarthria describes difficulty sounding words due to muscular weakness of the tongue, lips or jaw.

Examination of the vocal cords requires direct visualisation via fine nasendoscopy (where a very fine camera is passed through the nostrils and nasal cavity and down the pharynx). This should only be performed by a trained specialist and is not part of the routine ENT examinations.

If available, and there are no clear concerns about swallowing safety, ask the patient to sip some water to see if they struggle to swallow. If they do, they should be advised to avoid eating and drinking until a formal swallowing assessment is performed.

3.10 Legs and feet

3.10.1 Legs

Examination of the peripheral vascular system concentrates on examination of the lower limbs, because vascular problems rarely manifest in the upper limb. It is described in detail in *Chapter 4* (*Section 4.7*). However, when performing any one of the systems examinations, you should always also assess the legs and feet for signs of cardiovascular disease.

Start by feeling the temperature of the patient's feet with the back of your hand. If the feet are cool, move up the leg to find the point at which they become warm (indicating the point at which the arterial blood supply is impaired). Note any skin changes and whether the temperature changes over these areas.

Next, assess for oedema by pressing a finger into the skin. If an indentation remains after the finger is removed, this is evidence of fluid

in the subcutaneous tissues – pitting oedema. Repeating this higher up the leg highlights the extent of oedema and the severity of fluid overload.

Look for muscle wasting (from impaired development, damaged innervation or muscle underuse), limb deformities or scars. Be particularly alert for long scars on the inner calf which reflect previous vein harvesting for coronary artery bypass grafting (which is confirmed by the presence of a central sternotomy scar).

Finally, palpate the femoral, popliteal, posterior tibial and dorsalis pedis arterial pulses (**Figure 3.17**). Compare each side for volume and character. When palpating the femoral arterial pulse, use your other hand to palpate the radial arterial pulse. These should occur at the same time; if they do not then there is an impedance in the flow through one of the vessels.

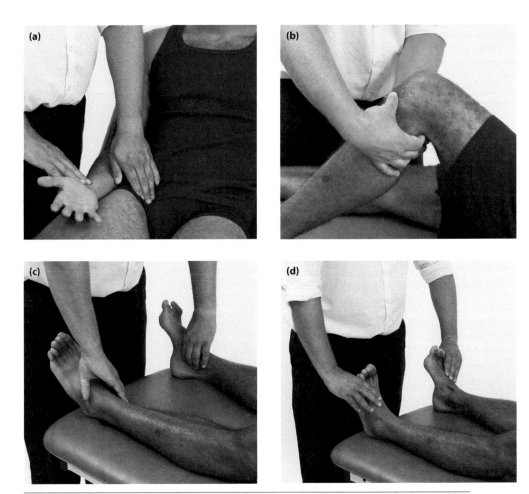

Figure 3.17 Palpating pulses: (a) femoral (whilst checking for radio-femoral delay); (b) popliteal; (c) posterior tibial; (d) dorsalis pedis arterial.

3.10.2 Feet

Look at the toes for evidence of clubbing and any nail changes (the causes are the same as for the hands). Always check the heels, soles and between the toes for skin injuries, ulcers and evidence of infection such as a white coating of fungus ('athlete's foot'), red and inflamed skin from bacterial cellulitis or ulcers.

3.11 Skin and hair

Dermatological diseases occur for a variety of reasons; they can be primary problems of the cells of the skin or hair follicles, or a clinical sign of illness elsewhere in the body.

3.11.1 Dermatological history

Dermatological conditions are difficult to tell apart. Patients present with rashes, focal lesions (an area of infarction, degeneration, inflammation, infection, haemorrhage or trauma), lumps, pigment changes and growths. The differential diagnoses are vast so a clear history gives focus and guides further investigation. The mnemonic 'DOCS MATCH2' is useful to cover the key components:

- **D**istribution – what areas of skin are affected? Does the problem involve the eyes or mouth?
- **O**nset – when did the problem start?
- **C**ourse – is the problem there all the time or does it come and go? Has it changed over time?
- **S**un exposure – does it get better, worse or is it unchanged when exposed to sunlight? Often a person notices lesions change when on sunny holidays.
- **M**edications – have they tried any medications (including creams) and have they affected the lesion? Have any OTC or herbal remedies helped?
- **A**ssociated symptoms – does the rash or lesion have any pain, itching, bleeding or discharge? Are there any other systemic symptoms such as a fever, tiredness, weight loss or joint aches?
- **T**riggers – are there any clear triggers that caused the lesions or make them worse?
- **C**ontacts – has the patient been in contact with anyone with a similar rash, suggesting a contagious element (such as chickenpox)? Has the patient travelled anywhere recently and if so, have they noticed any bites or skin injuries whilst they were away?
- **H**istorical lesions – have they had anything like this before? If so, was it ever diagnosed?
- **H**air changes – has the hair (both on the head and the body) changed also? If so, how? Has it fallen out? Is it growing back? Has it changed in coarseness or colour?

Past medical history

A clear past medical history is essential, as some diseases cause stereotypical skin lesions (**Table 3.11**). At times, skin lesions develop before the underlying disease becomes apparent. A full systems enquiry allows seemingly disparate or mild symptoms to be explored to point towards an underlying diagnosis.

Drug history

Ask the patient about any drugs they are taking, particularly ones that were initiated just prior to the skin problem developing – this could indicate a drug reaction. Always ask about any OTC or herbal remedies.

Table 3.11 *Skin lesions associated with systemic disease*

Skin lesion	Systemic disease	Description
Necrobiosis lipoidica diabeticorum	Diabetes mellitus	Tender, yellow-brown patches over lower limbs / shins
Acanthosis nigricans	Diabetes mellitus Polycystic ovarian syndrome Cushing's disease Acromegaly	Dark velvety hyperpigmentation in body folds
Pyoderma gangrenosum	Inflammatory bowel disease Rheumatoid arthritis Seronegative arthritis Haematological diseases (rare)	Deep ulcerating lesions and chronic wounds
Erythema nodosum	Inflammatory bowel disease Behçet's disease Infection Pregnancy	Tender nodules over shins caused by fat cell inflammation

Ask also about anything that comes in contact with their skin such as creams, lotions, cosmetics, soaps, body washes or hair dyes. Sometimes a change in fabric conditioners and detergents can cause skin irritation.

Enquire if the patient has any established allergies. Sometimes there are cross-reactions with other substances.

> **Latex fruit syndrome is the phenomenon whereby people with a latex allergy also develop intolerance or allergy to certain fruits.** This includes strawberries, bananas and kiwi fruit. It is caused by the fruits containing a protein similar to the allergen in latex, which cross-reacts with the body's immune system.

Social history

Ask the patient what they do for a living. If the problem gets worse at work and better during times away, this could indicate an allergen at work. Do they work with any irritant chemicals and if so, do they wear protective clothing such as gloves and goggles?

Alcohol and smoking worsen some dermatological complaints. Ask about intravenous drug use, as injection sites provide potential points for skin infections such as cellulitis or abscess formation.

Ask about the patient's home and whether their housing is clean. Infestations of bed bugs or scabies lead to rashes developing.

Ask about their day-to-day functioning. Many treatments require regular application or creams and a less abled person might need extra support through carers or district nurses to ensure they receive their treatment properly.

Table 3.12 *Definition of common skin lesions*

Lesion	Diameter	Description
Macule	<1.5cm	Small, flat and well circumscribed lesion that cannot be felt
Papule	<0.5cm	Well circumscribed lesion raised from the skin surface that can be felt
Vesicle	<0.5cm	Raised, fluctuant and fluid-filled lesion
Pustule	<0.5cm	Pus-filled vesicle
Bulla	>0.5cm	Raised, clear fluid-filled lesion
Nodule	>0.5cm	Solid, raised lesion that can be felt
Patch	>1.5cm	Flat area of abnormal skin colour
Plaque	>1cm	Flat palpable lesion that may be raised or thickened
Abscess		Collection of pus
Wheal		Papule or plaque swollen with localised oedema
Boil		Hair follicle infection (staphylococcal)
Carbuncle		Multiple adjacent boils merged together
Ulcer		Irregular area with loss of multiple layers of skin
Lichenification		Thickened skin with exaggerated skin lines
Scale		Fragments of shedding skin
Crust		Rough surface of blood, serum and cellular debris

3.11.2 Dermatology examination

When examining skin lesions, the more detail that is given, the easier it is to find the diagnosis. The patient should have as much or as many of the lesions exposed as possible.

General inspection

Begin by looking at the person as a whole and note the number of lesions (one, few or multiple). Note the distribution:

- Extensor: extensor surfaces, knees and elbows
- Flexural: flexural surfaces, cubital fossae, axillae, groins / genitals
- Acral: affecting hands and feet
- Dermatomal: affecting discrete dermatomal regions
- Follicular: affecting hair follicles
- Seborrhoeic: affecting areas with sebaceous glands (e.g. face and scalp).

Close inspection of lesion

Next take a closer look at a single lesion, paying attention to its size, shape, border, configuration, colour and morphology.

Size, shape and border

Assess the size of the lesion and the shape (i.e. round, oval or irregular). Coin-shaped lesions are referred to as 'discoid', ring-shaped as 'annular' and annular lesions with a central lesion as 'target lesions'. Pay attention to the border. Is it well demarcated from the rest of the skin or poorly defined?

Configuration

If the lesions are multiple, note how they are arranged on the skin. Lesions are:

- discrete: clearly separated from each other
- confluent: merged together
- linear: arranged in a line.

Colour

Note the colour of the lesion. It may be:

- erythematous: red lesions which blanch with pressure
- purpuric: red / purple lesions which do not blanch
- hyperpigmented: darkened lesion with increased melanin
- hypopigmented: lightened lesion with decreased melanin
- depigmented: white lesion with total loss of melanin.

Morphology

Different types of lesions have a distinct appearance or morphology. The commonest lesions are described in **Table 3.12**.

Hair

Hair changes can occur separately to skin lesions and may be the only presenting problem. Inspect the patient's hair noting the distribution of affected hairs, the presence and pattern of any balding or hair loss and the texture of remaining hair. Examples of clinical syndromes associated with changes to scalp hair are described in **Table 3.13** whilst those affecting body hair are described in **Table 3.14**.

Table 3.13 *Examples of clinical syndromes associated with changes to scalp / head hair*

Condition	Description
Male-pattern baldness	Hair loss from temples and vertex progressing to leave remaining rim of hair at sides and back of head
Female-pattern baldness	Diffuse hair thinning without hairline recession
Alopecia totalis	Total loss of hair
Alopecia areata	Hair loss in defined patches surrounded by normal hair growth
Telogen effluvium	Thinning and shedding of hair
Frontal balding	Associated with myotonia dystrophica

Table 3.14 *Common clinical syndromes associated with changes to body hair*

Condition	Change to body hair
Anorexia and bulimia nervosa	Fine, downy facial and body hair (lanugo hair)
Liver failure	Sparse chest hair in males secondary to higher-than-normal levels of circulating oestrogen
Polycystic ovarian syndrome (PCOS)	Thick, dark facial and body hair secondary to higher-than-normal levels of circulating androgens

3.12 Fluid / volume status and hydration

During the examination, you are able to estimate the patient's hydration or volume status. This is done by assessing the clinical signs listed in **Table 3.15**, and correlating their pattern with a status:

■ euvolaemic: volume status is normal
■ hypovolaemic: the patient is dehydrated

■ hypervolaemic (or overloaded or oedematous): the patient has too much fluid.

A patient's fluid status reflects the severity of underlying disease and an understanding of this aids decision-making regarding the rate and volume of intravenous fluid therapy.

Table 3.15 *Clinical signs associated with changes in volume status*

Clinical sign	Hypovolaemia	Euvolaemia	Hypervolaemia
Pulse	Tachycardia	Normal rate	Tachycardia
	Low volume	Normal volume	Large volume
	'Thready' character	Normal character	'Bounding' character
Blood pressure	Low	Normal	Normal or raised
Postural blood pressure drop present?	Yes	No	No
Mucous membranes	Dry	Wet	Wet
JVP	Absent or low	Normal	Raised
Other signs	Sunken eyes	–	Peripheral oedema
	Thirst		Pulmonary oedema
			Ascites

3.13 Systems examination

For any one patient, it is rarely necessary to examine every organ system. Usually the history indicates how you should proceed, pointing towards examination of specific system(s).

A full body examination is very time consuming, which is why you should try to identify the system or body region of interest during history-taking.

Examination of the main organ systems is done in four stages:
- Inspection
- Palpation
- Percussion
- Auscultation.

These are combined to form an overall impression, no matter which system is being examined (**Table 3.16**).

Table 3.16 *Using inspection, palpation, percussion and auscultation*

Method	Uses	Details
Inspection	Endobedogram	How does the patient look at rest?
	Hands / nails	Are there any nail changes, such as clubbing?
		Are there any signs of chronic liver disease?
		Are there any signs of chronic GI disease?
		Are there any signs of endocarditis?
	JVP	Is it elevated?
	Chest	Is the respiratory rate normal?
	Abdomen	Are there any visible masses?
Palpation	Peripheral and central pulses	What is the rate, rhythm, character and volume?
	Hands	Are they warm and well perfused, or cold?
	Chest	Are there any palpable heart sounds or murmurs?
	Breast	Are there any masses?
	Abdomen	Is there any pain?
		Are there any masses?
	Limbs	Is the muscular tone and power normal?
Percussion	Chest	Is the chest resonant or dull?
	Abdomen	Is there any organomegaly?
		Is there any ascites?
Auscultation	Chest	Are the breath sounds normal?
		Are the heart sounds normal?
	Abdomen	Are the bowel sounds normal?
	Central pulses	Are there any bruits?

Each of *Chapters 4–13* deals with a separate body system and the accompanying clinical examination. As you read them, and during clinical work, try not to let your attention to a particular system blind you to clinical signs relating to other systems. Always remain observant and vigilant; unexpected findings are common in clinical medicine. If you are performing a respiratory examination, for example, try not to be oblivious to the large inguinal hernia that the patient did not mention.

3.13.1 Inspection

This begins when the patient first walks through the door of the consulting room. Note whether the patient is able to walk unaided, or whether they require a walking aid, such as a stick or a frame, or even a wheelchair. Do they have a normal gait? What is your impression of their current psychological and emotional state?

In the hospital setting, observing the patient's condition as they lie in the bed provides important information. For example, is the patient able to greet you normally, or does a brain or speech problem make normal communication difficult?

When you look closely at a patient, tell them what you are doing; being stared at is uncomfortable if you don't know the reason.

3.13.2 Palpation

This is the 'laying on of hands' – pushing, pressing and manipulating areas of the patient's body to detect abnormalities. It requires a great deal of practice. It has the potential to cause the patient pain or discomfort, so proceed gently and respectfully.

> **If you do cause a patient pain, pause the examination and ask "is it all right if I continue?", and respect the answer**. Usually patients will allow the examination to continue but with use of a gentler touch.

Use palpation to determine the size and borders of the palpable internal organs, and detect any unusual masses. Palpation also incorporates parts of the examination which require the patient to move their limbs, either with or without your assistance, such as in the musculoskeletal and neurological examination.

3.13.3 Percussion

The percussion technique involves placing the fingers of your non-dominant hand over an area of the patient's body, and striking them firmly with the first or second fingers of your dominant hand (**Figure 3.18**). The striking motion and the following rebound are quick, like striking a note on a xylophone. The purpose is to produce a percussive sound, or 'note', which gives information about the underlying structures (**Table 3.17**).

Percussion notes sound:
- hollow, or 'resonant', indicating an air-filled structure
- dull, indicating a solid structure or collection of fluid.

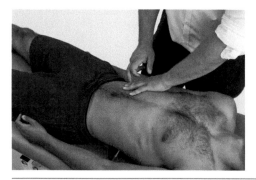
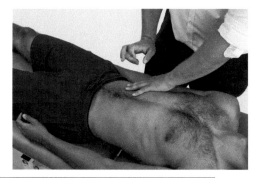

Figure 3.18 Percussing the abdomen: strike your fingers firmly with the finger of your other hand.

Table 3.17 *Using the percussion note to detect abnormalities*

Area of body	Percussion note	Interpretation
Chest	Resonant	Normal underlying lung
	Dull	Consolidated or collapsed lung
	'Stony' dull at lung bases	Pleural effusion
Abdomen	Resonant	Normal air-filled bowel
	Dull on right	Hepatic enlargement
	Dull on left	Splenic enlargement
	Dull in flanks	Ascitic fluid
Beneath thyroid mass	Dull over upper sternum	Posterior retrosternal extension of thyroid mass

Practice percussion on yourself, and notice the varying notes over different areas. For example, contrast the resonant note over your lungs with the dull note over your liver.

3.13.4 Auscultation

This is using your stethoscope to detect quiet sounds within the patient's body. The stethoscope has a use in examination of most body systems (**Table 3.18**). When using a stethoscope ensure that the earpieces are facing forward in line with your own ear canals (which run anteriorly). The end of the stethoscope has two sides, the diaphragm (covered side) and the bell (open side). The diaphragm acts to amplify high frequency sounds whilst the bell is used for low frequency sounds.

> **When using the bell of a stethoscope, do not press too hard.** Doing so stretches the underlying skin over the bell, effectively creating another diaphragm.

Table 3.18 *Uses of auscultation*

Body system	Use
Respiratory	Listening to breath sounds
	Listening for added sounds, such as crackles or wheeze
Cardiovascular	Listening to heart sounds
	Listening for heart murmurs
	Listening for bruits over the aorta, carotid or femoral arteries
	Listening for lung crackles that signify pulmonary oedema
GI	Listening to bowel sounds
	Listening for renal artery bruits
Thyroid	Listening for thyroid bruits

3.14 Answers to starter questions

1. In reality, the examination starts before the history, because the patient is observed at the beginning of the consultation, when any obvious abnormalities in appearance, speech or manner should be noted. It also proceeds in parallel with the history-taking, by watching the patient closely and noticing how they interact. This is especially true during a psychiatric assessment. The focused examination takes place after the history, because the patient's story guides you to the relevant system or systems that need to be examined.

2. There is no substitute for an experienced clinical examination, which draws on the healthcare professional's powers of analysis, insight, pattern recognition and observation. Whilst there are many advanced investigation and imaging options in modern medicine, they are of no use without the physician who selects the most appropriate one on the basis of sound diagnostic reasoning. When choosing an investigation, it is good practice to have a particular question in mind, which you would like the results to answer in order to confirm or rule out differential diagnoses.

3. There are cultural reasons for refusing an examination. Some women feel deeply uncomfortable being examined by a man, regardless of ethnicity, and they have the right to request a female professional. Similarly, some male patients prefer a male professional.

   Patients may refuse to be examined if they do not understand the reason for the examination, or disagree with the doctor's request. These disputes are usually resolved with careful communication of the healthcare professional's reasons for requesting an examination, and reassurance that a chaperone is available if they wish.

   Patients may refuse to be examined if they are confused – either due to dementia or delirium – and lack capacity to make informed decisions about their care. In these circumstances, the healthcare professional must decide whether to act in the patient's best interest and examine them against their wishes. These issues are explored in *Chapter 13*.

4. It is possible to estimate the systolic pressure by locating the furthest palpable pulse from the heart. As a rule of thumb:
   - If only the patient's carotid pulse is palpable, the systolic blood pressure is 60–70mmHg.
   - If the femoral pulse is palpable, the pressure is 70–80mmHg.
   - If the radial pulse is palpable, the systolic pressure is at least 80mmHg.
   - If the digital pulses are palpable on the lateral aspects of the fingers, then the systolic pressure is at least 100mmHg.

   These readings usually underestimate the systolic pressure, so an accurate reading with a sphygmomanometer is mandatory.

5. Transcutaneous oxygen saturation is a useful surrogate for arterial oxygenation. However, it only assesses the oxygen level, and therefore only detects hypoxia (type 1 respiratory failure). It does not assess the arterial carbon dioxide level, which is a major determinant of respiratory function. It is therefore possible to have completely normal transcutaneous oxygen saturation but have profound hypercapnia. Arterial blood gas analysis is therefore essential to guide oxygen therapy and to ensure that oxygen and carbon dioxide levels are within normal parameters.

Chapter 4
Cardiovascular system

Starter questions

1. What can holding a patient's hand tell you about their heart?
2. Why might a person who has suffered a heart attack walk with a limp?
3. Why is coronary heart disease (CHD) so common? And why is it increasing globally?
4. How can the respiratory symptoms of cardiac disease be differentiated from primary respiratory diseases?
5. Is heart failure solely due to poor lifestyle choices?
6. Why must diabetic patients be careful on the beach?

Answers to questions are to be found in *Section 4.9*.

4.1 Introduction

The cardiovascular system comprises the heart and blood vessels. Blood is pumped around the body, delivering oxygen, nutrition and immune cells to tissues, and removing waste products.

Cardiovascular disease is the biggest contributor to morbidity and mortality in the developed world. Disorders present as:

- **'plumbing'** problems, such as impaired blood flow through vessels (e.g. CHD)
- **'electrical'** problems, where the pacemaking and coordination of the heart's electrical system are affected (i.e. arrhythmias)
- **'pumping problems'**, where the heart no longer works effectively as the cardiovascular pump (i.e. heart failure).

Clinical assessment of the cardiovascular system includes assessing a patient's cardiovascular risk, i.e. quantifying their risk of CHD by the presence of risk factors. This estimates the likelihood that their presentation is cardiovascular, and their risk of long-term complications.

Case 4.1   30 minutes of central chest pain

Presentation

Mr Jefferson is 68 years old. He presents to the emergency department with 30 minutes of unresolving central chest pain.

Initial interpretation

Central chest pain is cardiovascular, oesophageal, musculoskeletal or respiratory in origin. Cardiovascular causes include myocardial ischaemia (angina pectoris and myocardial infarction), pericarditis and dissections. Respiratory causes include pleural irritation, pneumothorax, pneumonia and pulmonary embolus. Other important causes are gastro-oesophageal reflux and musculoskeletal injury / inflammation.

At this point, it is impossible to reach a differential diagnosis. Being male and 68 years old places Mr Jefferson at slightly higher risk of CHD, but we need more information.

History

Mr Jefferson's pain started suddenly after eating breakfast. It was heavy, did not radiate and was associated with sweating and nausea. It was constant and 8/10 in severity (10 being the worst he has ever experienced). It did not change with deep breathing or changing position. He has had similar chest pain 'on and off' for some years but this only occurs when walking uphill and is relieved by using his wife's 'angina spray'. His pain did not improve after receiving a spray under his tongue given by a paramedic.

Interpretation of history

Chest pain that develops after eating could be cardiac or gastroenterological in origin. Patients describe cardiac pain in terms of pressure: tight, squeezing, heavy or crushing. Radiation of pain to different areas helps discriminate between causes (e.g. angina pain often radiates down the left arm), so the lack of radiation in this case is not helpful in making a diagnosis. The sweating and nausea imply activation of the sympathetic nervous system (SNS), which is common in severe pain of any cause.

The pain is not 'positional', i.e. it does not change when moving his ribcage, back or arms,

so it is probably not musculoskeletal in origin. The absence of respiratory symptoms such as cough, or worsening of the pain on breathing, make respiratory disease less likely.

The exertional pain that he has been having for years which is relieved by his wife's 'angina spray' strongly suggests angina. This spray is likely to be glyceryl trinitrate (GTN) which dilates the blood vessels, relieving anginal pain (myocardial ischaemia) usually within 30 seconds; however, it also relieves oesophageal spasm after a few minutes. Having pre-existing angina makes Mr Jefferson at high risk for acute coronary syndrome (ACS), the destabilising and rupture of a plaque within the coronary vessels, causing a sudden impairment of blood flow to myocardium. The similarity of his current pain to the previous angina pain strongly implies that they are of the same aetiology. However, that this current pain is not relieved by GTN suggests ACS rather than stable angina.

Further history

Mr Jefferson takes ramipril 2.5mg and simvastatin 40mg daily for hypertension and high cholesterol, respectively. He has smoked 20 cigarettes a day for 30 years and works as a long-distance lorry driver.

Examination

He looks unwell, pale and clammy. His blood pressure is 167/99mmHg and oxygen saturations are 97% on air. Cardiac and respiratory examinations are normal. Peripheral vascular examination finds reduced pedal pulses.

Interpretation of findings

In summary, this patient has central chest pain which is not exertional and not relieved by rest or GTN. His normal oxygen saturations suggest the problem is not respiratory in origin. Most people who are acutely unwell, especially with pain, will appear pale and clammy, so this is a non-specific sign.

Mr Jefferson has many risk factors for CHD including hypertension, hypercholesterolaemia, smoking, sedentary occupation and evidence of peripheral vascular disease (PVD), which

Case 4.1 *continued*

often co-exists with CHD. Although he is on antihypertensive and cholesterol-lowering medications, his elevated blood pressure implies suboptimal control. A normal cardiovascular examination does not exclude ACS but a normal respiratory examination makes pulmonary oedema, pleural effusions, pneumothorax and pneumonia much less likely.

Considering his risk factors, signs and symptoms, ACS is the likely diagnosis: a medical emergency requiring prompt management. Diagnosis is confirmed with:

- electrocardiography (ECG) to detect signs of cardiac ischaemia
- blood tests for cardiac enzymes to detect myocardial cell death
- chest X-ray to detect signs of cardiac failure.

Investigations

Mr Jefferson's chest X-ray is normal. His ECG shows deep ST depression in leads V4–V6 and leads I and II (**Figure 4.1**). His blood results show a raised troponin T level of 68ng/ml and a random glucose of 14mmol/L. His full blood count and renal profile are normal.

Diagnosis

Mr Jefferson has ischaemic changes on his ECG and evidence of myocardial damage on his blood tests; troponins are cardiac enzymes released during myocardial damage. Mr Jefferson has had a non-ST elevation ACS (NSTEACS). He should be treated with two antiplatelet agents (aspirin and either clopidogrel or ticagrelor) and fondaparinux or a low molecular heparin (injectable anticoagulants). He requires angiography in order to assess his coronary arteries, and balloon angioplasty and stenting of areas of severe disease. His high random serum glucose indicates diabetes mellitus, which will require its own treatment to prevent further diabetic-related morbidity.

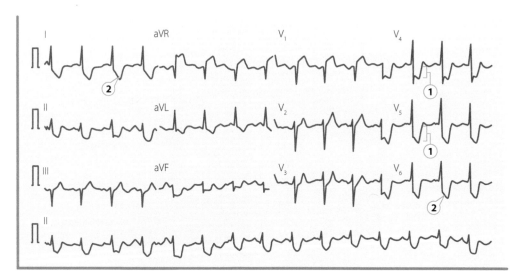

Figure 4.1 Mr Jefferson's electrocardiogram, showing signs of significant ischaemia. Note the depression of the ST segments in leads I, II, aVF and V3–V6 (1) and the inverted T-waves also seen (2).

In the UK, the Driver and Vehicle Licensing Agency (DVLA) mandates that patients suffering ACS must not drive for up to 6 weeks (although this varies if the patient has had an angioplasty). It is the patient's responsibility to tell the DVLA.

4.2 System overview

4.2.1 The heart and valves

The heart is composed of four chambers: two atria and two ventricles. The left atrium receives oxygenated blood from the lungs and the right atrium receives deoxygenated blood from the lower body (via the inferior vena cava) and the upper body (via the superior vena cava) (**Figure 4.2**).

The coronary arteries arise from the aortic root and supply oxygenated blood to cardiac muscle.

> **CHD is disease of coronary arteries** due to the deposition of fat-laden inflammatory cells.

The right ventricle ejects blood across the pulmonary valve into the pulmonary artery. The pulmonary artery carries blood into the lungs, where carbon dioxide is exchanged for oxygen. Oxygenated blood passes via the pulmonary vein into the left atrium.

In the left side of the heart, blood flows from the left atrium across the mitral valve into the left ventricle. The muscular left ventricle must generate enough pressure with each heartbeat to eject blood across the aortic valve into the aorta.

4.2.2 Blood vessels

The aorta is the largest artery in the body, and carries oxygenated blood from the heart to the systemic circulation. It divides in the pelvis into the left and right iliac arteries (**Figure 4.3**).

'Central pulses' are the carotid, axillary, brachial, and femoral pulses and 'peripheral pulses' are the radial, popliteal, posterior tibial and dorsalis pedis pulses (**Figure 4.4**).

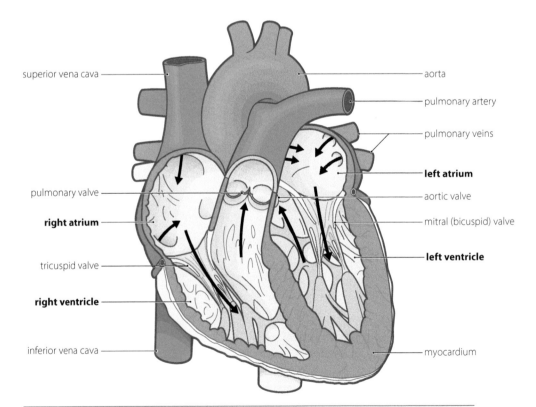

Figure 4.2 Cross-sectional anatomy of the heart, showing the communication between the four chambers and the direction of blood flow.

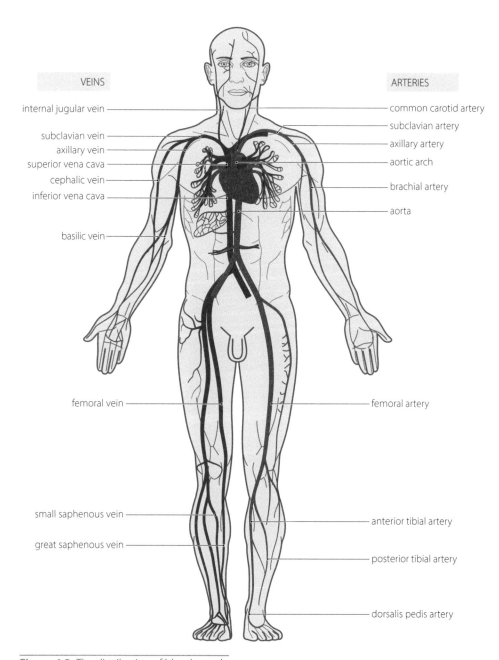

Figure 4.3 The distribution of blood vessels.

VEINS	ARTERIES
internal jugular vein	common carotid artery
subclavian vein	subclavian artery
axillary vein	axillary artery
superior vena cava	aortic arch
cephalic vein	brachial artery
inferior vena cava	aorta
basilic vein	
femoral vein	femoral artery
small saphenous vein	anterior tibial artery
great saphenous vein	posterior tibial artery
	dorsalis pedis artery

> **During examination, central arteries are used to assess blood pressure as they have similar pressures to the aorta.**

Systemic circulation

Arterioles

Arterioles are small diameter arteries; they are also known as 'resistance vessels' as they are capable of contracting and dilating to influence the total

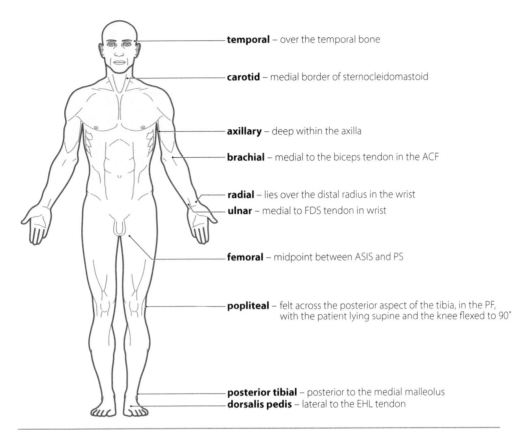

temporal – over the temporal bone

carotid – medial border of sternocleidomastoid

axillary – deep within the axilla

brachial – medial to the biceps tendon in the ACF

radial – lies over the distal radius in the wrist
ulnar – medial to FDS tendon in wrist

femoral – midpoint between ASIS and PS

popliteal – felt across the posterior aspect of the tibia, in the PF, with the patient lying supine and the knee flexed to 90°

posterior tibial – posterior to the medial malleolus
dorsalis pedis – lateral to the EHL tendon

Figure 4.4 Location of the common pulses. ACF = antecubital fossa, FDS = flexor digitorum profundus, PF = popliteal fossa, EHL = extensor hallucis longus, ASIS = anterior superior iliac spine, PS = pubic symphysis.

peripheral resistance and overall blood pressure (BP) (see *Section 3.4.2*).

Veins

Veins are 'capacitance vessels' as they carry most of the circulating blood volume. They are much less muscular than arteries, and have a reduced effect on BP. Venous blood is under a constant pressure, unaffected by ventricular contraction, and contains valves that prevent backflow of blood.

> **Atherosclerosis is the hardening and thickening of arteries due to the deposition of fat-laden immune cells within the vascular wall**. It is associated with non-modifiable and modifiable risk factors.

> Non-modifiable risk factors are:
> - advanced age
> - male sex
> - genetic susceptibility.
>
> Modifiable risk factors are:
> - smoking
> - elevated serum lipids including cholesterol
> - impaired glucose metabolism
> - obesity.

Fluid movement

The walls of blood vessels are semi-permeable, allowing fluid to move between the vessel lumen and the interstitium. The hydrostatic pressure is the intra-luminal pressure that pushes fluid into tissues. The oncotic pressure refers to the concentration gradient between the bloodstream and interstitium, due to the presence of large protein molecules in the blood. The oncotic pressure draws fluid back into the vessel.

4.2.3 The cardiac cycle

The cardiac cycle is the rapid sequence of events that take place over the course of one heartbeat. The cardiac cycle has two parts: systole and diastole.

Systole

During systole the ventricles contract, generating high pressures to push blood into the pulmonary artery (from the right ventricle) and the aorta (from the left ventricle). The tricuspid and mitral valves close at the beginning of systole to prevent backflow to the atria, creating the first heart sound (S1). This occurs at the time the central pulse is palpable.

Diastole

During diastole, the ventricles relax and fill with blood. The tricuspid and mitral valves open, and the pulmonary and aortic valves close, creating the second heart sound (S2). The closure of the pulmonary and aortic valves prevents backflow of blood from the pulmonary artery and aorta.

Cardiac conduction pathway

The heartbeat is generated when a wave of electrical charge (depolarisation) spreads through the individual cells of the heart muscle, called cardiomyocytes. As cardiomyocytes are depolarised, they contract. When enough cardiomyocytes contract together, the entire ventricle contracts, generating a heartbeat.

SA node

The sinoatrial (SA) node is a cluster of cardiomyocytes in the right atrium able to generate an electrical impulse, a property called automaticity. This impulse travels down around the atria, causing atrial contraction and the flow of blood into the ventricles (**Figure 4.5**).

AV node

The atrioventricular (AV) node is at the junction of the right atrium and right ventricle. It detects the

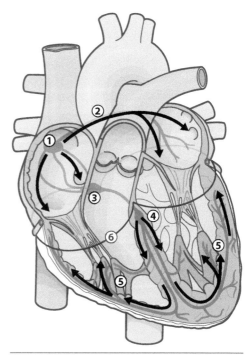

Figure 4.5 The conduction pathways of the heart. 1 = the sinoatrial (SA) node, 2 = Bachmann's bundle, 3 = atrioventricular (AV) node, 4 = bundle of His, 5 = Purkinje fibres, 6 = fibroannular rings (shown in pink) insulate the ventricles from the atria.

incoming electrical impulse and passes it to the ventricles.

Bundle of His

The impulse moves down the short bundle of His, a collection of highly conductive fibres, which divide into left and right branches supplying the ventricles. The resulting depolarisation of the ventricles causes ventricular contraction.

Control of heart rate

The heart rate is controlled by manipulation of SA node automaticity.

Sympathetic activation

The sympathetic nervous system (SNS) directly increases electrical activity at the SA node, resulting in a more rapid heart rate. The SNS also triggers the release of catecholamines (adrenaline and noradrenaline) from the adrenal glands. These hormones also increase the heart rate and force of the ventricular contraction, causing the classic 'thumping heartbeat' during an adrenaline response.

Parasympathetic activation

The parasympathetic nervous system influences the SA node via the vagus nerve, which decreases the frequency of impulse generation, thus lowering the heart rate.

Blood pressure

The continuous pumping action of the heart creates the systemic blood pressure (BP), an estimate of the intravascular pressure applied to the vessel wall.

The systolic BP is the maximum pressure generated by the ventricles during systole, and the diastolic pressure is the minimum pressure generated in diastole.

Factors affecting BP

BP is dependent on:
- **stroke volume (SV)**: the volume of blood ejected from the left ventricle with each contraction, in millilitres (ml)
- **heart rate (HR)**: the number of beats per minute (bpm)

- **cardiac output (CO)**: the volume of blood ejected from the heart per minute
- **total peripheral resistance (TPR)**: the mean pressure of the peripheral arteries.

These interact in the following way:
$$CO = SV \times HR$$
$$BP = CO \times TPR$$

The body controls HR and SV via the autonomic nervous system. TPR is modulated via arteriolar constriction / dilation, and by varying the total circulating blood volume.

> **Severe hypotension is treated with drugs that raise BP by increasing HR, SV and vasoconstriction.** Hypertension is treated by blocking catecholamines and renal hormones, reducing the circulating volume with diuretics, and inducing vasodilatation.

BP is controlled by three pathways:
- regulation of the SNS and PNS in response to pressure receptors (baroreceptors) in the large arteries.
- the release of renal hormones (e.g. renin), causing arteriolar constriction, and salt and fluid retention.
- the release of antidiuretic hormone (ADH) in the pituitary, causing fluid retention.

4.3 Symptoms of cardiovascular disease

History and examination assess for the features of the main cardiovascular diseases (**Table 4.1**) as well as risk factors for CHD and PVD.

The key symptoms are chest pain, palpitations, collapse, leg swelling, breathlessness, leg pain on exertion and ulcers.

4.3.1 Chest pain

This is due to cardiac, respiratory, gastro-oesophageal or musculoskeletal disease (**Figure 4.6**).

Cardiovascular causes

Stable angina

Stable angina pectoris (usually simply called 'angina') is chest pain caused by ischaemia (poor

blood supply) to the heart muscle, occurring when oxygenated blood fails to meet demand. Stable angina occurs on exertion, when the heart needs more oxygenated blood to match its increased workload.

Acute coronary syndrome

Cardiac ischaemic pain that occurs at rest, and is not relieved by GTN, indicates an ACS, a medical emergency (**Figure 4.7**):
- ST elevation myocardial infarction (STEMI)
- non-ST elevation MI
- unstable angina.

Pericarditis

Pericarditis is inflammation of the pericardium, the sac surrounding the heart, causing a sharp central

Table 4.1 *The main clinical features of cardiovascular disease*

Disease	Symptoms	Signs
CHD	Chest pain (angina)	Increased adiposity
		Tar staining
		Xanthelasma / xanthomata
		Corneal arcus
		Coronary artery bypass graft scar
Valvular disease	Breathlessness	Displaced cardiac apex
	Chest pain	Cardiac murmur
	Decreasing exercise tolerance	
Arrhythmias	Palpitations	Irregular pulse
	Chest pain	
	Breathlessness	
	Syncope	
Heart failure	Breathlessness	Elevated JVP
	Decreased exercise tolerance	Pulmonary oedema
	Orthopnoea	Peripheral oedema
	PND (paroxysmal nocturnal dyspnoea)	
	Ankle swelling	
PVD	Claudication	Lower limb hair loss
	Peripheral numbness	Lower limb soft tissue infections
	Cold limbs	Leg ulcers
		Cold extremities
		Weak / absent peripheral pulses

chest pain. It is relieved by leaning forward, and worsened by lying flat.

Aortic dissection

Thoracic aortic dissection is a tear in the intimal layer of the aorta, causing blood pooling within the vascular wall. It is a rare cause of chest pain, with a high mortality. It causes a tearing central chest pain that radiates to the back, and often also causes aortic regurgitation (when the aortic valve becomes leaky, allowing backflow of blood from the aorta into the left ventricle during diastole) or an ACS if it involves the proximal aorta.

Respiratory causes

Pleuritis – inflammation of the pleural lining of the lungs – causes pleuritic pain, a sharp intercostal pain worsened on deep inspiration and coughing. Causes include infection and systemic inflammatory diseases.

A pneumothorax is a collapsed lung due to collection of air in the pleural space, causing acute pleuritic pain and breathlessness.

Gastro-oesophageal causes

Gastro-oesophageal reflux disease (GORD) is the chronic regurgitation of stomach acid into the oesophagus. It causes heartburn (see *Section 6.3.1*).

Musculoskeletal causes

Injury to muscles and connective tissue in the ribcage causes pain of any part of the thorax. Musculoskeletal pain usually:

■ is aggravated by moving the back or thorax

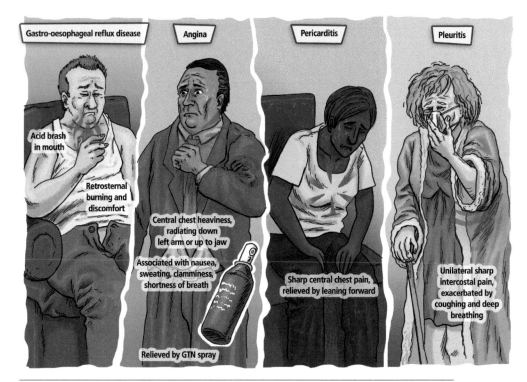

| Gastro-oesophageal reflux disease | Angina | Pericarditis | Pleuritis |

Acid brash in mouth

Retrosternal burning and discomfort

Central chest heaviness, radiating down left arm or up to jaw

Associated with nausea, sweating, clamminess, shortness of breath

Sharp central chest pain, relieved by leaning forward

Unilateral sharp intercostal pain, exacerbated by coughing and deep breathing

Relieved by GTN spray

Figure 4.6 The character of chest pain helps differentiate the cause between cardiac, gastro-oesophageal or pleuritic aetiologies.

■ causes a tender chest wall that is painful to palpation.

Differentiation

Diagnosis requires obtaining an accurate history of the pain, e.g. by using the mnemonic SOCRATES (**Table 4.2**).

4.3.2 Palpitations

Palpitations are an uncomfortable awareness of one's own heartbeat. Patients sense their heart beating quickly, slowly, regularly, irregularly, or describe extra beats.

Palpitations mean different things to different patients: ask them to tap out the rhythm of their heartbeat on a table to help understand their experience. For example, a fast, irregular rhythm would indicate atrial fibrillation.

Causes

A normal heart rate is 60–100 beats per minute. Sinus tachycardia is a regular tachycardia from the sinus node. It is a common cause of palpitations. Causes include:

■ emotional and psychological arousal: anxiety, excitement, fear
■ pain
■ exercise
■ fever and sepsis
■ endocrine disorders also cause sinus tachycardia (see *Section 4.5.4*).

Ventricular ectopic beats are 'extra' beats originating in the ventricles. They are considered normal and do not require treatment. Patients experience them as a pause followed by a forceful beat.

Differentiation

Diagnosis is aided by establishing the timing, nature and associated symptoms of palpitations

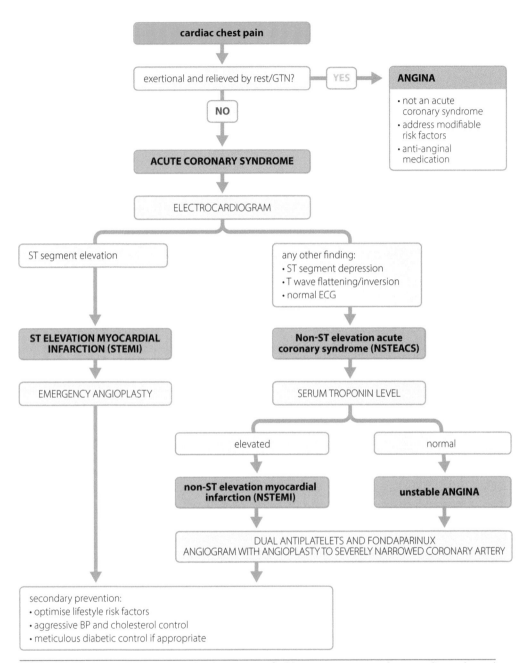

Figure 4.7 Differentiating between the three types of ACS, using symptoms, electrocardiography and cardiac enzymes (troponin).

(**Table 4.3**). Palpitations associated with syncope imply compromise of BP and require urgent investigation.

Exacerbating and relieving factors
Atrial fibrillation and flutter are exacerbated by excessive caffeine and alcohol, as is the frequency

Table 4.2 *Differentiating between potential causes of chest pain using the SOCRATES mnemonic*

	Cardiac	Gastro-oesophageal	Musculoskeletal	Respiratory
Site	Central chest Less commonly: epigastric, left side / right side of chest	Epigastric Retrosternal	Intercostal Unilateral	Intercostal Usually unilateral
Onset	Usually sudden onset	Variable	Sudden onset	Acute or subacute onset
Character	Squeezing Pressure Crushing	Burning Spasm	Aching Sharp	Pleuritic
Radiation	May radiate down left arm, up neck to jaw, or to epigastric region	Retrosternally to throat, or to epigastrium	Along muscles / tendons	May be single point pain, or radiate through ribs
Associated symptoms	Sweating Nausea Breathlessness	Nausea Belching Water or acid brash	Variable	Breathlessness
Timing	Angina typically lasts <20 minutes	During or shortly after food	During movement only	Usually constant
Exacerbating and relieving factors	Exacerbated by exertion Relieved by rest and nitrate therapy	Exacerbated or alleviated by eating Heartburn worse on lying flat Relieved by antacids	Exacerbated by certain positions / movements Chest wall tender to pressure Relieved by rest and simple analgesia	Exacerbated by deep inspiration and coughing Relieved by shallow breathing
Severity	Doctors often ask patients to score the pain out of 10 (10/10 being the worst pain imaginable). Whilst severity doesn't help differentiate between possible causes, it helps us understand how the pain is affecting the patient.			

of ventricular ectopics. Tachycardias are either chronic, or occur in discrete episodes ('paroxysms') lasting minutes, hours or days. An example is paroxysmal atrial fibrillation.

Palpitations due to anxiety-provoked sinus tachycardia generally correlate with mood and anxiety levels.

Associated symptoms

Both tachy- and bradyarrhythmias have the potential to cause a decrease in cardiac output, resulting in syncope. If the cardiac output drops significantly, perfusion of the coronary vessels deteriorates and ischaemic chest pain ensues – a serious sign of shock, requiring urgent medical attention.

Table 4.3 *Causes and symptoms of common arrhythmias, with associated symptoms*

Underlying rhythm	Feeling	Causes	Associated symptoms
Bradycardia	Dizziness Presyncope	Rate-slowing medications Beta blockers Rate-limiting CCBs Digoxin Sinus node disease AV node disease	Syncope Chest pain Confusion Yellow vision (digoxin) Hypothermia Low blood sugar
Sinus tachycardia	Heart racing Heart 'thudding'	Emotional / psychological arousal Thyrotoxicosis Sepsis Pain Exercise Drugs including illicit (such as cocaine or amphetamines) or legal (caffeine)	Tremor Anxiety, agitation
Ventricular ectopics	Sudden 'thud' 'Dropped beat'	Normal in isolation	None
Atrial fibrillation and flutter, atrioventricular nodal re-entry tachycardias	Rapid pulse 'Fluttering' in chest	Ischaemic heart disease Sepsis Thyrotoxicosis Alcohol excess Caffeine excess	Syncope Chest pain
Ventricular tachycardia	'Fluttering' in chest	Structural heart disease Myocardial ischaemia Severe heart failure	Syncope Chest pain Confusion / decreased consciousness

4.3.3 Collapse

Collapse means sudden and unpreventable loss in muscle tone, leading to a fall. Patients describe either:

- light-headedness and near collapse (presyncope), or
- total loss of consciousness (syncope).

Collapse and palpitations are often terrifying experiences for the patient. Reassure the patient and provide them with clear explanations to minimise their distress, and explain that whilst frightening, they can be treated.

Causes

The commonest causes of collapse are cardiogenic, neurocardiogenic, epileptic, metabolic, drug-induced and psychological (**Table 4.4**).

Terms of collapse can be subjective, e.g.:

- '**Light-headedness**' may mean presyncope, headache, vertigo or severe nausea.
- '**Vertigo**' – a sensation of the room spinning – is a symptom of vestibular or cerebellar disease, but may describe presyncope.
- '**Dizzy**' is common but highly ambiguous.

Table 4.4 *Common causes of syncope and associated symptoms, illustrating how exploration of the history, context and associated symptoms is crucial in making the diagnosis*

Cause	Speed of onset	Speed of recovery	Potential triggers	Associated symptoms
Neurocardiogenic (vasovagal)	Sudden	Rapid	Heat Change in posture Venesection Micturition Excessive cough	Light-headedness Weakness Tunnel vision
Tachyarrhythmia	Sudden	Rapid	Cardiac disease	Palpitations Chest pain
Bradyarrhythmia	Sudden	Minutes	None	Palpitations Chest pain Decreased consciousness or confusion
Left ventricular outflow tract obstruction	Sudden	Rapid	Exercise, increased cardiac output	Chest pain
Epileptic	Sudden; may have an aura	Slow	Sleep deprivation Non-compliance with anticonvulsant medication Alcohol excess Infection	Tongue biting (often lateral) Incontinence
Non-epileptic attack ('pseudoseizure')	Sudden	Rapid	Psychological	Psychiatric illness Often coexisting epilepsy
Hypoglycaemia	Gradual	Gradual	Hypoglycaemic medications including insulin	Pallor Sweating Tremor Confusion
Encephalopathic	Gradual	Slow	Severe liver failure Severe renal failure Chronic alcohol abuse	Mental clouding Agitation Tremor
Drug-induced	Dependent on dosage and type of drug	Slow	Excessive opiates, benzodiazepines, recreational drugs, alcohol	Pinpoint pupils (opiates) and hypoventilation

To clarify, ask: 'what did the dizziness feel like?', or 'did you feel that you were about to lose consciousness, or that the room was spinning around you?'

4.3.4 Leg swelling

Bilateral ankle swelling usually results from oedema, the accumulation of fluid in tissues. This is a sign of serious disease, including heart, liver and kidney failure. Fluid collects in gravity-dependent areas, i.e. the ankles and lower limbs in mobile patients and the sacral area in bed-bound patients.

Untreated peripheral oedema accumulates up to the level of the thighs, the abdominal wall, or even the chest. Oedema of any cause shows evidence of 'pitting' – when the skin is firmly depressed by a finger, an indentation remains for several minutes (**Figure 4.8**).

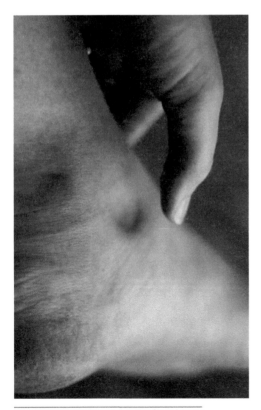

Figure 4.8 Pitting oedema of the lower extremities. A thumb is pressed firmly over the oedematous skin, leaving a pit or dimple.

Causes

The PEDAL mnemonic helps to differentiate causes (**Table 4.5**) which are divided into cardiac and non-cardiac (**Table 4.6**).

Cardiac

Oedema develops in right ventricular failure due to increased hydrostatic pressure. Isolated right ventricular failure is usually due to chronic lung disease (known as cor pulmonale), but the commonest cause is secondary to left ventricular failure. This is called biventricular or congestive cardiac failure (CCF), and occurs due to CHD, severe valvular disease, chronic atrial fibrillation or diseases of the myocardium (cardiomyopathies).

Non-cardiac

Peripheral oedema develops in low-protein states, due to low intravascular oncotic pressure. In renal failure, the kidney loses excessive protein in the urine (i.e. protein-losing nephropathy, or nephrotic syndrome if >3g per day). Patients with nephrotic syndrome also develop oedema of the hands and face. Liver failure causes decreased synthesis of albumin, the main circulating protein.

Lymphoedema is impaired lymphatic drainage of the interstitial fluid. It occurs predominantly in the lower limbs, and is either genetic, idiopathic or secondary to surgery, cancer or chronic infection.

Myxoedema is a rare cause of bilateral lower limb oedema. It is caused by severe hypothyroidism (see *Section 13.6.4*).

Unilateral leg swelling

This is usually due to a localised disease process.
Deep vein thrombosis. This is a clot formation in the lower limb veins, causing unilateral swelling and tenderness in the calf muscle.

Risk factors include:
- oral contraceptive pill
- personal history of venous thromboembolism (VTE)
- family history of clots
- recent long-haul travel
- recent period of immobility
- recent surgery
- diagnosis of cancer.

Cellulitis. This soft tissue and skin infection results in erythema, pain and swelling of the

Table 4.5 *The PEDAL mnemonic to take a history of ankle swelling*

	Questions	Relevance
Presence	"Do you have any swelling in your ankles or your feet?"	Identifies the presence of swelling
Exacerbating and relieving factors	"Does anything make the swelling better or worse?"	Oedema is worse in the evening and slightly better in the morning It is ameliorated by elevating the legs Swelling due to cellulitis or DVT does not have diurnal variation
Development	"When did the swelling start?"	If the swelling developed suddenly, it is more likely to be a popliteal cyst rupture, DVT, or due to trauma Insidious onset implies oedema or lymphoedema
Associated symptoms	"Do you have any other symptoms?"	In CCF, patient will have signs of pulmonary oedema (see 'Breathlessness', *Section 4.3.5*) In renal failure, the patient may notice periorbital puffiness, hand swelling, or frothy urine In liver failure, the patient may be jaundiced or have other signs of liver disease
Legs: unilateral or bilateral?	"Are both legs swollen or just one?"	Bilateral swelling implies oedema or lymphoedema Unilateral swelling is more likely to be due to local disease processes

Table 4.6 *Cardiac and non-cardiac causes of ankle swelling*

	Mechanism	Clinical features
Cardiac cause	Right ventricular failure causes increased hydrostatic pressure in the systemic circulation	Oedema develops in dependent areas Usually accompanied by signs of left ventricular failure, e.g. pulmonary oedema
Non-cardiac causes		
Renal failure	Protein loss from the kidney	Generalised oedema including hands and face Frothy urine
Liver failure	Decreased albumin manufacture in liver	Oedema develops in dependent areas Accompanied by other signs of liver failure, e.g. ascites, jaundice
Lymphoedema	Impaired lymphatic drainage	Thickening and hardening of skin May not be pitting oedema
Myxoedema	Severe hyperthyroidism leading to increased dermal fibroblast activity	Pretibial areas May not be pitting oedema
Medications, e.g. CCBs	Vessel dilatation and fluid leak	Often around ankles, may be unilateral

affected skin. The patient may have other signs of sepsis.

Local soft tissue injury. Local trauma due to a sports injury or a fall, for example, results in soft tissue pain and swelling. The skin is usually normal in colour, and often warm to touch.

Popliteal cyst. This is a swelling of the synovial bursa behind the knee. It is either primary (idiopathic), or secondary to rheumatological disease.

If the cyst ruptures, it causes severe pain and swelling to the popliteal fossa and calf muscle.

4.3.5 Breathlessness

Breathlessness (i.e. dyspnoea) is the unpleasant sensation of not being able to breathe enough to meet the body's demands, despite increasing the respiratory rate. It is a cardinal feature of respiratory problems.

Causes

The mnemonic AEROS is useful when differentiating causes of breathlessness (**Table 4.7**).

Respiratory

Sudden onset breathlessness may signify a pneumothorax, a PE, or an acute exacerbation of chronic airways disease. Chronic breathlessness is common to all respiratory diseases (see *Section 5.3.1*).

	Questions	Relevance
Associated symptoms	"What other symptoms are you having?"	Ischaemic chest pain points to angina attacks
		Productive cough with coloured sputum implies infection, including infective exacerbations of airways disease
		Wheezing is associated with asthma and COPD
		Sharp pleuritic pain may indicate a pneumothorax or PE
Exacerbating factors	"What makes it worse?"	Dyspnoea on lying flat is orthopnoea, and is a sign of pulmonary oedema or possible diaphragmatic insufficiency
		Asthma attack triggers include allergens, aerosols, cold weather, exercise and non-compliance with inhalers
Relieving factors	"What makes it better?"	Patients with airways disease obtain benefit when they use their salbutamol inhaler
		Patients with orthopnoea find their breathlessness improves when they sit upright
Onset	"When did it start?"	Sudden onset breathlessness with coughing frothy sputum is a sign of acute left ventricular failure
		Sudden onset dyspnoea with unilateral pleuritic pain is in keeping with a pneumothorax or PE
		Gradual onset breathlessness may signify developing heart failure; if accompanied by coughing and wheezing, it is related to airways disease
		Acute onset breathlessness coinciding with palpitations is associated with tachyarrhythmias
Severity	"How bad is the breathlessness?"	This indicates the effect on daily life, and is also useful to monitor symptom response to treatment (e.g. new inhaler or a diuretic)

Table 4.7 *Use the mnemonic AEROS when taking a breathlessness history*

Cardiovascular

Pulmonary oedema is the accumulation of fluid in the pulmonary interstitial space, causing breathlessness. It is due to left ventricular failure. It either worsens over a period of weeks and months (with chronic heart failure) or develops suddenly following an ACS. When severe, it causes:

- **paroxysmal nocturnal dyspnoea (PND)**: waking during the night with severe breathlessness. Patients often feel the urge to get out of bed and walk around until the symptoms abate.
- **orthopnoea**: the onset of breathlessness on lying flat, due to redistribution of pulmonary blood flow. Affected patients sleep upright on several pillows. Ask breathless patients how many pillows they have, and what happens when they lie flat.

4.3.6 Exertional leg pain

Pain in the lower limbs on exertion is classified as vascular or non-vascular in origin (**Table 4.8**), as investigation and treatment are very different.

Vascular causes

Vascular claudication is ischaemic muscular pain, most often of the lower limb, due to PVD (i.e. atherosclerosis). It is aggravated by walking, and relieved by rest. GTN has minimal effect on the pain.

Severe PVD often causes pain whilst lying in bed, as sufficient lower limb blood flow is gravity-dependent. The pain is usually relieved by hanging the leg over the side of the bed.

Non-vascular causes

Lumbar spinal stenosis

Neurogenic claudication is lower limb pain due to lumbar spinal stenosis, an age-related degenerative spinal disease. Vascular claudication must be differentiated from vascular claudication as the two are managed very differently (**Table 4.9**).

4.3.7   Lower limb ulcers

Patients with PVD often present with arterial or venous ulcers. Ulcers are differentiated by location, presence of pain and associated skin changes (**Table 4.10**).

	Aetiology	Distribution of pain	Exacerbating factors	Relieving factors
Vascular cause	Peripheral arterial disease	Muscles of lower leg, radiating proximally	Exertion	Rest Lowering legs
	DVT	Posterior leg muscles	Exertion	None
Non-vascular cause	Degenerative spine disease	Buttocks and thighs, radiating to lower leg	Standing / lying flat Exertion	Bending forwards Sitting Rest
	Joint disease	Within joints	Exertion Worse in morning	Rest Gentle mobilisation
	Myositis	Proximal muscles	None	None
	Polymyalgia rheumatica	Proximal muscles	Worse in mornings	None

Table 4.8 *Vascular and non-vascular causes of lower limb pain*

Table 4.9 *Differentiating between vascular and neurogenic claudication*

Vascular claudication	Neurogenic claudication
Pain begins in calf and radiates up to thigh and buttock	Pain begins in thigh and buttock and radiates down to calf
Pain worsened by exertion	Pain worsened by exertion
Pain relieved by rest	Pain relieved by changing position
Pain rapidly relieved on rest	Pain slowly abates on rest and position change

Table 4.10 *Comparing lower limb ulcers: clinical features and location*

Type	Location	Other signs	Pulses	Pain
Venous	Gaiter area (medial aspect shin)	Haemosiderin deposition Varicose veins	Usually present	Yes
Arterial	Pressure areas (heel, lateral malleolus, between toes)	Dry skin Nail changes Cool	Absent	Yes
Neuropathic	Pressure areas (heel, lateral malleolus, between toes)	Charcot joints Altered sensation	Usually present	No

4.4   The cardiovascular history

4.4.1   Past medical history

In addition to eliciting past medical and surgical illnesses, clarify the patient's risk factors for CHD. This provides context in which to judge whether or not their symptoms are cardiovascular in origin. Ask about conditions that predispose to CHD:

- Have you ever been told that you have high blood pressure?
- Have you ever had your blood cholesterol levels measured? Were they high?
- Do you have diabetes?

4.4.2 Medications

Be aware that many medications used in cardiovascular medicine (**Table 4.11**) are used in other conditions:

- **Propranolol**, a beta blocker used to treat hypertension, is also used in thyrotoxicosis, benign essential tremor and anxiety.
- **Doxazosin**, an alpha blocker used to treat hypertension, is also used to treat prostatic hypertrophy.
- **Verapamil**, a calcium channel blocker (CCB) used to treat hypertension, is also used to treat cluster headaches.

> **Avoid miscommunication when discussing past medical history by clarifying the patient's response to questions.** For example, a patient might answer 'no' when asked if they have high blood pressure, when they mean that their blood pressure is currently well controlled with antihypertensives.

Table 4.11 *Common medications used in cardiovascular medicine*

Drug group	Nomenclature and examples	Uses in cardiovascular medicine	Common side-effects
Antiplatelets	Aspirin Clopidogrel Ticagrelor Prasugrel	Prevent platelet aggregation	GI ulcers Bleeding Dyspnoea (ticagrelor)
Nitrates	Isosorbide mono- / dinitrate GTN	Anti-anginal	Headache Hypotension
Alpha-1 blockers	have the suffix *-zocin* Doxazocin Alfuzocin	Antihypertensive	Postural hypotension
Beta blockers	have the suffix *-olol* Bisoprolol Atenolol Sotolol	Anti-anginal Controlling tachyarrhythmias Antihypertensive (less commonly) Prognostic benefit in heart failure and post-MI	Bradycardia Bronchospasm Fatigue Impotence
CCBs:			
Dihydropyridines	have the suffix *-dipine* Nifedipine Amlodipine	Antihypertensive	Peripheral oedema Skin flushing Perianal ulcers
Non-dihydropyridines	Verapamil Diltiazem	Anti-anginal Controlling tachyarrhythmias	Bradycardia
Renin–angiotensin system blockers:			
Angiotensin-converting enzyme (ACE) inhibitors	have the suffix *-pril* Perindopril Ramipril	Antihypertensive Renal protection in diabetes Prognostic benefit in heart failure	Cough (more common in ACE inhibitors) Renal impairment Hyperkalaemia Angioedema
Angiotensin receptor blockers (ARBs)	have the suffix *-sartan* Losartan Candesartan	Antihypertensive Renal protection in diabetes Prognostic benefit in heart failure	Cough (more common in ACE inhibitors) Renal impairment Hyperkalaemia Angioedema

Drug group	Nomenclature and examples	Uses in cardiovascular medicine	Common side-effects
Other anti-arrhythmics	Amiodarone Flecainide Digoxin	Treatment of arrhythmias	Widely variable, includes nausea, electrolyte disorders, skin disorders, thyroid disorders, lung fibrosis, bradycardia
Diuretics:			
Loop diuretics	Furosemide Butenamide	Fluid overload in cardiac failure	Electrolyte disorders Dehydration Renal impairment
Thiazide diuretics	have the suffix -*thiazide* Bendroflumethiazide Hydrochlorothiazide	Antihypertensive	Electrolyte disorders, especially hyponatraemia Gout Dehydration, renal failure
Potassium-sparing diuretics	Spironolactone Eplerenone	Fluid overload in cardiac failure	Hyperkalaemia Dehydration, renal impairment
Anticoagulants	Warfarin Heparin Rivaroxaban Dabigatran Apixaban	Prevention of thrombosis in arrhythmias	Bleeding Skin necrosis
Statins	have the suffix -*statin* Simvastatin Atorvastatin	Reduce cholesterol	Muscle aches Myositis Rhabdomyolysis

4.4.3 Social history

This focuses on establishing the presence of modifiable risk factors and how the patient's health is impacting on their life.

Smoking

Tobacco smoking is the single most important predictor of cardiovascular disease and a smoking history should be obtained (see *Section 1.5.6*).

Alcohol

High alcohol intake may lead to hypertension, arrhythmias or cardiomyopathy (see *Section 1.5.6*).

Caffeine

Ask about caffeine intake, including energy drinks, especially in patients with palpitations. Excessive caffeine exacerbates tachyarrhythmias, and causes a sinus tachycardia in most people.

Illicit drugs

Ask about illicit drugs such as cannabis (which may be smoked with tobacco) or heroin. Repeated cocaine use accelerates atherosclerosis, tachyarrhythmias or an ACS.

Employment

Find out whether the patient is in employment, and whether they have a sedentary job or one that involves physical activity.

Physical activity

Enquire whether the patient is active in their daily life, and whether they take any exercise. A sedentary lifestyle greatly increases the risk of cardiovascular disease, and exacerbates the venous stasis associated with DVT.

Diet

Establish whether the patient's diet contains a healthy amount of fruit and vegetables, or excessive fats or sugar.

Functional capacity

Establish functional capacity and how this has changed in recent weeks in patients with breathlessness or fatigue. This helps quantify symptoms of chronic disease, such as congestive heart failure or COPD, and monitor response to treatment.

Ask if symptoms have affected:

- their daily life
- ability to work
- enjoyment of hobbies and interests.

For example, patients with severe angina may be reluctant to leave the house for fear of provoking an attack, and therefore not able to shop for themselves or visit loved ones.

4.4.4 Family history

Ask about:

- lipid disorders, e.g. familial hypercholesterolaemia: "Do people in your family tend to struggle with high cholesterol?"

- CHD under the age of 60 (more strongly associated with genetic cardiovascular diseases): "Is there a history of heart attacks in the family? At what sort of age?"
- sudden unexpected death – this may be due to congenital heart disease: "Has there ever been a member of your family who died suddenly and unexpectedly, maybe due to a heart defect?"
- endocrine disorders, such as diabetes, which accelerate cardiovascular disease.

4.4.5 Cardiovascular risk assessment

The patient's risk factors are used to calculate their cardiovascular risk, e.g. using the Joint British Societies' risk calculator. This uses evidence-based data to estimate 10-year risk of a cardiovascular event.

Risk factor variables include:

- age
- presence of hypertension
- presence of hyperlipidaemia
- smoking status
- previous CHD (ACS or angina)
- family history of CHD
- presence of diabetes
- body mass index (BMI).

Different calculators produce different risk scores, so the same (locally recommended) one should be used for consistency.

4.4.6 Systems review

Ensure to ask about other symptoms patients have, as they are often connected with cardiovascular disease (**Table 4.12**).

4.5 Signs of cardiovascular disease

Look for signs of CHD, valvular disease, arrhythmia and heart failure, as well as risk factors for CHD (**Table 4.2**).

4.5.1 Hand and nail changes

Bacterial endocarditis causes:

- splinter haemorrhages – small dark red-brown dots or dashes seen in the nails of the hands or feet; they are tiny embolic clots (**Figure 4.9**)
- Osler's nodes (**Figure 4.10**)– tender red lesions on the palm or soles
- Janeway lesions – painless red lesions to the palms and soles.

Table 4.12 *A full system review related to cardiovascular disease*

System	Symptoms	Cardiovascular causes
Respiratory	Cough	Infection, pulmonary oedema
	Haemoptysis	Pulmonary embolism, severe pulmonary oedema, right heart endocarditis
Endocrine	Change in weight or energy levels	Thyroid disease
	Excessive thirst and urination	Diabetes mellitus
Gastrointestinal	Weight gain	Worsening generalised oedema in cardiac failure, including ascites
	Acid reflux	Gastro-oesophageal disease worsened by long-term aspirin use
	Nausea and vomiting	Symptoms of ACS
Neurological	Syncope	Cardiac disease Arrhythmia Orthostatic hypotension
	Headache	Side-effect of GTN
	Stroke	Often associated with atrial fibrillation, or concomitant CHD
Genitourinary	Impotence	Signifies peripheral arterial disease or medication, e.g. beta blockers
	Proteinuria	Nephrotic syndrome causing peripheral oedema

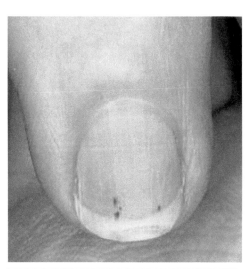

Figure 4.9 Splinter haemorrhages are small dark flecks in the nail bed.

Clubbing
Cardiac causes of nail clubbing (see *Section 3.6* and **Figure 3.5**) include
- benign cardiac tumours
- cyanotic congenital heart disease
- subacute endocarditis.

Peripheral cyanosis
This is a bluish discolouration of the fingers and nails and indicates hypoxia.

Tar staining
This is a brown discolouration of the fingers, indicating long-term cigarette smoking.

Capillary refill time:
This is prolonged when tissues are poorly perfused, e.g. in hypotension or PVD (see *Section 4.7.4*).

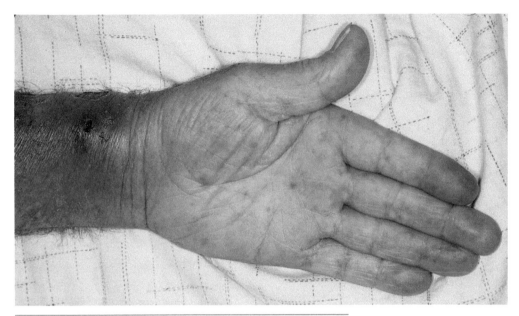

Figure 4.10 Osler's nodes are painful red bumps on the palms or soles.

4.5.2 Eyes

There are two signs of cardiovascular disease in the eyes: corneal arcus and conjunctival pallor.

Corneal arcus

This is a common sign in the elderly, but indicates hyperlipidaemia in younger patients (**Figure 4.11**). It looks like a white ring in the iris of the eye.

Conjunctival pallor

This is seen when lowering the patient's lower eyelid and examining the interior skin. A pale appearance of the skin indicates anaemia, which may be the cause of a hyperdynamic clinical state.

4.5.3 Xanthomata

Xanthomata are cholesterol-rich skin deposits strongly associated with hyperlipidaemia, representing lipid accumulation in macrophages. They look like pale papules on the skin. They occur at different sites:

- Tendon xanthomata occur in the skin over areas of tendons and are associated with familial hypercholesterolaemia.
- Xanthelasma around the eyes is associated with all hyperlipidaemias (**Figure 4.12**).
- Palmar xanthoma of the hand is associated with hyperlipidaemia, particularly hypercholesterolaemia.

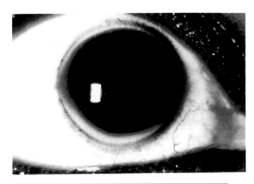

Figure 4.11 Corneal arcus is a hazy white line around the iris of the eye.

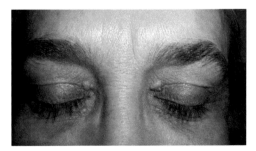

Figure 4.12 Xanthelasma are whitish-yellow collections under the skin, usually seen around the eye.

4.5.4 Abnormal heart rates

Bradycardia

This is a heart rate <60bpm. Bradycardia could be the result of SA node disease (i.e. impaired automaticity), or AV node disease (i.e. impaired conduction). It is often caused by drugs.

Tachycardia

This is a rate >100bpm.

Atrial fibrillation

This causes an irregular rhythm. Both atria experience chaotic electrical activity, rather than ordered impulses from the sinus node.

Atrial flutter

Atrial flutter causes a regular tachycardia with atria depolarising at around 300bpm. The ventricular rate depends on how many of these are conducted by the AV node to the ventricles:

- 1 in 2 = 150bpm (most common)
- 1 in 3 = 100bpm
- 1 in 4 = 75bpm.

Ventricular tachycardia

Ventricular tachycardia is a tachycardia originating in the ventricles and is a medical emergency. It occurs in patients with severe CHD, severe heart failure or congenital abnormalities.

4.5.5 Abnormal respiratory rates

A normal resting respiratory rate is 10–20 breaths per minute.

Tachypnoea

Tachypnoea is an increased respiratory rate, often the earliest sign in any acutely unwell patient. Cardiac causes include:

- angina attacks
- ACS
- untreated heart failure.

Alternatively, it is a sign of respiratory disease (see *Section 5.3.1*) or metabolic abnormalities.

Bradypnoea

Bradypnoea (less than 10 breaths per minute) is normal in a sleeping patient but may be a clinical sign of a side-effect of certain drugs (**Table 5.7**).

4.5.6 Unequal pulses

Diseases of the proximal aorta cause pulses of unequal volume, or a delay between pulses:

- Coarctation of the aorta is a congenital narrowing of the aortic lumen.
- Aortic dissection causes bleeding into the vascular wall, which occludes the lumen.

If the affected area is proximal to the left subclavian artery, there is delay from the right to left radial pulses (a 'radio-radial delay') and a low volume left pulse (**Figure 4.13**). If the affected

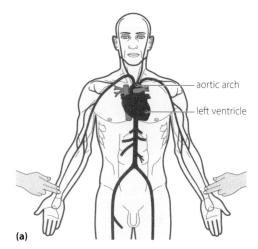

aortic arch

left ventricle

(a)

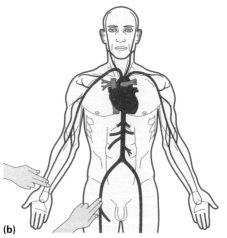

(b)

Figure 4.13 Assessing for (a) radio-radial delay, indicating pathology of the aortic arch proximal to the left subclavian artery; (b) radio-femoral delay, indicating pathology of the descending aorta.

area is distal to the left subclavian artery, there is a delay between the radial and femoral pulse ('radio-femoral delay').

4.5.7 Abnormal pulse volume / character

Palpation of the carotid artery provides information about the pulse volume and character. Pulse volume corresponds to the left ventricle stroke volume.

Low volume pulse

This is a weak, or thready, pulse, and reflects decreased cardiac output. It is found in hypovolaemia, circulatory shock (dangerously low BP leading to poor perfusion of the body's tissues with oxygenated blood), and conditions that restrict the ejection of blood from the heart, such as aortic stenosis.

High volume pulse

This is described as 'bounding', or hyperdynamic, and signifies high cardiac output states, such as fever and sepsis, pregnancy, anaemia and aortic regurgitation.

Pulse character

The character of the pulse correlates with the pulse pressure; the difference between systolic and diastolic pressures (**Figure 4.14**).

Slow rising pulse

This corresponds to a narrow pulse pressure and is found in aortic stenosis, as the left ventricle struggles to eject blood into the aorta. The carotid fills slowly, resulting in a slow expansion of the carotid pulse with each beat. It is difficult to palpate if severe.

Collapsing pulse

This corresponds to a wide pulse pressure and is found in aortic regurgitation. The carotid pulse peaks quickly and forcefully, and then 'falls away'.

4.5.8 Displaced apex beat

The apex beat is the most inferior and lateral point on the chest in which the heartbeat is palpable. It should be in the 5th intercostal space, in the mid-clavicular line. It is displaced laterally when the heart is enlarged (i.e. cardiomegaly). The commonest causes are mitral and aortic regurgitation, both of which result in left ventricular failure.

4.5.9 Heaves

Parasternal heave occurs in right ventricular failure, chiefly in cases of pulmonary hypertension and cor pulmonale. When the examiner's palm is laid firmly over the left parasternal area, a heave is felt as a forward 'thump', which seems to forcefully push the palm up from the chest wall.

4.5.10 Murmurs

Murmurs are audible blood flow, usually due to abnormal flow caused by valvular pathologies. Valves are either narrow (stenosis), or fail to close properly, allowing backflow of blood (regurgitation) (**Table 4.13**). If the patient has

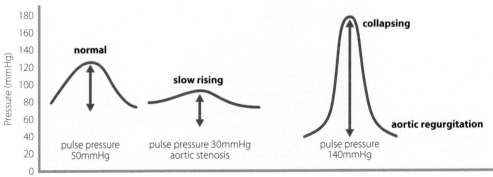

Figure 4.14 Comparing pulse character and pulse pressure.

Table 4.13 *Common left-sided murmurs*

	Aortic stenosis	Aortic regurgitation	Mitral stenosis	Mitral regurgitation
Clinical features	Slow rising pulse Narrow pulse pressure Low volume pulse if severe Quiet S1	Collapsing pulse Wide pulse pressure	Malar flush Usually in atrial fibrillation Tapping apex (palpable S1)	Often associated with connective tissue disorders, e.g. rheumatoid arthritis
Part of stethoscope used	Diaphragm	Diaphragm	Bell	Diaphragm
Character of murmur	Harsh ejection systolic murmur	Early diastolic murmur	Mid-diastolic rumble	Pansystolic 'blowing' murmur
Radiation of murmur	Up to carotids	Towards tricuspid area	No radiation	Into the axilla
Apex beat	Not displaced but forceful	Displaced laterally	Not displaced	Displaced laterally

had a metallic valve replacement, you will hear the clicking of the valve from the end of the bed. Increased flow across a normal valve may cause a 'flow murmur' in high output cardiac states (see high volume pulse, above).

4.5.11 Thrills

A thrill is a palpable murmur. Thrills are detected over the aortic and pulmonary areas of the precordium, as these valves are closest to the chest wall. A thrill feels like a vibration with each systole, or like the purring of a cat.

4.5.12 Bruits

Bruits are noises heard on auscultation of arteries, and represent turbulent blood flow. Turbulence is most often due to vessel stenosis, which in turn is usually due to atherosclerosis.

Patients with carotid bruit are at high risk of stroke. Renal artery bruit represents renal artery stenosis, a cause of hypertension, whilst an aortic bruit, along with a palpable pulsatile mass, indicates an abdominal aortic aneurysm where the enlarged vessel facilitates turbulent flow.

4.5.13 Fluid overload

Fluid overload manifests as generalised oedema. A patient with CCF develops fluid overload via the following mechanisms:
- Reduced blood flow to the kidney activates hormones which cause fluid and sodium retention.
- CCF leads to increased hydrostatic pressure, favouring movement of fluid into the interstitium.

These patients will have peripheral oedema, pulmonary oedema, and an elevated jugular venous pressure (JVP) (see **Figure 3.8**). A raised JVP and peripheral oedema without pulmonary oedema signifies isolated right heart failure.

> **The incidence of heart failure is increasing as people live longer.** This implies that the ageing heart will invariably fail if given enough time. However, with regular exercise, abstaining from smoking, and no genetic susceptibility to diabetes or CHD, there is good evidence that the heart will retain normal function for life.

4.5.14 Hypovolaemia

Hypovolaemia is a state of decreased circulating blood volume. Hypovolaemic patients have non-specific signs of dehydration: dry mucous membranes, decreased skin turgor, sunken eyes, and cool, poorly perfused extremities.

4.5.15 Crackles

These are crackling sounds heard on lung auscultation during inspiration, and represent pulmonary oedema or respiratory causes (see *Section 5.5.16*).

4.5.16 Reduced breath sounds

In addition to pulmonary oedema, fluid collects in the pleural space, causing pleural effusions. They cause reduced breath sounds at the lung bases.

4.5.17 Ulcers

Ulcers are lesions with a break in the epithelium.

Arterial ulcers

These are found on the lower limbs in peripheral vascular disease and develop due to ischaemia of the dermal capillary bed. They have a 'punched-out' appearance and are intensely painful.

Venous ulcers

Venous ulcers are the commonest type and occur due to impaired venous draining of the lower limbs. They are related to local inflammatory response to venous hypertension. They are very painful.

Neuropathic ulcers

These are a complication of diabetic peripheral neuropathy. They begin as trivial injuries undetected by the patient and progress as wound healing is impaired by diabetic vascular disease. They are often painless.

4.5.18 Limb ischaemia

Signs of arterial insufficiency to the lower limbs include (**Figure 4.15**):
- absent dorsalis pedis, posterior tibial and popliteal pulses

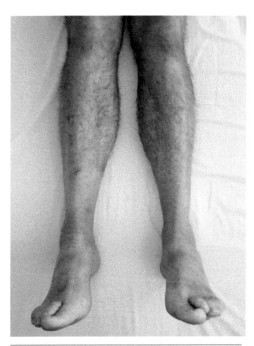

Figure 4.15 Chronic ischaemia of the legs. Notice the decreased hair distribution and pale feet.

- cold extremities, with signs of peripheral cyanosis
- loss of hair on lower legs, with dry skin and poor condition of nails
- evidence of arterial ulcers or non-healing wounds
- chronic foot infections
- gangrene (necrotic tissues) of the toes.

Ischaemia of the upper limbs is rare due to abundant collateral blood flow.

4.5.19 Hypertension

This is a syndrome of BP consistently above 140/90mmHg.

Essential hypertension

Essential or idiopathic hypertension accounts for 80–90% of all hypertension diagnoses. It has a complex pathophysiology, incorporating genetic and environmental factors.

Secondary hypertension

This is elevated BP due to other disease processes, including:

- **endocrine**: some endocrine diseases cause hypertension (see *Section 13.5.2*)
- **renovascular**: renal artery stenosis results in excess renal hormones which increase fluid retention and vasoconstriction.

> **White coat syndrome is when a patient's anxiety gives either a falsely high or low blood pressure reading.** A diagnosis of abnormal blood pressure should be made on 24-hour BP reading with the patient in their home environment.

If hypertension is identified, look for signs of end-organ damage:
- left ventricular hypertrophy and failure
- hypertensive retinopathy (see **Table 10.9**)
- hypertensive nephropathy – manifests as chronic kidney disease and proteinuria.

4.5.20 Diabetes

Diabetes is a major cause / accelerant of CHD and therefore signs of diabetes must be closely sought (see *Section 13.7.3*).

4.6 The cardiovascular examination

Like all examinations, a consistent and thorough approach is required (**Table 4.14**).

4.6.1 'ID CHECK'

This is detailed in *Section 3.2*.

4.6.2 Endobedogram

Have a good look at the patient:
- Are they dyspnoeic or uncomfortable?
- Are they overweight?
- Around the bedside (if they are in a hospital bed) are there oxygen masks, medications or tobacco products?
- Are there scars (**Figure 4.16**)? If there is a midline sternotomy scar, they may have had a coronary artery bypass graft, so check the legs for scars of vein harvesting.

4.6.3 Inspection

Hands

Ask the patient to hold them out in front of them.
- Look for tar staining and peripheral cyanosis.
- Take their hands in your own and note the perfusion of the hand and fingers. Are they warm and well perfused or cool and shut down?
- Look for the peripheral stigmata of cardiovascular disease (see *Section 4.5.1*).

Radial pulse

Assess the radial pulse rate and rhythm.

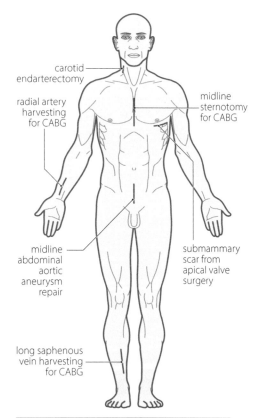

Figure 4.16 Common cardiovascular surgical scars. CABG = coronary artery bypass graft.

Table 4.14 *The sequence of the cardiovascular examination*

Element	Details
General inspection	Appearance: does the patient look systemically well or unwell?
	Environment: are there any clues suggesting disease?
	Face: is the patient centrally cyanosed?
	Chest: is the patient visibly breathless at rest?
	Is the patient over- or underweight?
Hands	Are there any nail abnormalities?
	Is there any evidence of vasculitis?
Wrist	What is the heart rate and rhythm?
Elbow / knee / ankle	Are there any tendon xanthomata?
Arm	What is the blood pressure?
Neck	Is the JVP elevated?
	What is the character of the carotid pulse?
Face	Is there evidence of xanthelasma or corneal arcus?
	Is there conjunctival pallor?
	Is there any flushing of the face?
	Is there central cyanosis?
	How is their dentition?
Chest	Inspection: are there any scars or deformities?
	Palpation: is the apex beat displaced? Are there any heaves or thrills?
	Auscultation: are the heart sounds audible? Are there any murmurs?
	Lung bases: are there any crackles?
Legs	Is there any peripheral oedema?
Abdomen	Is the abdominal aorta palpable? Is it enlarged?
	Are there any renal bruits?
Fundi	Is there evidence of hypertensive or diabetic retinopathy?

In atrial fibrillation (AF), the heart rate at the radial pulse may be lower than that at the apex as each ventricular contraction may not be strong enough to produce an arterial pulse wave, similar to small waves being overtaken by larger ones before reaching a seashore.

Assess for a collapsing pulse and slow rising pulse by pressing the fingertips of your right hand over the patient's left brachial pulse, then lift their forearm above their head (**Figure 4.17**). A collapsing pulse feels like the impulse is 'falling down' their forearm toward their elbow, and a slow-rising pulse feels like the blood is rising slowly toward the hand.

Elbows

Check the extensor aspect of the elbow for xanthomata.

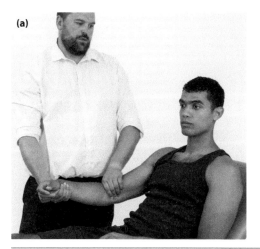
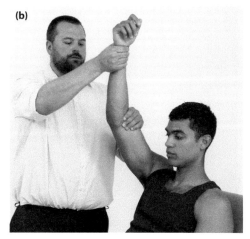

Figure 4.17 Assessing for (a) slow rising; (b) collapsing pulse in the forearm.

Blood pressure

Measure the blood pressure (see *Section 3.4.2*), noting the absolute values, pulse pressure and any variance between lying and standing, or between left and right arms.

Face and eyes

Inspect the face and around the eyes for:

- corneal arcus
- conjunctival pallor, indicating anaemia
- xanthelasma
- malar flush (erythema across cheeks and nasal bridge associated with mitral stenosis).

Check under the patient's tongue for central cyanosis, and assess their dentition.

Neck

Examine the jugular venous pulse, looking for the elevated JVP of right heart failure.

Carotid pulse palpation

Assess the character and volume of the carotid pulse.

4.6.4 Palpation

Apex beat

Feel for the apex beat. Note if it is displaced. In the rare condition of dextrocardia, the heart is on the right side of the chest.

Heaves

Lay the palm of your hand vertically across the left parasternal area and feel for a parasternal heave.

Thrills

Lay your hand horizontally across the aortic and pulmonary areas of the precordium and feel for thrills.

Delay

Assess for radio-radial and radio-femoral delay (**Figure 4.18**).

4.6.5 Auscultation

You may already suspect to hear a murmur if associated signs are present (**Table 4.13**).

Chest

Listen with the diaphragm of the stethoscope at each of the areas, finishing at the apex for S1, S2 and any added sounds, whilst palpating the carotid pulse; S1 occurs with the pulse, and S2 occurs after the pulse. Then use the bell to listen for mitral stenosis, which is a low-pitched murmur undetectable by the diaphragm.

S1 (first heart sound):
> T1 – closure of tricuspid valve
> M1 – closure of mitral valve

S2 (second heart sound):
> A2 – closure of aortic valve
> P2 – closure of pulmonary valve

Pericarditis manifests itself as a squeaky 'rub' with each heartbeat.

In addition to S1 and S2, you may detect a third or fourth heart sound.

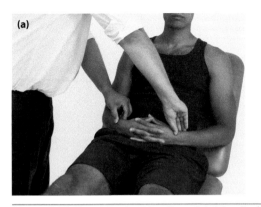
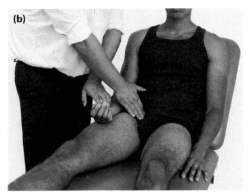

(a)   **(b)**

Figure 4.18 Examining for (a) radio-radial; (b) radio-femoral delay.

S3

The third sound (S3) comes straight after S2 in early diastole, and it occurs in severe heart failure and volume overload. The combination of S1 + S2 + S3 is often called a 'gallop' rhythm.

S4

S4 is the fourth heart sound and occurs immediately before S1. It signifies a hypertrophic and failing left ventricle.

Valve areas

Valve sounds are best heard in particular valve areas (**Figure 4.19**). Ask the patient to roll onto their left side and auscultate over the apex to hear the mitral valve (**Figure 4.20**). Left-sided murmurs are heard louder in held expiration, whilst right-sided murmurs are louder in inspiration (**Figure 4.21**). All valvular murmurs radiate in the direction of blood flow.

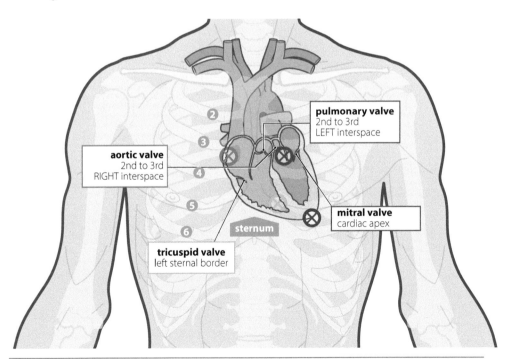

pulmonary valve
2nd to 3rd
LEFT interspace

aortic valve
2nd to 3rd
RIGHT interspace

mitral valve
cardiac apex

sternum

tricuspid valve
left sternal border

Figure 4.19 Areas of the precordium used to auscultate the heart valves. These areas do not correlate with anatomical placement in the thorax.

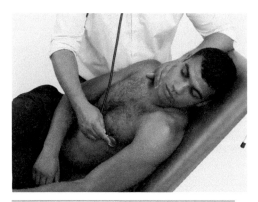

Figure 4.20 To accentuate mitral murmurs, roll the patient (still lying at a 45° angle) onto their left side.

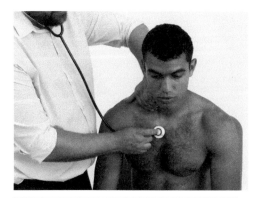

Figure 4.21 To accentuate aortic murmurs, ask the patient to lean forward, exhale fully then pause their breathing.

Give clear instructions when trying to accentuate left-sided murmurs during respiration:
- To optimise aortic valve murmurs: 'Breathe in, breathe out, stop'
- To optimise pulmonary valve murmurs: 'Breathe out, breathe in, stop'

Most patients will only be able to stop breathing for a few seconds.

Abdomen

Abdominal aortic aneurysm

Place the diaphragm of the stethoscope firmly against the patient's epigastrium and listen for aortic bruits. Ascertain aorta size by palpating the furthest left and right limits of the pulsation; more than 3cm between these points indicates an aortic aneurysm (**Figure 4.22**).

Renal bruit

With the diaphragm of the stethoscope, auscultate over the area to the left and right of the aorta in the upper abdomen, listening for bruits.

Neck

Listen to the carotid pulse with the diaphragm of the stethoscope for a carotid bruit. Ensure any noise heard is not the radiation of an ejection systolic murmur of aortic stenosis (**Table 4.13**).

4.6.6 Finishing off

Auscultate the lung bases for the crackles of pulmonary oedema. Check for sacral oedema, and peripheral oedema, commenting on its severity: to the level of the mid-shins, knees, mid-thighs, abdominal wall or above.

"To complete my examination, I would like to perform fundoscopy, examine an ECG, perform a urine dipstick test and examine the peripheral vascular system."

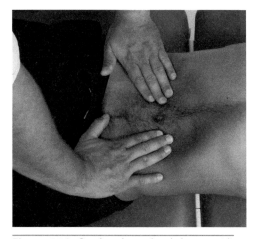

Figure 4.22 Gently palpate the abdomen with both hands to check for an abdominal aortic aneurysm.

4.7 Examination of the peripheral vascular system

Chronic venous disease causes unsightly and painful conditions such as varicose veins and ulcers. Peripheral arterial disease causes limb-threatening ischaemia and amputation. The peripheral vascular system is normally considered to be of the lower limbs; vascular disease of the arms is relatively rare.

4.7.1 'ID CHECK'

This is detailed in *Section 3.2*.

4.7.2 Endobedogram

Does the patient look unwell?
Are there any limb prostheses or walking aids?
Are there any amputations?
Are there medications or tobacco products?

4.7.3 Inspection

Dressings must be taken down so that important findings are not overlooked.

Signs of arterial disease

Ask if the patient has any pain; areas affected by arterial insufficiency are very painful when touched.

  Examine the colour of the lower limbs:
- Pink / red skin implies adequate perfusion.
- Pale, white or bluish skin corresponds with increasing severity of arterial disease.
- Look for areas of necrosis (black, dead tissue) or ulcers (active or healed).

Look for amputations:
- Toes are amputated for chronic infection and necrosis.
- Below- and above-knee leg amputations imply a heavy atherosclerotic burden.
- Look for any scars of femoral-popliteal bypass surgery or saphenous vein harvest.

> **The changes seen in the hands with cardiovascular disease (such as splinter haemorrhages, clubbing and Osler's nodes) are often also seen in the toes.**

Signs of venous disease

Look for swelling.
- Bilateral swelling implies peripheral oedema (see *Section 4.5.13*).
- Unilateral swelling is more likely due to localised pathology.

Look for signs of chronic venous stasis:
- Are there varicose veins?
- Are there scars suggesting previous varicose vein stripping?
- Is there evidence of varicose eczema? This is itchy and inflamed skin overlying varicose veins.
- Are there venous ulcers?

Look for haemosiderin deposits in the skin. Haemosiderin is an iron storage complex, and manifests as brown pigmentation, usually on the shins.

4.7.4 Palpation

Temperature

Run both hands down the legs, comparing left to right. A temperature gradient down the leg indicates either peripheral ischaemia or generalised hypovolaemia.

Capillary refill time

Test capillary refill time in the great toe. A prolonged time suggests impaired blood supply.

Deep vein thrombosis

Measure and compare the circumference of both calves at the tibial tuberosity; a difference of >2cm circumference is a sensitive marker for deep vein thrombosis (DVT).

Thrombophlebitis

Thrombophlebitis is a superficial tender vein with surrounding erythema and has the potential to progress to a DVT.

Varicose veins

These are dilated, bulky veins usually due to incompetent venous valves.

Sensation

Assess the lower limb sensation (see *Section 3.10*). Peripheral neuropathy and peripheral arterial insufficiency usually coexist. Assess sensation with a microfilament; pinprick testing with a sharp needle may pierce the skin, causing injury and infection.

Pulses

Start by palpating the most peripheral pulse (**Figure 4.4**), then move proximally:

- Dorsalis pedis
- Posterior tibial
- Popliteal
- Femoral
- Abdominal aortic.

4.7.5 Auscultation

Listen over the abdominal aorta and the renal and femoral arteries for bruits. This would suggest atherosclerosis, stenosis or an aneurysm.

4.7.6 Buerger's test

Raise the leg until the foot becomes dusky. The angle of elevation required to achieve this from the bed is 'Buerger's angle'. The smaller Buerger's angle is, the more severe the arterial disease.

Allow the leg to hang off the bed and assess for the time taken to recolour. Severe arterial disease has a longer reperfusion time.

4.7.7 Finishing off

Thank the patient and inform them that they can get dressed, offering help if needed. Complete the examination by washing your hands.

4.8 Common investigations

'Spot' tests, such as an electrocardiogram, may not capture intermittent cardiac problems. Prolonged (or 'ambulatory') tests better provide a comprehensive picture of the patient's signs and symptoms (**Table 4.15**).

4.8.1 Cardiac investigations

Electrocardiography

Electrocardiography (ECG):

- evaluates electrical evidence of heart rate and rhythm
- provides a visual representation of cardiac electrical activity
- locates areas of focal ischaemia and conduction defects.

24-hour ECG monitoring can identify intermittent arrhythmias.

Echocardiography

Echocardiography uses ultrasound (US) to view the heart. It visualises valves and measures the severity of stenosis or regurgitation. It measures the degree of heart failure and diagnoses pericardial effusions.

Chest radiography

Chest radiography demonstrates cardiomegaly, pericardial effusions, and pulmonary oedema or pleural effusions.

Blood tests

Serum blood testing is used to diagnose:

- anaemia
- renal function
- clotting disorders
- serum lipid levels
- diabetes mellitus.

Serial blood cultures, from various sites, are essential in infective endocarditis to prove the diagnosis and guide antimicrobial treatment.

> **X-ray and CT imaging involves a small dose of ionising radiation**, which fractionally increases the lifetime risk of cancer, whereas US and ECG do not.

Table 4.15 *Choosing investigations in cardiovascular disease*

	Indications	Benefits	Limitations
ECG	Assess heart rhythm Diagnose ACS	Non-invasive	Snapshot view May be normal even in presence of disease, or abnormal when no new changes
Echocardiogram	Examine the structure and function of the heart	Non-invasive	2D representation of 3D structure Inter-user variability Limited by body habitus, e.g. obese or hyperinflated lungs
Chest X-ray	Assess heart size Look for pulmonary oedema	Quick, easy to do	Radiation required (minimal)
24-hour ECG	Diagnose arrhythmias	Captures intermittent arrhythmias	Dependent on arrhythmia occurring within 24-hour window
24-hour BP monitoring	Diagnose hypertension or hypotension	Minimises white coat hypertension Gives trend of BP over time	Patients may find repeated BP measurements uncomfortable

Testing for complications of heart disease

Urine dipstick
Proteinuria is abnormal and could indicate nephropathy secondary to hypertension or diabetes.

Glycosuria signifies diabetes, an important risk factor for cardiovascular disease.

Fundoscopy
Eye examination (fundoscopy; see *Section 10.6.4*) is performed yearly in people with diabetes to assess for diabetic retinopathy. Fundoscopy is performed in cases of uncontrolled hypertension, to evaluate for hypertensive retinopathy.

4.8.2 Peripheral vascular investigations

Arterial system

Arterial duplex scan
This is a US assessment of the blood vessels. The direction and velocity of blood flow through arterial vessels is assessed, and areas of stenosis identified.

Ankle brachial pressure index (ABPI)
The BP of the leg and the arm are compared using the following formula:

$$ABPI = \frac{\text{systolic pressure of leg (mmHg)}}{\text{systolic pressure of arm (mmHg)}}$$

- A ratio of <0.9 indicates arterial disease
- A ratio of <0.5 indicates critical ischaemia.

Angiography
Angiography utilises intravascular contrast to image vessels, highlighting atherosclerosis, stenosis or aneurysm. The images are often generated with computed tomography (CT). It requires IV contrast, which carries a small risk of causing contrast nephropathy.

Venous system

Ultrasound Doppler scan
Whilst the superficial veins of the leg are visible, the deep veins are assessed with US techniques.

Venous US Doppler studies assess the direction and velocity of flow, and diagnose a DVT.

CT venography
CT venography is used when the clinician has a strong suspicion for DVT, despite negative US Doppler scans.

4.9 Answers to starter questions

1. Many cardiovascular diseases manifest clinical signs in the peripheral circulation, where the smallest vessels are. These clinical signs are therefore observable in the peripheral anatomy, i.e. the hands and feet. Endocarditis causes immune complex deposition in the peripheries, leading to Osler's nodes, Janeway lesions, and splinter haemorrhages in the hands. Subacute endocarditis causes clubbing. In hypovolaemic states and severe anaemia, the hands are cold and poorly perfused, and have a prolonged capillary refill time. Tar staining between the second and third fingers of the dominant hand equates to a significant smoking history, a strong risk factor for cardiovascular disease.

2. There are two potential causes for this. Patients with severe CHD often had peripheral arterial disease, as the pathology of these diseases is the same: atherosclerosis. Complications of peripheral arterial disease include painful leg ulcers, soft tissue infections of the feet and intermittent claudication. All of these conditions may lead to limping. A second potential reason involves diabetes. Diabetes is a strong risk factor for atherosclerosis, and therefore CHD and PVD. PVD is associated with peripheral neuropathy – disease of the peripheral sensory and motor nerves. Diabetic neuropathy affecting the common peroneal nerve causes 'foot drop' – inability to dorsiflex the foot. This causes gait disturbances.

3. CHD is the leading cause of death worldwide. Unhealthy diets, smoking and increasing levels of obesity are the most likely causes in both the developed and developing world. As humans live longer, they are more likely to be diagnosed with heart disease. Whilst modifiable risk factors play a huge role, there is a genetic burden; people from the Indian subcontinent in particular have a strong genetic susceptibility for type 2 diabetes and heart disease.

4. A careful history is the greatest method for differentiating between cardiac and respiratory causes of symptoms such as breathlessness and chest pain. Patients with a respiratory condition often have accompanying symptoms of wheeze, cough and sputum production, and chest pain is pleuritic in nature. Patients with cardiac pathologies experience exertional chest pain, which is tight and constrictive, and relieved by rest and GTN.

5. The commonest cause of heart failure is CHD, which is largely dependent on lifestyle factors: smoking, drinking, obesity and poor diet. However, there are other risk factors that are out of patients' control. Hereditary hyperlipidaemias, type 1 diabetes, essential hypertension, structural heart disease and a host of other genetic factors place certain individuals at high risk of cardiovascular disease, despite addressing all modifiable risk factors. Additionally, post-viral dilated cardiomyopathy affects people of any risk profile.

6. People with diabetes are prone to peripheral neuropathy, due to microvascular disease of the nerves themselves. This means they are much less likely to notice small skin breaks, cuts and scrapes. Due to the poor wound healing and immune suppression associated with diabetes, these trivial injuries become infected and develop into neuropathic ulcers, which require intensive treatment. Many patients with long-term diabetes are forced to undergo amputation of toes, feet or whole lower limbs, due to severe ulceration. Therefore, people with diabetes are advised to never walk barefoot. Walking barefoot on a beach leaves the diabetic foot extremely vulnerable to small injuries and infection.

Chapter 5
Respiratory system

Starter questions

1. Why do some non-tobacco smokers develop lung cancer yet some tobacco smokers do not?
2. What can looking at a patient's skin tell you about their COPD?
3. Why do patients with stable respiratory disease become more breathless?
4. Why does tuberculosis (TB) continue to cause problems after it is treated?
5. Why are some hypoxic patients not given oxygen?

Answers to questions are to be found in *Section 5.8.*

5.1 Introduction

The respiratory system comprises the lungs and airways. Inhaled oxygen diffuses into the blood whilst waste gases, e.g. carbon dioxide, diffuse out and are exhaled.

The burden of respiratory disease is high. It kills more people in the UK than cardiovascular disease, with lung cancer having the second highest mortality rate of all cancers (after pancreatic cancer). Disorders affect:

- airways (e.g. asthma and COPD)
- alveoli (e.g. pneumonia and pulmonary oedema)
- lung interstitium (i.e. interstitial lung disease)
- pulmonary blood flow (e.g. pulmonary emboli and pulmonary hypertension)
- pleurae (e.g. pneumothorax and pleural effusion)
- chest wall movement (e.g. motor neurone disease and obesity hypoventilation syndrome).

Clinical assessment of the respiratory system includes quantifying the severity of disease and the impact on the patient's day-to-day life.

Case 5.1: Breathlessness and wheeze

Presentation

Jacinta Begum is 19 years old. She presents to her GP with worsening breathlessness and wheeze.

Initial interpretation

Breathlessness has many causes. Respiratory causes can be any of those listed in *Section 5.1*. Non-respiratory causes include:

- cardiac causes such as myocardial ischaemia (including angina pectoris and myocardial infarction)
- metabolic disturbances such as metabolic acidosis, including diabetic ketoacidosis
- psychogenic breathlessness.

Being young makes certain chronic diseases such as COPD, coronary artery disease and malignancy less likely, but we need more information.

History

Jacinta has suffered intermittent breathlessness since childhood but this has worsened in the last year. Her chest feels tight when waking. After exercise or being in the cold, her breathing sounds wheezy. She has a harsh cough at night which affects her sleep. She denies any chest pain.

Interpretation of history

Breathlessness with wheeze could be respiratory or cardiac. A wheeze that comes and goes indicates bronchial inflammation. Cardiac wheeze is due to excess fluid in the alveoli. It tends to be continuous and accompanied by other cardiac (chest pain) or sympathetic stimulation symptoms (sweating and nausea).

Breathing difficulty changing through the day is termed 'diurnal' and is a key asthma symptom. Common triggers include cold weather, exercise and irritants (e.g. dust or pet hair). However, these triggers can irritate the airways in other lung diseases such as pulmonary fibrosis and bronchiectasis. She describes a nocturnal cough which is a classical symptom of asthma but may represent gastro-oesophageal reflux that worsens when lying flat.

The lack of pain makes myocardial ischaemia and pulmonary embolism less likely but we cannot totally exclude them. Painless myocardial ischaemia, termed 'silent', can affect some women, the elderly and those with diabetes. Pulmonary emboli that do not infarct the pleurae can be painless.

Further history

Jacinta suffers from eczema and seasonal hay fever. She uses topical emollient creams and antihistamines in the spring and summer months. She has no other medical history. She smokes 5 cigarettes a day and has done for 1 year since starting at fashion college. There is no family history of cardiac disease at a young age. She was born in the UK and has not recently travelled abroad.

Examination

She looks well and is breathing comfortably at rest. Her respiratory rate is 14 and her peripheral oxygen saturations are 99% on room air. There is no clubbing or tar staining of the fingers. Respiratory and cardiovascular examination is normal. She has dry skin affecting her hands and elbows.

Interpretation of findings

A normal respiratory examination makes pleural effusions, pneumothorax and infection much less likely. Her age and lack of cardiovascular risk factors also make primary cardiac disease unlikely. She has no risk factors for pulmonary embolism. She was born in the UK and so she is less likely to have TB. However, if a close family member has it, or she has recently travelled to a high-risk area, this could be a possibility.

Jacinta has worsening breathlessness and wheeze which has been the case since childhood, but it has been more apparent recently. Her symptoms exhibit diurnal variation and have clear triggers. Her symptoms have worsened recently which may reflect starting smoking or being exposed to fabric dust at college. She has atopy (a tendency towards

Case 5.1 *continued*

hypersensitivity reactions) which has a strong association with asthma.

The likeliest diagnosis is asthma. This is common but if left uncontrolled can present as a medical emergency.

To confirm the diagnosis, we must demonstrate a reduction in airway compliance associated with her symptoms, and an improvement with bronchodilating medications (e.g. salbutamol). This is done by keeping a diary of peak expiratory flow rate (PEFR) when both symptomatic and well. A chest X-ray (CXR) to rule out structural abnormalities and signs of severe infection, and an electrocardiogram (ECG) to investigate for myocardial ischaemia, are also necessary.

Investigations

Jacinta's CXR and ECG are normal. Her peak flow diary shows a diurnal variation which is more marked on the days she attends college (**Figure 5.1**). Her PEFR increases if she takes salbutamol when she is symptomatic.

Diagnosis

Jacinta has asthma. When exposed to allergens her PEFR decreases then increases with inhaled bronchodilators – a phenomenon termed 'reversibility'. She should be started on long-term inhaled therapy with inhaled corticosteroids (the 'preventer' medication) with additional inhaled short-acting bronchodilators (the 'reliever' medication). She should be taught to use these medications properly and provided with alternative equipment such as a spacer device to ensure that she takes her dose effectively. Quitting smoking will not only help her asthma but reduce her risk of cancer and COPD in the future. Measures to avoid exposure to allergens, such as wearing a mask whilst working, should be explored.

> **In the UK, employers have a duty to offer protective equipment or alternative roles to employees with hypersensitivity to certain allergens.** In some cases, prolonged exposure can lead to irreparable lung damage that can be severely disabling or even life-threatening.

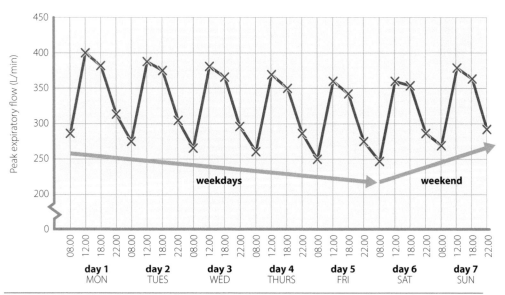

Figure 5.1 Jacinta's peak expiratory flow rate diary showing diurnal variation that is markedly worse on weekdays.

5.2 System overview

5.2.1 Airways

The upper respiratory tract runs from pharynx to trachea (**Figure 5.2**). The trachea divides to the main bronchi which marks the beginning of the lower respiratory tract (also known as the bronchial tree). These bronchi undergo multiple divisions, becoming smaller until they eventually communicate with the alveoli.

The upper tract is kept open with the support of the bones, muscles and cartilage that surround it. The lower tract contains cells producing surfactant that reduces surface tension to keep the airways open. Both the upper and lowers tracts contain ciliated and mucus-producing cells which trap and expel microbes, allergens and pollutants.

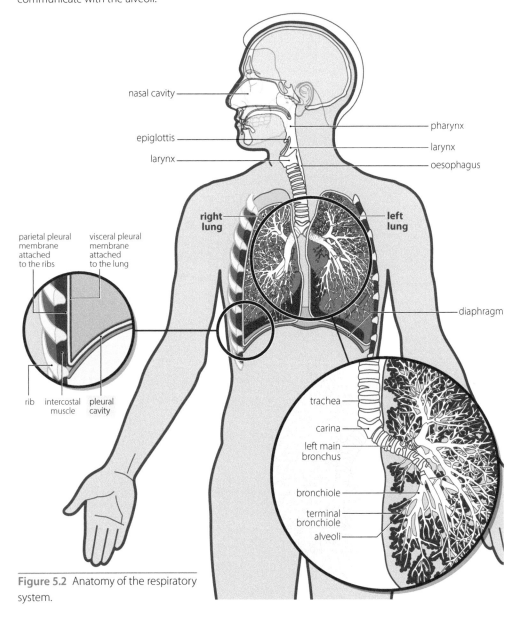

Figure 5.2 Anatomy of the respiratory system.

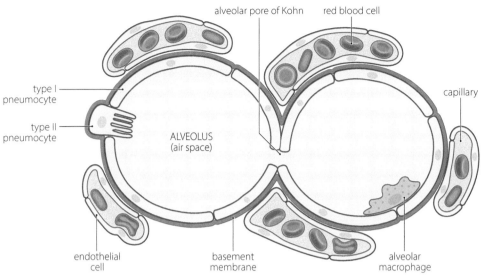

Figure 5.3 The structure of the alveoli.

5.2.2 Alveoli and interstitium

Alveoli are hollow sacs in which gas exchange occurs (**Figure 5.3**). Oxygen enters the alveoli where it is absorbed into the blood stream and blood carries carbon dioxide to the capillaries surrounding the alveoli, where it is released by diffusion. Their walls are single layers of pneumocytes supported by a thin elastic basement membrane. The space between alveoli (the interstitium) contains collagen and elastin fibres. In healthy lungs, the alveoli provide around 75m² total surface area for gas exchange; a little larger than a squash court.

> In interstitial lung disease, the interstitial space expands, leading to loss of alveolar volume and reduced lung function.

5.2.3 Pulmonary blood flow and lymphatics

Deoxygenated blood from the right ventricle is supplied to capillaries in the lungs by the pulmonary artery (**Figure 5.4**). Once oxygenated

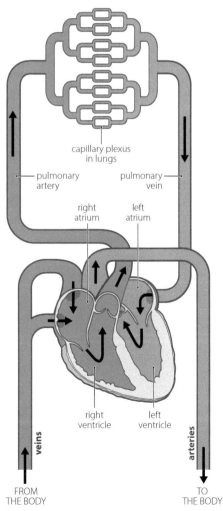

Figure 5.4 Anatomy of the pulmonary circulation.

in the alveoli, blood travels in the pulmonary vein to the left side of the heart to enter the systemic circulation. The pulmonary arterial pressure is low (around 8–20mmHg at rest) due to the large calibre of the vessels.

> **Shunts, such as a patent foramen ovale or patent ductus arteriosus, are congenital anatomical anomalies through which deoxygenated blood bypasses the pulmonary circulation.** This causes low systemic oxygen concentrations, breathing difficulties and developmental problems.

Extracellular fluid from air spaces and interstitial tissues in each lung drains via lymphatic vessels and lymph nodes into the subclavian veins on the same side.

5.2.4 Pleurae

The outer surface of the lungs and inner surface of the thoracic cage are each covered by a membrane called a pleura (*visceral* and *parietal* pleura, respectively). These are separated by a few millilitres of lubricating fluid to help the lungs to expand freely.

5.2.5 Chest wall

The thoracic cage comprises skeletal bones (ribs, sternum and thoracic spine), cartilage and muscle (**Figure 5.5**). The base is formed by a large dome-shaped muscle, the diaphragm. Intercostal muscles lie between the ribs.

5.2.6 Mechanics of ventilation

During inspiration, the thoracic muscles (except the internal intercostals) contract, expanding the thoracic cage and flattening the diaphragm. Intrathoracic pressure falls, drawing air into the lungs. This causes the lungs to inflate and alveoli to open. This requires:
- adequate thoracic muscle strength
- low airway flow resistance
- elastic lung compliance
- low alveolar surface tension (provided by surfactant from pneumocytes).

In expiration, these muscles relax (whilst internal intercostal and abdominal muscles contract),

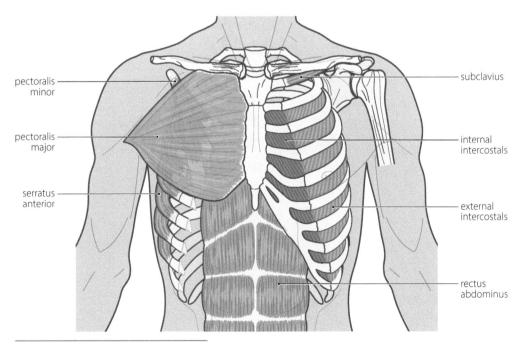

pectoralis minor

pectoralis major

serratus anterior

subclavius

internal intercostals

external intercostals

rectus abdominus

Figure 5.5 Anatomy of the thoracic cage

releasing tension on interstitial elastin fibres, reducing intrathoracic pressure and expelling air from the lungs.

5.2.7 Control of ventilation

Respiratory centres in the brainstem control breathing via the autonomic nervous system.
- Central chemoreceptors in the medulla respond to changes in pH which are indicative of changes in carbon dioxide concentration in the blood.
- Peripheral chemoreceptors in the aortic arch and carotid bodies respond to oxygen concentrations in the blood.

If low oxygen and/or high carbon dioxide concentrations or low pH are detected by the chemoreceptors, they stimulate an increased respiratory rate by activating the nerves within the respiratory centres.

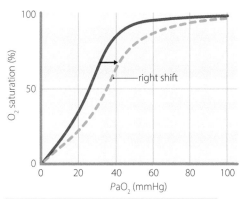

Figure 5.6 Oxygen dissociation curve. As the partial pressure of oxygen in the tissues decreases, the affinity for oxygen to haemoglobin decreases causing oxygen to be released. Right shift occurs when carbon dioxide levels are increased or pH levels are decreased. The affinity of oxygen to haemoglobin is reduced therefore delivering more oxygen to the tissues. Red = normal oxygen dissociation curve. Blue = right shift

5.2.8 Gas transfer

Oxygen

Oxygen travels from alveolar space to the blood via passive diffusion. A small amount of oxygen dissolves in the plasma but the majority binds to haemoglobin in red blood cells.

In the tissues, oxygen dissociates from haemoglobin and diffuses from the blood into tissues to be used by mitochondria. More active tissues (e.g. muscles during exercise) use more oxygen, reducing the oxygen concentration in nearby capillaries. The lower the concentration of oxygen, the more readily haemoglobin releases its bound oxygen molecules (**Figure 5.6**). As each molecule is unbound, the shape of the haemoglobin molecule changes to allow the next to release more easily.

> **In the Bohr effect ('right shift'; Figure 5.6) an increase in carbon dioxide concentration or decrease in pH (e.g. caused by active tissues) lowers the affinity of oxygen to bind to haemoglobin, causing the oxygen dissociation curve to shift to the right.** This lowers the threshold for oxygen to be released.

Carbon dioxide

Carbon dioxide is a toxic waste product of aerobic respiration. The majority reacts with water molecules in the blood plasma and red cells to produce carbonic acid (H_2CO_3). A hydrogen ion then dissociates from the molecule to create the less-toxic bicarbonate (HCO_3^-), which travels dissolved in the blood back to the lungs:

$$H_2CO_3 \rightleftharpoons H^+ + HCO_3^-$$

The remaining carbon dioxide either dissolves directly in plasma or binds to haemoglobin. Once in the pulmonary capillaries, carbon dioxide diffuses across the alveolar wall and is exhaled.

5.2.9 Respiratory buffering

Respiratory buffering is the process through which the respiratory system adapts to changes in blood pH. This is achieved by altering carbon dioxide levels in the blood. Excess hydrogen ions bind to bicarbonate ions in the serum to form carbonic acid (see equation below). This then dissociates to carbon dioxide and water. Increasing respiration allows for increased carbon dioxide excretion and thus helps to lower blood pH. This happens over minutes or hours.

$$H^+ + HCO_3^- \rightleftharpoons H_2CO_3 \rightleftharpoons CO_2 + H_2O$$

When carbon dioxide is retained in chronic respiratory diseases, the kidneys compensate for this by retaining bicarbonate ions to maintain normal blood pH. This renal compensation takes days to weeks to occur.

5.2.10 Ventilatory failure

When pathology occurs, the lungs can lose their ability to support adequate oxygen absorption or carbon dioxide excretion. This is called respiratory failure.

> **Respiratory failure can only be diagnosed on arterial blood gas sampling because this is closely representative of the blood exiting the lungs.** Venous blood gas sampling underestimates oxygen concentrations and overestimates carbon dioxide concentrations.

Type 1 respiratory failure

This describes low oxygen concentrations in the blood (hypoxia) and occurs whilst carbon dioxide levels remain normal. The main symptom of type 1 respiratory failure is breathlessness and the patient may be cyanosed (see below).

Type 2 respiratory failure

This describes raised carbon dioxide concentrations in the blood (hypercapnoea) with either normal or low oxygen concentrations. The kidneys are able to compensate for this over time by reabsorbing more bicarbonate in to the blood. If there is no renal compensation, the patient will have a low or normal bicarbonate concentration and thus a low blood pH (acidosis) – this is called a decompensated type 2 respiratory failure. If the type 2 respiratory failure has been present for some time, the kidneys will compensate, producing a raised bicarbonate concentration and normal pH.

5.2.11 Lung immunity

The lung mucosa and blood supply contain immune cells that attack and digest inhaled microbes, pollutants and allergens to prevent lung damage. Severe (such as in pneumonia) or abnormally prolonged (such as in asthma and hypersensitivity) immune responses reduce lung function over time.

5.3 Symptoms of respiratory disease

History and examination assess for the features of the main respiratory diseases (**Table 5.1**) and their impact on quality of life.

The key symptoms are breathlessness, cough, sputum production, haemoptysis, chest pain and wheeze.

5.3.1 Breathlessness

Breathlessness (dyspnoea) is the unpleasant sensation of not being able to breathe enough to meet the body's demands. Breathlessness is the commonest presentation of respiratory disease. It is distressing, disabling and can lead to depression, social isolation and physical deconditioning. Understanding the cause of the breathlessness is the first step to treating the underlying condition.

Causes

Use the mnemonic AEROS to differentiate causes of breathlessness (see **Table 4.7**). The degree of breathlessness and its impact is quantified in the UK using the Medical Research Council (MRC) scale (**Table 5.2**).

Respiratory

The presentation of breathlessness will identify the cause (**Table 5.3**). It can have preceding symptoms (like chest pain or leg swelling). Acute episodes can either fully resolve or have ongoing (but less severe) breathlessness in between.

Table 5.1 *The main features of respiratory disease*

Disease	Definition	Symptoms	Signs
Asthma	Long-term airway inflammation with reversible bronchospasm and airway obstruction	Intermittent dyspnoea	Atopy Normal examination when well Wheeze when symptomatic
COPD	Progressive airway inflammation with bronchospasm, chronic cough and airway obstruction	Progressive dyspnoea Acute exacerbations Cough ± sputum	Cough ± sputum Hyperexpanded chest Wheeze when symptomatic May have signs of cor pulmonale
Pneumonia	Lower respiratory tract infection with consolidation	Acute dyspnoea Productive cough ± haemoptysis May have pleuritic chest pain	Temperature Tachycardia Coarse crackles May have signs of pleural effusion
Bronchiectasis	Permanent enlargement of airways with excessive mucus production	Chronic productive cough Acute exacerbations	Clubbing Bronchial breathing May have signs of cor pulmonale
Lung fibrosis	Scarring of lungs resulting in excessive connective tissue accumulation	Progressive dyspnoea Acute exacerbations	Fine crepitations May have signs of cor pulmonale
Lung cancer	Cancer originating from lung tissue	Progressive dyspnoea Cough ± haemoptysis Weight loss	Clubbing Horner's syndrome if sympathetic chain affected Lymphadenopathy May have normal examination May have signs of pleural effusion
Pleural effusion	Excess fluid within the pleural cavity due to irritation, infection, bleeding or trauma	Dyspnoea Pleuritic chest pain	Tracheal deviation Stony dull percussion note Absent breath sounds Coarse crackles just above fluid level
Pneumothorax	Air within the pleural cavity	Dyspnoea Pleuritic chest pain	Tracheal deviation Hyper-resonant percussion note Absent breath sounds

Score	Degree of breathlessness
0	Normal
1	Able to walk and keep up with people of similar age but not when walking up hills or stairs
2	Able to walk 1.5km on the level at own pace but unable to keep up with people of similar age
3	Able to walk about 100m on the level without stopping
4	Breathless at rest or on minimal effort (e.g. when undressing or moving around the room)

Table 5.2 *The Medical Research Council scale for dyspnoea*

Table 5.3 *Patterns of dyspnoea*

Onset	Conditions
Sudden	**No warning:** Pulmonary embolism, Pneumothorax
	Preceding symptoms: Asthma, Lobar collapse, Pulmonary embolism, Pulmonary oedema
Episodic	**Normal between episodes:** Asthma, Hyperventilation, Ischaemic heart disease
	Persisting dyspnoea between episodes: COPD, 'Chronic' asthma, Cardiac failure, Valvular heart disease
Progressive (over weeks)	Pleural effusion, Lobar collapse, Pulmonary embolism, Cardiac failure, Neuromuscular disease, Extensive malignancy, Lymphangitis carcinomatosis, Anaemia
Progressive (over months to years)	COPD, Interstitial lung disease, Pulmonary embolism (months rather than years), 'Chronic asthma', Bronchiectasis, Pneumoconiosis, Chest wall disease

Cardiovascular

Pulmonary oedema is the accumulation of fluid in the alveoli. It is often caused by left ventricular failure. Characteristic symptoms include orthopnoea (increased breathlessness on lying flat) and paroxysmal nocturnal dyspnoea (severe breathlessness or coughing attacks at night).

Metabolic

In states of acidosis (low blood pH), such as metabolic acidosis, including diabetic ketoacidosis, the respiratory system compensates by increasing the respiratory rate to 'blow off' carbon dioxide and buffer the acidosis.

Musculoskeletal

Deformities of the thoracic cage (e.g. scoliosis, kyphosis or trauma) can reduce the maximum volume of the lungs. As such, the amount of air that can be inspired is reduced so the respiratory rate is increased to compensate.

Psychological

Panic attacks can manifest as an inability to breathe and chest discomfort, thus causing hyperventilation.

5.3.2 Cough

Cough is a reflex manoeuvre that sharply increases intrathoracic pressures to help clear mucus and foreign bodies from airways.

Causes

Respiratory

Coughs are defined by duration and whether they produce mucus or not.

- Acute (occurring within 1 week) and subacute (lasting between 1 and 4 weeks) cough can be caused by acute infection, asthma or inhaled foreign bodies.
- Chronic coughs (lasting longer than 4 weeks) have many causes (**Table 5.4**).
- A cough with large volumes of sputum (a mixture of saliva and mucus) indicates increased mucus production which tends to indicate airway diseases.

A cough can occur during the day, at night or both. In asthma, the cough is usually worse in the morning but can also wake people up at night.

In some cases, they can make a particular sound (such as a barking cough with croup or a staccato cough with *Chlamydia* pneumonia).

Upper airway irritation, such as pharyngitis, viral infections and post-nasal drips, cause a non-productive cough.

Cardiovascular

The accumulation of pulmonary oedema can cause cough. It is typically productive of pink frothy sputum.

Musculoskeletal

Irritation of the diaphragm by either pleural inflammation, such as in pleural effusions (excess fluid within the pleural space), or from lesions below the diaphragm, such as abscesses between the liver and diaphragm, can stimulate the cough reflex.

Gastrointestinal

Gastro-oesophageal reflux (see *Section 6.3.1*) can initiate the cough reflex. This is worse on lying flat when the effect of gravity on gastric contents is lost.

Psychological

'Cough habit' is the development of a cough without an irritant or cause. It is more common in children and adolescents than in adults. The cause is unclear but it can be improved with psychological therapy and behaviour modification.

5.3.3 Sputum

Sputum is a normal part of the respiratory system's defence against pathogens and irritants. Excessive

Table 5.4 *Causes of a persisting cough*		
	Persisting cough with no or minimal sputum	**Persisting cough with sputum**
Common causes	Asthma	Asthma (yellow sputum)
	Post-nasal drip	Smoking
	Gastro-oesophageal reflux	COPD
	Cough habit	
	Smoking	
Uncommon causes	Lung cancer	Lung cancer
	Interstitial lung disease	Bronchiectasis
	Whooping cough	Interstitial lung disease
	Foreign body inhalation	Lung abscess
	Mediastinal lymphadenopathy or lesions	Occupational dust exposure
	Occupational dust exposure	

quantities are produced when there is underlying disease. Ask about colour, consistency and quantity to help identify the underlying cause. Also check whether the quantity or colour of the sputum has changed if they have chronic symptoms.

Mucoid
- White or clear sputum.
- Thin.
- Produced in viral infections and chronic lung diseases without superadded infections (e.g. COPD, interstitial lung disease and bronchiectasis).

Purulent
- Green or brown sputum.
- Thick.
- Produced in acute bacterial infections including those exacerbating underlying chronic diseases.

Mucopurulent
- White sputum mixed with discoloured sputum.
- Produced in mild bacterial infections or during the recovery phase of more severe infections.

5.3.4 Haemoptysis

Haemoptysis (coughing blood) is always abnormal. Ask about the amount (in flecks,

teaspoons, cups or bowls), colour and duration (**Table 5.5**). A small amount of haemoptysis is common in infections or conditions with a chronic cough. If a patient has a large volume haemoptysis, think about pulmonary haemorrhage (life-threatening bleeding) – a medical emergency.

5.3.5 Chest pain

The differentials for chest pain are numerous (see *Section 4.3.1* and **Table 4.2**); respiratory causes give a pleuritic pain.

Pleuritic chest pain

Pleuritic chest pain is classically sharp, localised and worse on inspiration. Pain can be so severe that it limits the depth of breathing. Pleural disease is the main cause of pleuritic chest pain because it affects the pleural membranes, which are highly innervated and sensitive to pain.

Pneumothorax

Air between the pleural membranes (called a pneumothorax) causes the pleura to stretch (**Figure 5.7a**). These can be:
- spontaneous (typically in tall, fit, young males)
- secondary to external damage (including iatrogenic)
- due to rupture of underlying bullae.

Table 5.5 *Main causes of haemoptysis*

Cause	Amount of blood	Colour	Acute vs. chronic
Bronchitis	Small (5–20ml)	Dark red	Acute
Pneumonia	Small (5–20ml)	'Rusty'	Acute
Tuberculosis	Small to moderate (5–100ml)	Dark and bright red mixed with purulent sputum	Chronic
Aspergilloma	Small to moderate (5–100ml)	Dark and bright red mixed with purulent sputum with plugs	Chronic
Pulmonary embolus	Small (5–20ml)	Frothy and pink	Acute
Lung cancer	Variable	Dark and bright red ± mucoid sputum	Chronic
Bronchial arterial damage / pulmonary haemorrhage	Massive (>200ml)	Bright red blood	Acute

A pneumothorax is said to be a 'tension' pneumothorax when more air accumulates in the pleural space with each breath, leading to significant ventilatory and haemodynamic compromise. This is a medical emergency and requires immediate treatment.

Pleural effusion

The accumulation of fluid within the pleural cavity can stretch and irritate the pleura and also compress the underlying area of lung (**Figure 5.7b**). An effusion that is infected is called an empyema and a bloody effusion is called haemothorax.

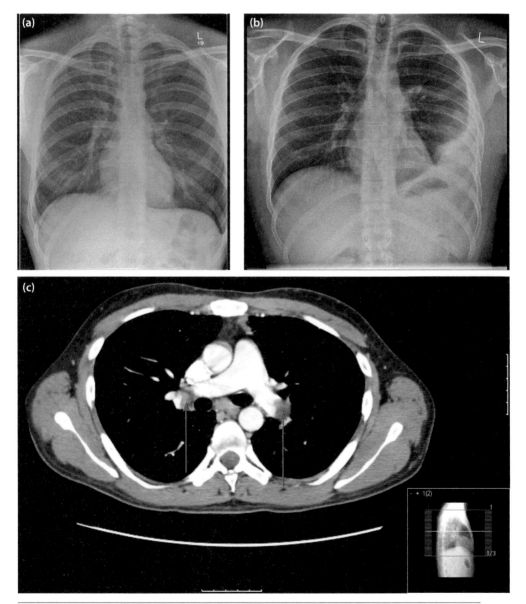

Figure 5.7 (a) Chest radiograph with a pneumothorax. (b) Chest radiograph with a pleural effusion. (c) Computed tomography (CT) scan with a pulmonary embolus (red arrow).

Pulmonary embolus

A clot in the pulmonary artery blocks the blood supply to the pleura, causing painful ischaemia (**Figure 5.7c**). These usually embolise from a clot elsewhere in the body such as a deep vein thrombosis (DVT).

Musculoskeletal

The cartilaginous joints of the anterior thoracic cage become inflamed, either through trauma or overuse, which gives a pleuritic-type chest pain due to irritation with chest wall movement.

5.3.6 Wheeze

Wheeze is a sound produced by air moving through an obstructed airway. A wheeze louder

> **Stridor is a harsh inspiratory wheeze that indicates a potentially life-threatening obstruction of the upper airway.** Acute stridor is a medical emergency.

on inspiration implies upper airway obstruction whilst an expiratory wheeze indicates lower respiratory obstruction. The causes of wheeze are listed in **Table 5.6**.

5.3.7 Ankle swelling

'Cor pulmonale' is a severe right-sided heart disease caused by chronic hypoxic lung disease, and causes bilateral leg oedema.
Unilateral leg swelling with calf pain could indicate a DVT which has the potential to embolise to the lungs.

Other causes of ankle swelling are discussed in *Section 4.3.13*.

5.3.8 Upper airway symptoms

Rhinitis (inflammation of the nasal passages) and sinusitis (inflammation of the cranial sinuses) are associated with viral infections (such as the common cold and influenza), bacterial infections, asthma and vasculitis.

Table 5.6 *Main causes of wheeze*

Pathophysiology	Wheeze	Causes
Laryngeal or tracheal obstruction	Harsh inspiratory wheeze = stridor	Inhaled foreign body
		Epiglottitis
		Anaphylaxis
Bronchial obstruction	Monophonic	Tumour (intrinsic or extrinsic obstruction)
	Expiratory	Foreign body
Bronchoconstriction	Polyphonic	Asthma
	Expiratory	COPD
		Infection

5.4 The respiratory history

5.4.1 Past medical history

Many diseases have respiratory complications, so the medical history is key to establishing the cause. Always ask about childhood asthma which can resolve then recur in later adulthood. Hay

fever, eczema and asthma are all atopic conditions (immune hypersensitivity to allergens) and often occur together.

Previous tuberculosis infection can damage lungs; the resulting cavities can become infected with the *Aspergillus* fungus and cause chronic inflammation of the airways that leads to bronchiectasis. Partially treated or untreated tuberculosis can reactivate, causing a more acute infection. Ask about travel to high risk areas (**Figure 5.8**).

Cardiac disease is the main differential for breathlessness and chest pain. Enquire about risk factors such as hypertension, ischaemic heart disease, diabetes or hypercholesterolaemia.

5.4.2 Medications

Inhaled medications (such as salbutamol, salmeterol and tiotropium) are often not taken properly. Ask the patient to demonstrate how they take their inhaler to check their technique. Ask about other medications because some may cause or worsen respiratory diseases (**Table 5.7**).

5.4.3 Family history

Some respiratory diseases are inherited or are more likely to occur if there is a family history. Ask about:
- asthma and atopy in family members
- any inherited respiratory disorders (i.e. cystic fibrosis)
- any household contact with current or previous TB infection.

5.4.4 Social history

This focuses on establishing the presence of modifiable risk factors and how their health is impacting on their life.

Smoking
Tobacco smoking is the main predictor of respiratory disease. Obtain a smoking history (see *Section 1.5.6*) including exposure to smoke at home or work.

Alcohol
High alcohol intake is a risk factor for aspiration (food, drink and oral secretions passing into the lungs) and community-acquired pneumonia (see *Section 1.5.6*).

Illicit drugs
Ask about illicit drugs such as cannabis (which may be smoked with tobacco), heroin or crack cocaine smoking. Inhaled drugs accelerate underlying lung disease and increase the risk of bullae (abnormal air pockets replacing normal lung tissue) formation. Intravenous drug injection is a risk factor for developing HIV which can lower immunity and increase the risk of acquired infections.

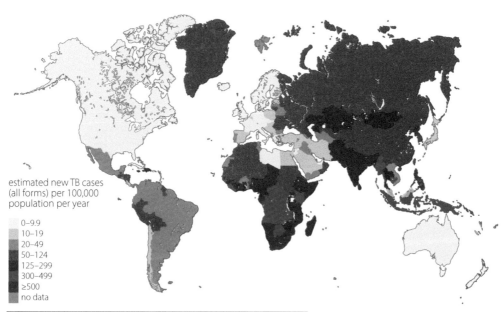

estimated new TB cases (all forms) per 100,000 population per year

- 0–9.9
- 10–19
- 20–49
- 50–124
- 125–299
- 300–499
- ≥500
- no data

Figure 5.8 Map depicting areas of high tuberculosis prevalence.

Table 5.7 *Drug therapies with respiratory side-effects*

	Disease or respiratory effect	Drugs
Common	Asthma	Beta blockers (worsening symptoms) NSAIDs (exacerbation in 5%) Muscle relaxants
	COPD	Beta blockers (worsening symptoms)
	ACE inhibitors	Dry cough
	Increased risk of pulmonary embolism	Oral contraceptive pill Tamoxifen
	Increased risk of infection	Corticosteroids (oral and inhaled) Biological therapies Immunosuppressants Chemotherapy
	Respiratory depression	Opiates Anxiolytics Antidepressants Antipsychotics
Uncommon	Interstitial lung disease	Amiodarone Cytotoxic chemotherapy Gold Nitrofurantoin
	Pulmonary eosinophilia	Nitrofurantoin Sulfonamides Sulfasalazine Chlorpropamide
	Non-cardiogenic pulmonary oedema	Opiates NSAIDs
	Pleural disease	Practolol Methysergide Bromocriptine
	Lupus-like syndrome	Hydralazine Isoniazid Procainamide

Employment

Ask if the patient is employed and what they do. Exposure to occupational allergens (such as fabric fibres or coal dust) is a major cause of hypersensitivity disorders. Ask if their symptoms get worse when at work because this indicates an allergen in their workplace. Always ask if the patient has ever been exposed to asbestos because asbestos-related lung diseases can present many years after exposure.

Physical activity

Enquire whether the patient is active in their daily life, and whether they take any exercise.

A sedentary lifestyle (minimal mobilisation with long periods of inactivity) greatly reduces lung function, and exacerbates the venous stasis (blood pooling in the legs) associated with DVT.

Hobbies and pets

Ask if the patient has any pets or whether their symptoms worsen around animals. Pet hair is a common allergen exacerbating asthma. Ask if they have ever come into contact with birds and/or their droppings which could suggest exposure to proteins causing lung hypersensitivity. A wide range of bacteria and moulds causing lung hypersensitivity are associated with many hobbies such as beer brewing, gardening and using hot tubs or saunas.

Social circumstances

Damp, mouldy and overcrowded housing conditions increase the risk of fungal lung infections, especially in those with already established respiratory disease. Additionally, those who are limited by breathlessness, such as COPD or bronchiectasis, may not be able to climb stairs, which could affect their ability to leave the house.

Functional capacity

Establish functional capacity (how far they can walk, what activities of daily living they can perform independently and whether they can climb stairs) and how this has changed in recent weeks in patients with breathlessness or fatigue. This helps quantify symptoms of chronic disease, such as congestive heart failure, or COPD, and monitor response to treatment.

5.4.5 Systems review

Ask about other symptoms associated with respiratory disease that the patient might have (**Table 5.8**).

Table 5.8 *Systemic symptoms associated with respiratory disease*		
Body system	**Systems review finding**	**Relevance to respiratory system**
Neurological	Daytime somnolence (sleepiness)	Carbon dioxide retention
	Headaches	
	Small hand muscle weakness	Malignant invasion of cervical plexus
Cardiovascular	Fluid overload	Right heart failure from chronic respiratory disease
	Palpitations	Atrial fibrillation from right atrial dilatation
Gastrointestinal	Reduced oral intake	As a consequence of breathlessness and/or chronic respiratory disease
	Weight loss	Underlying cancer or burden of chronic breathlessness
	Weight gain	Causing obstructive sleep apnoea; obesity can cause wheeze and worsen asthma
Psychological	Depression	Social isolation or reduced functionality
	Anxiety	Can be both a cause or symptom of breathlessness
Other	Loss of libido	From carbon dioxide retention

5.5 Signs of respiratory disease

Look for signs of emergency problems such as respiratory distress and hypoxia which need urgent treatment. Always look for evidence of right-sided heart failure because this indicates that a respiratory disease is more likely to be chronic than acute. For ease, the signs below are discussed in the order found during the routine respiratory system examination.

5.5.1 Dyspnoea

Breathlessness can occur on exertion (such as when the patient is walking into the examination room), when talking or whilst at rest.

Accessory muscle use

When breathlessness is severe, it is associated with the use of muscles that are not commonly utilised in respiration but can be recruited for additional respiratory movement:
- prominence of the trachea when inspiring (tracheal tug) from accessory neck muscle use
- excessive recession of the intercostal muscles
- leaning forward and placing hands on a flat surface with the arms held in extension ('tripod' posture).

5.5.2 Hand and nail changes

Cyanosis

A blue discolouration of the nails ('peripheral cyanosis') indicates low oxygen concentrations in the blood. This is due to high levels of deoxyhaemoglobin which has a blue/purple colour compared to the bright red of oxygenated haemoglobin.

Clubbing

Respiratory causes of nail clubbing include:
- lung cancer
- bronchiectasis and cystic fibrosis
- interstitial lung disease.

Tar staining

This is a brown discolouration of the fingers, indicating long-term cigarette smoking.

Capillary refill time

Capillary refill time (see *Section 4.7.4*) is prolonged (greater than 3 seconds) when tissues are poorly perfused, e.g. in severe infections and heart failure.

Rash

Some systemic diseases which affect the respiratory system can present with skin changes, for example, lupus and scleroderma.

Tremor

A fine tremor (with a frequency of around 10Hz) is a side effect of β_2-agonist (e.g. salbutamol) overuse. This is best seen with the patient's arms outstretched and palms facing down (**Figure 5.9a**).

Flap

A coarse pushing movement of the hands can be seen when the arms are outstretched and palms facing forwards. This is caused by carbon dioxide retention in decompensated type 2 respiratory failure (**Figure 5.9b**).

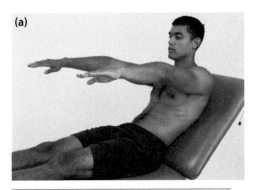
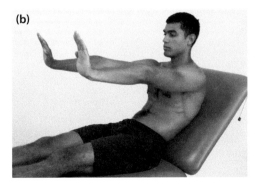

Figure 5.9 Assessing for (a) tremor and (b) flap.

5.5.3 Pulse

High carbon dioxide concentrations associated with type 2 respiratory failure give a 'bounding' (forceful and large volume) pulse. Patients with chronic respiratory diseases can develop atrial fibrillation due to the effect on the sinoatrial node in the overloaded right atrium.

5.5.4 Blood pressure

Tension pneumothorax, severe pneumonia and massive pulmonary embolism present with shock (systolic blood pressure <100mmHg) and tachycardia (pulse rate >100bpm). This relies on clinical correlation of the patient as a whole. Chronic high blood pressure is a key cause of heart disease, which presents with dyspnoea.

5.5.5 Eyes

Conjunctival pallor

A pale appearance of the conjunctiva is the result of anaemia which is a cause of breathlessness.

Horner's syndrome

Apical lung tumours can invade the cervical sympathetic chain causing Horner's syndrome (see *Section 10.7.3*) with ptosis, miosis and anhydrosis (**Figure 5.10**).

5.5.6 Lips and tongue

Central cyanosis produces blue discolouration of the lips and tongue and is a sign of hypoxia (deoxyhaemoglobin concentrations >50g/L).

5.5.7 Lymphadenopathy

Palpable cervical lymphadenopathy (enlargement of the lymph nodes of the neck) is felt in:
- lung cancer
- infections (including HIV)
- multisystem inflammatory diseases.

5.5.8 Raised jugular venous pressure

A raised jugular venous pressure (see *Section 3.7.1*) is a sign of raised right-sided heart pressure. This can be acute, such as in a large pulmonary embolus, or chronic as with cor pulmonale.

5.5.9 Chest wall deformity

Deformities of the chest wall reduce the ability to fully expand the lungs.

Kyphoscoliosis

Scoliosis is a lateral curvature of the spine, kyphosis is an anteroposterior curvature. These changes develop either in childhood or later as a result of vertebral damage from osteoporosis, metastatic disease or infections such as TB.

Pectus carinatum

Known as a 'pigeon chest', a protruding sternum is a normal finding, but it is also a sign of severe childhood asthma (**Figure 5.11**).

Pectus excavatum

A concave anterior chest wall is not associated with any respiratory disease but can reduce lung capacity if severe (**Figure 5.11**).

Hyperexpanded chest

A 'barrel chest' is a sign of chronic lung hyperexpansion such as with long-standing COPD.

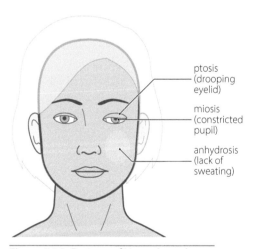

ptosis (drooping eyelid)

miosis (constricted pupil)

anhydrosis (lack of sweating)

Figure 5.10 Features of Horner's syndrome.

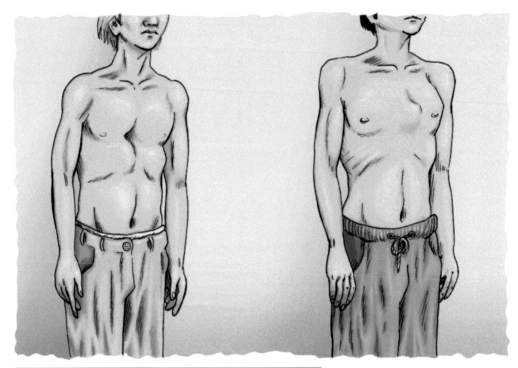

Figure 5.11 Pectus carinatum (right) and pectus excavatum (left).

Flail segment

Trauma to the chest wall involving multiple rib fractures causes a flail segment of the chest wall which does not move with the rest of the thoracic cage. This is painful and leads to localised reduced lung expansion as well as an increased risk of secondary lung infection.

5.5.10 Tracheal deviation

When lung tissue collapses, traction pulls the mediastinum and trachea towards the affected side (indicating upper mediastinal shift). Large effusions or pneumothoraces push the trachea away from the affected side.

5.5.11 Chest expansion

Chest expansion is reduced locally, unilaterally or bilaterally. Reduced expansion reflects an inability of alveolar expansion in the underlying area. It is due to:
- excess fluid within the alveoli
- lung volume loss either through bronchial obstruction and segment collapse, pneumothorax or extrinsic pressure from a pleural effusion
- reduced interstitial elasticity as in interstitial lung disease
- pain limiting movement.

5.5.12 Tactile vocal fremitus

Tactile vocal fremitus is the ability to feel transmitted airway sounds on the chest wall whilst the patient is talking. It is increased or decreased depending on the cause (**Table 5.9**).

5.5.13 Displaced apex beat

High pulmonary artery pressure strains the right ventricle, causing the muscle to hypertrophy. If severe, this causes lateral displacement of the apex beat with lower mediastinal shift (similar to tracheal deviation).

5.5.14 Parasternal heave

Hypertrophic right ventricular muscle is felt as a parasternal heave (thrusting sensation felt whilst palpating next to the sternum). When associated

Table 5.9 *Causes of abnormal tactile vocal fremitus and vocal resonance*

Tactile vocal fremitus or vocal resonance change	Causes
Increased	Consolidation
	Large cavities
	Top of pleural effusion
	Dense local fibrosis
Decreased	Pleural effusion
	Pneumothorax
	Lobar collapse / obstruction
	Pleural thickening
	Raised hemidiaphragm
	Pneumonectomy / lobectomy
	Bullae
	Severe airways disease (generalised)
	Obesity (generalised)

with a loud second heart sound it signifies pulmonary hypertension.

5.5.15 Percussion

Normal lungs give a hollow sound ('resonance') when percussed. Abnormally large amounts of air, such as in a pneumothorax or large bulla, give a 'hyper-resonant' note. A 'dull' percussion note is heard with fluid, collapse or consolidation. The dullest note ('stony dull') is heard with pleural effusions.

> **Consolidation is a build-up of fluid within the interstitium**. This can be pus (pneumonia or inflammation), interstitial fluid (pulmonary oedema), blood (pulmonary haemorrhage) or cells (bronchoalveolar carcinoma).

5.5.16 Abnormal breath sounds

Vesicular breath sounds

Normal breath sounds are 'vesicular' and indicate unimpeded airflow. There is a pause between the audible inspiratory and expiratory phases.

Bronchial breath sounds

Harsh breath sounds are normal if heard over the trachea. If heard within the lungs, they indicate transmitted sounds from larger central airways through an area of fibrosis or consolidation. The gap between inspiratory and expiratory phases is lost.

Wheeze

Wheeze represents turbulent airflow through narrowed airways. If the airways affected are the same size, the wheeze is monophonic (single note); if the airways are different sizes, the wheeze is polyphonic (multiple notes). They are usually heard during expiration.

Crackles

Crackles are also known as crepitations. They are crackly sounds heard over the different areas of the chest and are best heard on inspiration.
- Coarse crackles are heard in airways disease.
- Interstitial lung diseases and pulmonary oedema give a softer sound.

Rubs

Pleural irritation causes a rubbing sound, much like the noise produced when walking on fresh snow.

5.5.17 Vocal resonance

Like tactile vocal fremitus, vocal resonance relates to the transmission of sounds increasing through the lungs when there is consolidation present. The changes depend on the underlying pathology (**Table 5.10**).

5.5.18 Signs of cor pulmonale

Severe lung disease can lead to increased right-sided heart pressure and failure. The signs of this are:

■ raised jugular venous pressure (see *Section 3.7.1*)

Table 5.10 *Summary of examination findings in common respiratory disease*

Presentation	Trachea	Expansion	Percussion	Auscultation	Vocal resonance
Pneumothorax	Central (small) or deviated away (large)	Reduced on affected side	Hyper-resonant	Absent breath sounds No added sounds	Reduced or absent
Pleural effusion	Central (small) or deviated away (large)	Reduced on affected side	Stony dull	Absent breath sounds Pleural rub Bronchial breathing at top of effusion	Reduced or absent
Lobar consolidation	Central (small) or deviated away (large)	Reduced on affected side	Dull	Bronchial breathing (if dense) Coarse crackles	Increased
Lobar collapse	Deviated towards	Reduced on affected side	Dull	Absent breath sounds No added sounds	Reduced
Pulmonary fibrosis	Central	Reduced bilaterally	Resonant	Fine inspiratory crackles	Normal
Bronchiectasis	Central	Reduced bilaterally	Resonant	Coarse inspiratory crackles	Normal or increased
COPD or asthma	Central	Reduced bilaterally	Resonant	Prolonged expiration Quiet breath sounds Expiratory wheeze	Normal or reduced
Apical scarring (post-TB)	Deviated towards	Reduced unilaterally	Resonant or dull	Bronchial breathing Focal crackles	Normal or increased

- loud second heart sound
- murmur of tricuspid regurgitation (pansystolic murmur louder on inspiration)
- hepatomegaly due to venous congestion
- systemic fluid overload with peripheral oedema (and ascites if severe).

5.6 The respiratory examination

5.6.1 'ID CHECK'

This is detailed in *Section 3.2*.

The patient should be reclined at 45° and have their top removed (*Section 3.2.1*).

5.6.2 Endobedogram

Have a good look at the patient:

- Are they dyspnoeic or uncomfortable?
- Is there a sputum pot at the bedside? If so, look at the colour and consistency.
- Are they overweight?
- Around the bedside, are there oxygen masks, medications or tobacco products?
- Are there scars (**Figure 5.12**)?
- Are there any chest wall deformities?

5.6.3 Inspection

Hands

Ask the patient to hold their hands out in front of them.

- Look for tar staining and peripheral cyanosis.
- Hold their hands and note the perfusion of the hand and fingers. Are they warm and well perfused or cool and shut down?

- Look for the peripheral stigmata of respiratory disease (*Section 5.5.2*)
- Note any joint changes that indicate other systemic diseases.
- Assess for a tremor and flap (see **Figure 5.9**).

Radial pulse

Assess the radial pulse rate and rhythm (*Section 3.4.1*). A tachycardia or arrhythmia can cause breathlessness.

Blood pressure

Measure the blood pressure (see *Section 3.4.2*).

Face and eyes

Inspect the face and around the eyes for:

- conjunctival pallor
- Horner's syndrome.

Ask the patient to raise their tongue to the roof of their mouth to check for central cyanosis (see **Figure 3.12**).

Neck

Examine the JVP and palpate the cervical lymph nodes (see **Figure 3.12** and *Section 3.7.3*).

ANTERIOR

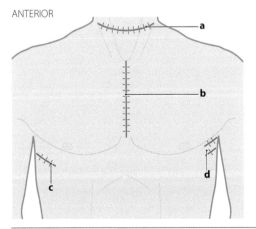

POSTERIOR

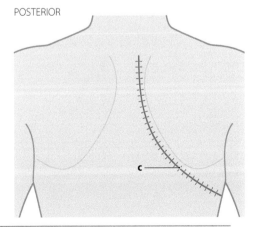

Figure 5.12 Thoracic scars: (a) tracheostomy; (b) midline sternotomy; (c) lobectomy/pneumonectomy; (d) thoracoscopy.

5.6.4 Palpation

Trachea

Assess the tracheal position by placing your index and ring fingers either side of the trachea and trace the position and direction with your middle finger. This can be uncomfortable so warn the patient first and do not press hard. The trachea is displaced sideways by either being pushed or pulled to a particular side by and underlying disease process (**Figure 5.13a**).

Apex beat

Feel for the apex beat. Note if it is displaced.

Heaves

Lay the palm of your hand vertically across the left parasternal area (the left border of the sternum) and feel for a parasternal heave.

Chest expansion

Place your hands around the patient's chest with your fingers around the sides and your thumbs almost touching in the middle. Your thumbs should not be touching the chest but resting just above it (**Figure 5.14**). Ask the patient to take

(a)

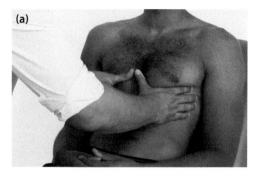

(b)

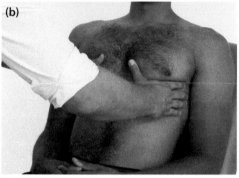

Figure 5.14 Assessing chest expansion.

a deep breath and note whether both thumbs move apart symmetrically. Repeat this in the upper and lower zones of the chest.

> **For descriptive purposes, the areas of the thorax are split into zones**. The upper zones relate to the areas from the supraclavicular area to the level of the 3rd rib, the middle zones from 3rd to 6th ribs and the lower zones from the 6th ribs down.

(a)

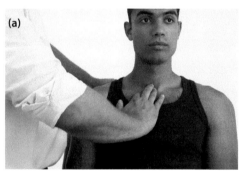

(b)

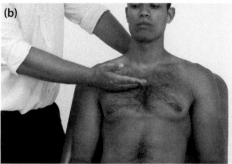

Figure 5.13 (a) Palpating the trachea.
(b) Assessing tactile vocal fremitus.

Tactile vocal fremitus

Place your hands horizontally on the patient's chest and ask them to say '99' (**Figure 5.13b**). Repeat in the upper, middle and lower zones and in the axillae. Note whether it is increased or decreased.

> **Patients are asked to say '99' because it produces a nasal sound that is easily transmitted through the thorax.**

5.6.5 Percussion

Use your middle finger to sharply tap on the patient's clavicles, listening the sound generated. Warn the patient that this might be uncomfortable. Then, place the middle finger of one hand over a rib space running parallel to the rib and tap sharply with the other middle finger, again listening to the sound (**Figure 5.15**).

Perform this comparing each zone on each side before moving on to the next, i.e. percuss both upper zones then both middle zones, both lower zones and both axillae.

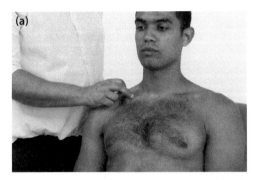

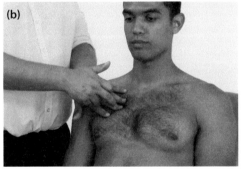

Figure 5.15 Percussing the thorax.

5.6.6 Auscultation

Breath sounds

Press the diaphragm of the stethoscope firmly against the patient's chest wall. Ask them to take a slow, deep breath in and out through their mouth. Note whether the breath sound is vesicular, bronchial or reduced.

As with percussion, auscultate the same area on each side, comparing side to side as you progress.

> **Ask the patient to cross their arms over their chest when auscultating the thorax.** This draws the scapulae up and around the chest wall to give you more area to examine.

Added sounds

Listen for added sounds whilst listening to the breath sounds:
- are there any added sounds such as wheeze, crackles or rubs?
- are they loud or soft?
- do they occur in inspiration or expiration?

Respiratory phases

Note the duration of inspiration and expiration. The normal ration is 1:2. A prolonged expiratory phase is found in airway and interstitial diseases.

Vocal resonance

In the same areas as auscultation, place the diaphragm of the stethoscope firmly on the chest and ask the patient to say '99'. Is the sound enhanced or inaudible?

> **Whispering pectriloquy is another test for underlying consolidation or fibrosis**. Ask the patient to whisper '101' whilst you listen over the chest wall with a stethoscope. It should be inaudible over normal areas but transmitted over abnormal areas.

Heart sounds

Listen to the heart sounds as described in the cardiovascular chapter (*Chapter 4*). Is there a loud second heart sound or the murmur of tricuspid regurgitation?

5.6.7 Finishing off

Check for sacral oedema and peripheral oedema by gently pressing on the legs and sacrum to assess for 'pitting' (see *Section 4.3.13*) and comment on its severity: to the level of the mid-shins, knees, mid-thighs, abdominal wall, or above.

Table 5.11 *The sequence of the respiratory examination*

Element	Details
General inspection	*Appearance*: does the patient look systemically well or unwell?
	Environment: are there any clues suggesting disease?
	Face: is the patient centrally cyanosed?
	Chest: is the patient visibly breathless at rest?
	Weight: is the patient over- or underweight?
Hands	Are there any nail abnormalities?
	Is there any evidence of tremor or flap?
Wrist	What is the heart rate and rhythm?
Arm	What is the blood pressure?
Face	Is there conjunctival pallor?
	Is there evidence of Horner's syndrome?
	Is there central cyanosis?
Neck	Is the jugular venous pressure elevated?
	Is there palpable lymphadenopathy?
	Is the trachea deviated?
Chest	Inspection: are there any scars or deformities?
	Palpation: does the chest expand symmetrically? Is tactile vocal fremitus normal? Is the apex beat normal?
	Percussion: is the percussion note normal?
	Auscultation: are the breath sounds normal? Are there any added sounds? Are heart sounds normal?
Legs	Is there any peripheral oedema?
Abdomen	Is there any ascites?

5.7 Common investigations

The tests used in investigating, diagnosing and monitoring respiratory disease are shown in **Table 5.12**.

5.7.1 Chest radiography

Chest radiography (CXR) gives a 2D view through the thorax (see **Figure 5.7**).
- Normal lung appears dark with faint white lines through it.
- Consolidation is patchy and white. Air bronchograms (a visible air-filled bronchiole within an area of consolidation) may be seen.
- Fluid is white. When in the pleural space it shows a meniscus.
- Air, as in pneumothorax, cavities and bullae, is dark.
- Heart size is approximated to assess for cardiomegaly.

> **As the chest radiograph is 2D, any change seen can be within or outside the lungs (e.g. a breast lump) and should correlate with the clinical findings.**

Table 5.12 *Choosing investigations in respiratory disease*

	Indications	Benefits	Limitations
Chest radiograph (CXR)	Look for consolidation, fluid or abnormal air	Quick Easy to perform	Two-dimensional Poor views of mediastinum Radiation (small dose)
Computed tomography (CT)	Look for interstitial diseases, cancer, mediastinal disease and vascular problems	Detailed 3D view Relatively quick	Requires patient to lie flat Radiation (moderate dose)
Spirometry	Assess and monitor lung function	Non-invasive Easy to perform Diagnostic	Requires good effort to obtain true reading
Arterial blood gas	Diagnose and monitor respiratory failure	Quick Reliable	Painful

5.7.2 Computed tomography

Computed tomography (CT) scans give a 3D view through the thorax. They can assess airways and interstitial tissues as well as the structures within the mediastinum that are less clear on radiographs. Injecting radiopaque dye into the bloodstream allows assessment of the vasculature.

5.7.3 Spirometry

Spirometry is a measure of lung function used to diagnose certain conditions (such as asthma and COPD) and monitor for progression.

5.7.4 Electrocardiography

An electrocardiogram (ECG) records electrical heart activity and can assess for evidence of right-sided heart strain and arrhythmia.

5.7.5 Echocardiography

Echocardiograms show heart structure and function and can diagnose right heart failure, tricuspid regurgitation and pulmonary hypertension.

5.7.6 Blood tests

Serum blood testing is used to diagnose:
- anaemia
- infection (both markers of infection or antigens to particular microbes)
- inflammatory disorders
- allergy.

5.7.7 Arterial blood gas

Arterial blood gas analysis measures the pH, carbon dioxide and oxygen concentrations, bicarbonate level, base excess and lactate of a patient's arterial blood. This is used to diagnose and monitor respiratory failure in both the acute and chronic setting.

5.7.8 Sputum analysis

Sputum is cultured in the laboratory for bacterial and fungal infections. Some infections require special sputum tests such as Ziehl–Neelsen staining used to detect TB.

5.8 Answers to starter questions

1. To develop cancer, a mutation must occur within a cell, leading to uncontrolled cell division forming a tumour. The cocktail of chemicals in tobacco smoke is the biggest cause of mutations but not the only ones: genetics, radiation exposure and other chemical damage can also contribute. The immune system includes cells that target and destroy abnormal or damaged cells such as cancer cells and can prevent these from developing into tumours. Some people are more resistant to the effects of tobacco smoke and so do not develop the mutations that others do. Finally, the more a person smokes, the more likely they are to develop cancer, so some people who smoke less are at a lower risk.

2. Part of the management of COPD includes treatment with inhaled corticosteroids to reduce the rate of acute exacerbations. Over time, the cumulative dose can be enough to give a systemic effect. Acute exacerbations of COPD are treated with short courses of oral steroids. For people with severe COPD and multiple exacerbations, the amount of steroids used can lead to the development of Cushing's syndrome (see *Section 13.2.3*). This leads to a thin, papery skin that is easily bruised.

3. Long-term respiratory disease causes a rise in the pulmonary arterial blood pressure. This puts strain on the right side of the heart leading to the development of cor pulmonale. The impact this has on reducing venous return to the left side of the heart and the increase in systemic blood pressure can cause hypertrophy and eventual failure of the left side of the heart (biventricular failure), therefore causing breathlessness.

   For some people, worsening breathlessness means breathlessness that worsens the more they move. In alveolar and interstitial diseases, the distance oxygen needs to diffuse to in order to reach the blood is increased. As the heartbeat quickens during exercise and the time a red blood cell travels through the pulmonary capillaries decreases, the amount of oxygen that can be taken up by each red blood cell is reduced, leading to reduced oxygen delivery to tissues, triggering the respiratory rate to increase and a feeling of breathlessness.

4. In the acute TB infection, the immune response is relatively small and many patients do not develop symptoms until the disease has progressed somewhat. During this time, the infection causes scarring and hypertrophy of mucus-producing cells. After the infection is gone, these changes remain, leaving the patient with bronchiectasis. Sometimes, the infection causes a cavity which is infected at a later date by organisms such as *Aspergillus fumigatus*. TB may spread to other parts of the body and cause infection elsewhere even when the respiratory infection is treated. Finally, TB can survive in a dormant state where it is kept under control by the immune system but not fully eradicated. When the immune system is suppressed, such as in HIV or with immunosuppressive medications, it 'reactivates' and causes renewed infection.

5. The exact cause is unknown, but some patients with chronic respiratory disease such as COPD develop type 2 respiratory failure when they are given oxygen. One theory is that people with chronic lung disease develop a relative resistance to body CO_2 levels and respiratory acidosis. These people rely solely on hypoxia stimulating their cerebral respiratory centres to maintain their respiratory effort (the 'hypoxic drive'). Administering oxygen eliminates the hypoxic drive and they develop respiratory failure. Another theory suggests that oxygen therapy shifts the haemoglobin–carbon dioxide dissociation curve to the right, thereby increasing carbon dioxide levels (the 'Haldane effect'). This results in increased CO_2 in the blood, which the patient is unable to excrete by increasing their respiratory effort.

Chapter 6
Gastrointestinal system

Starter questions

1. Is awareness of malnutrition still relevant in modern medicine?
2. Why might a patient who is constantly tired end up with a colostomy?
3. If alcohol was banned, would there be no liver disease?
4. Should I ask for a chaperone when performing an abdominal examination?
5. What is diarrhoea?

Answers to questions are to be found in *Section 6.8*.

6.1 Introduction

The gastrointestinal (GI) tract is the long, complex tube that begins at the mouth and terminates at the anus, which is responsible for the digestion and absorption of nutrients. It works in concert with the other abdominal organs of digestion: the pancreas, liver and gall bladder, all of which play roles in the endocrine and exocrine processes of metabolism. The interdependent nature of the individual organs of digestion is relevant to understanding digestive and nutritional disease, as problems with one component always affect another.

Various components of the digestive system are also responsible for:

- maintaining immunity
- glucose metabolism and homeostasis
- coagulation of blood
- regulation of cholesterol and triglycerides.

Case 6.1 Slowly worsening abdominal pain

Presentation

Mr Wilkins is a 57-year-old man who visits his GP with epigastric pain, which is getting slowly worse over a period of weeks. It usually occurs shortly after eating a meal.

Initial interpretation

Abdominal pain is the presenting symptom of a wide range of diseases. The location of pain helps determine the underlying disease process. Epigastric pain is commonly due to inflammation of the stomach lining (gastritis) or small bowel (duodenitis), pancreatic diseases or problems with the gall bladder and bile duct. Acute pancreatitis is associated with severe nausea and vomiting. Both gastritis / duodenitis and gallstones in the biliary system typically occur after eating, when the digestive system is activated, so they remain important differentials in this case.

History

Mr Wilkins describes his pain as being 'like a stabbing knife' in the central upper region of his abdomen. It usually develops after eating a meal, reaching maximum intensity after ten minutes. It doesn't radiate to any other area. It usually lasts about 60 minutes, after which it decreases to a dull ache. He has tried various OTC painkillers without success.

Interpretation of history

This description of the pain helps us narrow our differential somewhat. Pain associated with meals indicates gastric, duodenal or gall bladder disease. Pain secondary to gallstones is colicky, and focused in the right upper area of the abdomen. The sharp, stabbing nature of Mr Wilkins' pain is typical of peptic ulcer disease (PUD), an extreme form of GI inflammation. Pancreatic disease cannot be ruled out at this point, so further information is required.

A rare cause of episodic epigastric pain is atypical angina pectoris. Anginal pain can be precipitated by eating in severe CHD, but there would definitely be an exertional component as well, so it is not the diagnosis here.

Further history

Mr Wilkins has not experienced any vomiting. He does not think that he has lost any weight. He has not noticed any swelling of his abdomen. There is no history of bleeding from the rectum. He does not drink alcohol, although he does smoke 10 cigarettes a day. He takes simple OTC remedies for long-standing heartburn. He also takes regular ibuprofen for osteoarthritis of the knees.

Examination

General inspection of the patient reveals a slim, pale gentleman. He has some tenderness of the abdomen on deep palpation, but there are no masses. His heart rate, respiratory rate and blood pressure are all within normal parameters. A digital rectal examination does not reveal any masses or rectal blood.

Interpretation of findings

The absence of vomiting and weight loss now makes acute pancreatitis very unlikely. Diseases of the liver cause abdominal pain if the liver becomes enlarged and stretches its surrounding capsule, but no liver enlargement was detected on abdominal examination. The patient has three risk factors for developing PUD: acid reflux (heartburn), prolonged anti-inflammatory use and smoking. This is the most likely diagnosis.

Investigations

Mr Wilkins undergoes blood testing, which reveals a mild anaemia. He undergoes endoscopic examination, which reveals a large peptic ulcer on the greater curve of the stomach, and generalised inflammation of the gastric lining. The ulcer shows signs of chronic bleeding, which explains his anaemia.

Diagnosis

Mr Wilkins has PUD in the form of a bleeding gastric ulcer. He requires high dose acid

Case 6.1 continued

suppression therapy to promote ulcer healing. Untreated peptic ulcers lead to complications (**Figure 6.1**). If the ulcer shows signs of heavy bleeding, the endoscopist injects it, covers it in a thick adhesive, clips it to prevent bleeding or uses a heated probe to provide haemostasis. The endoscopist usually takes a biopsy of the ulcer, as a small minority of peptic ulcers are malignant. The biopsy is also used to diagnose *Helicobacter pylori* bacteria, a cause of peptic ulcers. If *H. pylori* is detected, it must be eradicated with antibiotics. Mr Wilkins requires a repeat endoscopy after 6–8 weeks to ensure the ulcer has healed.

In terms of secondary prevention of PUD, Mr Wilkins must stop smoking, and avoid gastrotoxic medications such as anti-inflammatory medications.

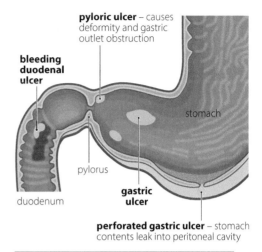

Figure 6.1 Long-term complications of peptic ulcer disease.

The majority of peptic ulcers cause pain but bleed very little. If they do bleed, it is usually a slow ooze over time, which goes unnoticed by the patient until they become clinically anaemic. Rarely, a peptic ulcer erodes into a blood vessel, causing devastating exsanguination.

6.2 System overview

The entire gastrointestinal system is divided into the upper and lower GI tracts and the hepatopancreaticobiliary system.

6.2.1 Upper GI tract

This extends from the mouth to the ileum. Key diseases of each section are listed in **Table 6.1**.

Mouth

The mouth is responsible for mastication and lubrication of food, and digestion begins in the form of carbohydrate breakdown by salivary amylase.

Oesophagus

The oesophagus is lined with a stratified squamous epithelium, which transitions to a columnar epithelium at the gastro-oesophageal junction located a few centimetres above the stomach. Muscular peristalsis moves the food bolus down the oesophagus into the stomach. The lower oesophageal sphincter (LOS) prevents regurgitation of stomach contents (**Figure 6.2**).

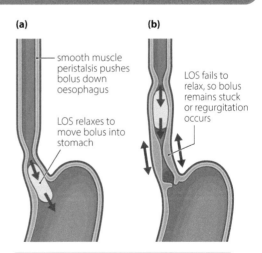

Figure 6.2 (a) Normal oesophageal peristalsis moves a food bolus towards the stomach, and the lower oesophageal sphincter (LOS) relaxes to allow entry into the stomach; (b) achalasia is the failure of the LOS to relax.

Table 6.1 *Common disease processes of the upper gastrointestinal tract in association with anatomic location*

Part of tract	Disease	Definition	Features
Mouth	Tumours	Squamous cell carcinomas affect mouth, pharynx or vocal cords	Obstruction to swallowing, loss of voice
	Sicca	Dry mouth due to autoimmune destruction of the salivary glands (Sjögren's syndrome)	Dry mouth, difficulty lubricating food and swallowing
Oesophagus	Tumour	Intrinsic obstruction, due to tumour, large ulcer or oesophageal spasm	Dysphagia Regurgitation Painful swallowing (odynophagia)
	GORD	Extrinsic compression due to mediastinal mass, e.g. thymoma, mediastinal lymphadenopathy	Dysphagia Regurgitation Heartburn
	Achalasia	Achalasia Scleroderma (CREST)	Dysphagia Regurgitation Painful swallowing (odynophagia)
Stomach	Autoimmune gastritis	Autoimmune destruction of the parietal cells causing achlorhydria and vitamin B12 deficiency	Malabsorption: weight loss and malnutrition GI infections Macrocytic anaemia
	Tumours	Gastric cancer usually presents late, as tumours grow to large size before they cause symptoms	Early satiety, vomiting, weight loss
	Gastric outlet obstruction	Tumours close to the pyloric sphincter obstruct movement of chyme into the duodenum	Vomiting, epigastric pain
	Gastroparesis	Loss of smooth muscle action due to autonomic failure	Vomiting, epigastric pain
	PUD	Spectrum of disease from mild gastritis to severe ulceration	Epigastric pain Haematemesis
Duodenum	PUD	Duodenal ulceration	Abdominal pain several hours after eating or at night
	Coeliac disease	Autoimmune destruction of duodenal lining	Abdominal pain, malabsorption, iron deficiency
Jejunum	Short bowel syndrome	Due to surgical resection of diseased bowel	Weight loss, malnutrition Diarrhoea

Part of tract	Disease	Definition	Features
Ileum	Ileal Crohn's disease	Inflammation and ulceration of ileum	These are all malabsorption syndromes, resulting in: ■ weight loss ■ malnutrition ■ diarrhoea ■ steatorrhoea ■ iron-deficiency anaemia ■ abdominal cramps ■ bloating
	Small bowel lymphoma	Malignancy of the intestinal lymphatic system	
	Small bowel bacterial overgrowth	Excessive growth of bacteria in the small bowel due to gut dysmotility or previous surgery	

Barrett's oesophagus is metaplastic change to the lower oesophageal lining due to chronic acid reflux. Metaplasia is the transformation of one cell type to another. In this case the squamous oesophageal epithelium becomes a columnar epithelium in response to chronic acid exposure. This places the patient at a higher risk of developing oesophageal carcinoma.

Stomach

The stomach secretes protein-cleaving enzymes, such as pepsin, which break down large protein molecules into smaller ones that are absorbed in the intestine. It secretes hydrochloric acid, which in turn activates digestive enzymes, and facilitates the breakdown of large protein molecules. The acidic environment of the stomach kills most swallowed bacteria.

There are multiple types of secretory cells in the gastric epithelium, which release various substances to aid digestion and maintain the integrity of the stomach lining (**Table 6.2**).

The gastric outlet is encircled by the pyloric sphincter. When stomach pressure overcomes the natural resistance of this sphincter, the partially digested food and gastric juices (this mixture is called 'chyme') pass into the duodenum.

Small intestine

This is the site for the majority of nutrient absorption. The small intestine is around 6 metres

Table 6.2 *Gastric epithelial cells and their function*

Cell type	Function
Foveolar cells	Both foveolar and goblet cells produce mucus, which forms a protective layer over the stomach lining and protects it from the corrosive effects of hydrochloric acid
Goblet cells	
Chief cells	Secrete pepsinogen, which is converted to pepsin by stomach acid; pepsin breaks down proteins into smaller peptides
Parietal cells	Secrete hydrochloric acid Produce intrinsic factor, a molecule that binds to vitamin B12 so it is absorbed in the ileum
G cells	Secrete gastrin, a hormone that activates enterochromaffin-like cells and parietal cells
Enterochromaffin-like cells	Secrete histamine, which aids hydrochloric acid secretion, and serotonin, which activates gastric peristalsis

long, in contrast to the large intestine, which is around 1.5 metres in length.

Duodenum

The duodenum is the first part of the small intestine, and is responsible for ongoing breakdown of macromolecules, such as proteins and complex carbohydrates. The presence of acidic chyme stimulates the secretion of hormones and electrolytes that neutralise acidity and promote bile flow from the gall bladder (**Table 6.3**).

Jejunum

The jejunum is the major absorption site of the small bowel, with the exception of:
- iron, which is absorbed in the duodenum
- vitamin B12, which is absorbed in the ileum.

The jejunal mucosa is covered in villi – tiny projections that dramatically increase the surface area available for nutrient absorption. The mucosa itself is lined with enterocytes. These are simple columnar cells capable of absorption. The cell membranes are lined with microvilli, which further increase the surface area. Absorbed nutrients enter the bloodstream, and drain to the liver via the portal vein.

Ileum

The ileum is also lined with enterocytes, which are covered in villi and microvilli, thereby facilitating ongoing nutrient absorption. The mucosa also contains specialised lymphoid tissue organised into follicles called Peyer's patches. This tissue acts as immune sensors, detecting and differentiating between normal commensal gut organisms and pathogenic organisms, and activating the immune system if infection is present.

Large intestine

The large bowel is composed of:
- the colon, which is responsible for absorbing water from digested food
- the rectum, where faeces is impacted and stored before defecation.

There is minimal nutrient absorption in the large intestine. The common diseases of both sections are listed in **Table 6.4**.

> **The colon is home to over a hundred species of bacteria, which aid digestion and fermentation of food.** Antibiotics kill off certain strains, modifying the ratio of particular strains, which disrupts the normal symbiotic relationship. This allows surviving pathogenic bacteria (e.g. *Clostridium difficile*) to flourish and cause infection.

Table 6.3 *Duodenal cells and their secretions that aid digestion*

Cell	Secretion	Function
S cells	Secretin	Switches off acid production by gastric parietal cells to diminish duodenal acidity
		Stimulates bicarbonate production in the pancreas
		Stimulates bile synthesis in the liver
I cells	Cholecystokinin	Acts on the CNS to promote satiety
		Causes contraction of the gall bladder to eject bile into the bile duct and duodenum
		Stimulates pancreatic digestive enzyme secretion
Brunner's glands	Alkaline mucus	Protects duodenal epithelium from stomach acid and provides alkaline environment needed for pancreatic enzyme function
	Enteropeptidase	Converts the inactive pancreatic digestive enzymes to active form, e.g. trypsinogen into trypsin

Table 6.4 *Common disease processes of the lower GI tract in association with anatomic location*

Part of tract	Disease	Cause	Definition	Features
Colon	Tumours	Multiple inherited forms exist, or may be sporadic	Usually adenocarcinoma	Diarrhoea Iron-deficiency anaemia
	Inflammatory bowel disease	Immune-mediated	Inflammation and ulceration of the mucosa	Macroscopic lesions on endoscopy Periods of remission punctuated by acute flares, incorporating: ■ diarrhoea ■ PR bleeding ■ abdominal pain ■ fever ■ extra-intestinal complications
	Microscopic colitis	Idiopathic Adverse effect of proton pump inhibitors (PPIs)	Microscopic inflammation of the colonic epithelium and connective tissue	Normal macroscopic appearances on endoscopy Chronic watery diarrhoea
	Ischaemic colitis	Atheromatous vascular disease	Colonic inflammation due to chronic ischaemia	Abdominal pain Bloody stools History of vascular disease Elderly patients
	Infective colitis	Infection with various bacteria, including: ■ *Escherichia coli* ■ *Salmonella typhi* ■ *Shigella* ■ *Campylobacter*	Acute infective inflammation	Acute onset abdominal pain Fever Diarrhoea, usually bloody Possible history of eating undercooked / reheated food
Rectum / anal canal	Tumours	Multiple inherited forms exist, or may be sporadic	Usually adenocarcinoma, although anal cancers may be squamous cell	Tenesmus Obstruction
	Anal fissures	Usually due to constipation and straining	Longitudinal breaks in the superficial epithelium	Pain on defecation PR bleeding
	Haemorrhoids	Low fibre diet, constipation Obesity	Dilated blood vessels inside or external to the anal canal	Pain on defecation PR bleeding Pruritus ani Palpable / visible mass extruding from anus

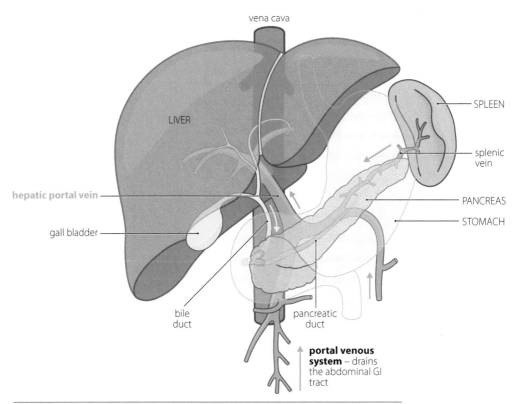

Figure 6.3 The interconnecting 'plumbing' of the hepatopancreaticobiliary system.

6.2.2 Hepatopancreaticobiliary organs

These organs are the liver, gall bladder, pancreas and spleen. They are grouped together as they are part of one 'plumbing' system (**Figure 6.3**). The liver synthesises bile, which is collected in the gall bladder and ejected down the bile duct. The pancreas makes digestive enzymes, which move down the pancreatic duct which then empties into the bile duct. This then drains into the duodenum via the sphincter of Oddi.

Liver
The liver plays a role in digestion, immunity, coagulation and metabolism (**Table 6.5**). It is susceptible to chronic impairment by infection, metabolic disorders and toxicity (**Table 6.6**).

> **The prevalence of non-alcoholic fatty liver disease (NAFLD) is increasing in line with obesity.** Whilst there is a genetic predisposition, the modifiable risk factors are high cholesterol and diabetes, meaning that it is often accompanied by coronary artery disease.

Pancreas
The pancreas has an exocrine and endocrine function. The endocrine function is discussed in *Chapter 13*. As an exocrine gland, the pancreas secretes enzyme-rich digestive juices (**Table 6.7**), which flow down the pancreatic duct into the duodenum.

Gall bladder
The gall bladder is a reservoir for bile, which is produced in the liver. The presence of food in the

duodenum stimulates the gall bladder to contract and eject bile down the common bile duct.

Obstruction of the common bile duct impairs biliary flow, and leads to jaundice. This obstruction is either intrinsic, such as gallstones or bile duct cancer (cholangiocarcinoma), or extrinsic pressure, due to lymph nodes or the close proximity to cancers of the pancreatic head.

Spleen

The spleen has two primary functions:
- It filters out and breaks down old red blood cells.
- It stores and activates immune cells that fight infection.

It is possible for people to live without a spleen, but they are more susceptible to infection, and therefore must take long-term antibiotics and have regular immunisations against severe bacterial infections such as pneumonia.

Table 6.5 *Roles of the liver, and the sequelae of liver dysfunction*

Role	Process	Sequelae of liver dysfunction
Emulsification of dietary fats	Synthesis of bile, which emulsifies fat, allowing it to be metabolised	Steatorrhoea
Regulation of glucose metabolism	Storage of glucose in the form of glycogen	Hypoglycaemia
Metabolism of protein, glycerol and lactate	Gluconeogenesis	Elevated lactate levels Hypoglycaemia
Blood coagulation	Synthesis of clotting factors	Coagulopathy
Hormone regulation	Breakdown of circulating hormones, including insulin and oestrogen	Elevated circulating hormone levels
Excretion of nitrogenous waste compounds	Conversion to urea, which is excreted in urine	Hepatic encephalopathy

Table 6.6 *Causes of chronic liver disease*

Cause	Pathology	Associations
Infective	Chronic hepatitis B and hepatitis C infection lead to inflammation and chronic damage	Other blood-borne viruses, e.g. HIV
Autoimmune		
Primary biliary cholangitis	Autoimmune destruction of intra-lobular bile ducts in the liver	Other autoimmune diseases
Primary sclerosing cholangitis	Fibrotic obliteration of bile ducts	UC Cholangiocarcinoma
Autoimmune hepatitis	Autoimmune destruction of hepatocytes	Other autoimmune diseases, especially SLE
Drug-induced	Direct hepatocyte toxicity or intra-hepatic cholestasis	Other unwanted systemic drug effects

Table 6.6 (cont'd)

Cause	Pathology	Associations
Alcohol-induced	Inflammation and fibrosis of hepatocytes via inflammatory pathways	Other alcohol-induced organ damage, e.g. cardiomyopathy, peripheral neuropathy, cerebellar disease
Non-alcoholic steatohepatitis (NASH)	Hepatic fat accumulation leading to inflammation then fibrosis	Obesity Type 2 diabetes
Metabolic		
Hereditary haemochromatosis	Genetic propensity to excessive iron deposition in the liver	Iron deposition in joints and pituitary gland
Wilson's disease	Genetic propensity to excessive copper deposition in the liver	Parkinsonism, due to copper deposition in the basal ganglia
Thrombotic	Thrombosis of the portal vein (Budd–Chiari syndrome)	Other thrombotic phenomena, e.g. DVT
Genetic	Alpha-1 antitrypsin deficiency is a rare inherited cause of cirrhosis	Advanced lung emphysema via same processes, favouring the lung bases
Heart failure	Right heart failure causes hepatic engorgement, leading to centrilobular necrosis	Signs and symptoms of cardiac failure

Table 6.7 Digestive enzymes secreted by the pancreas and their function

Enzyme	Function
Trypsin Chymotrypsin	Both trypsin and chymotrypsin break down protein molecules into peptide chains
Lipase	Breaks down fats into fatty acids and glycerides; fats must be emulsified by bile before they are broken down
Amylase	Breaks down carbohydrates into simple sugars

6.3 Symptoms of gastrointestinal disease

The main symptoms of GI disease include heartburn, abdominal pain, change in bowel habit, swallowing problems, vomiting, regurgitation, fatigue, gastrointestinal bleeding and weight loss.

6.3.1 Heartburn

This is a retrosternal burning that ranges from mild discomfort to severe pain. It is a symptom of gastro-oesophageal reflux disease (GORD). Patients with severe GORD cannot tolerate lying flat, as acid seeps up into the lower oesophagus, so they sleep sitting upright. Heartburn is associated with acid brash – the taste of acid at the back of the mouth.

> **Patients often use 'heartburn', 'dyspepsia', 'reflux' and 'indigestion' interchangeably**, so enquire what they mean.

6.3.2 Abdominal pain

The abdomen is divided into nine anatomical areas; pain in each area has different potential causes (**Figure 6.4**).

Colic is pain that comes in intense waves then dissipates for a short period, and is related to the intermittent action of smooth muscle peristalsis upon an obstructed system (**Table 6.8**). Renal colic is due to stones in the ureters. Patients draw their legs up in the foetal position, and feel compelled to keep moving, either rolling on the bed or pacing the room, to minimise the

pain. Biliary colic is due to obstruction to the bile duct, and causes right upper abdominal pain, occasionally radiating to the shoulder tip.

Peptic ulcer disease

Peptic ulcer disease (PUD) causes stabbing or burning pain. The patient often has a history of GORD. Smoking is also a risk factor.

The main causes of PUD are:

- prolonged use of non-steroidal anti-inflammatory drugs (NSAIDs, e.g. ibuprofen). They strip the gastric mucosa of its protective layer, rendering it vulnerable to strong gastric acid.
- *Helicobacter pylori* (*H. pylori*) infection.

PUD of the stomach causes abdominal pain during or immediately after eating. PUD of the duodenum causes abdominal pain two or three hours after eating, or during the night (whilst digesting the evening meal).

Pyelonephritis

This is infection of the kidney. It causes flank pain, fever, dysuria and rigors – generalised

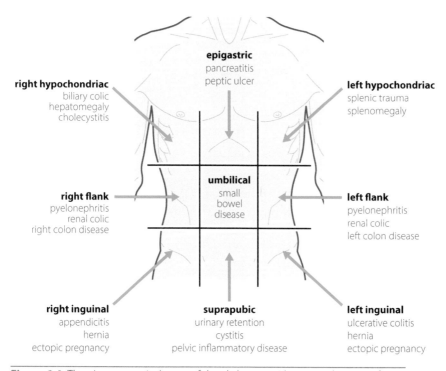

epigastric
pancreatitis
peptic ulcer

right hypochondriac
biliary colic
hepatomegaly
cholecystitis

left hypochondriac
splenic trauma
splenomegaly

umbilical
small
bowel
disease

right flank
pyelonephritis
renal colic
right colon disease

left flank
pyelonephritis
renal colic
left colon disease

right inguinal
appendicitis
hernia
ectopic pregnancy

suprapubic
urinary retention
cystitis
pelvic inflammatory disease

left inguinal
ulcerative colitis
hernia
ectopic pregnancy

Figure 6.4 The nine anatomical areas of the abdomen with potential causes of pain.

Type of colic	Cause	Features
Biliary colic	Presence of gallstones in the common bile duct (cholelithiasis)	Right upper quadrant and epigastric colic
		Worse after eating fatty meal
		Classically affects obese women in their 40s
		Gallstones often cause biliary obstruction, leading to jaundice
Renal colic	Presence of renal stones in the ureter (nephrocalcinosis)	Severe colic radiating from flank to groin ('loin to groin')
		Micro- / macroscopic haematuria
Bowel colic	Severe constipation	History of bowels not opening
		Impacted faeces on digital rectal exam
		Nausea and vomiting if severe

Table 6.8 *Causes of colicky pain and associated features*

uncontrollable shivering due to bacteraemia (the presence of bacteria in the bloodstream).

Inflammatory bowel disease

Abdominal pain associated with extra-intestinal signs (outside the digestive system) is the presenting symptom of inflammatory bowel disease (IBD). IBD comprises two separate conditions:

■ Crohn's disease
■ Ulcerative colitis (UC).

Both diseases lead to inflammation and ulceration of the intestinal mucosa (**Table 6.9**). They cause acute episodes of abdominal pain and diarrhoea, rectal bleeding and signs of systemic inflammation (such as fever, tachycardia and elevated white cell count (WCC)), followed by periods of remission that last between weeks and years.

Infection

Gastroenteritis is an acute infection of the digestive tract. Viral infections are more common than bacterial infections. Norovirus is a highly infectious disease which causes severe abdominal pain, vomiting and loose stools.

Irritable bowel syndrome

This is a functional bowel disorder. It is common, with a prevalence of around 10% in the UK. It comprises several key symptoms in addition to cramping abdominal pain:

■ Alteration in bowel habit between diarrhoea

and constipation, or a propensity for one extreme; diarrhoea is more common
■ Flatulence
■ Bloating.

Patients with irritable bowel syndrome (IBS) are usually able to identify foods that exacerbate their symptoms and avoid them. There are no micro- or macroscopic changes detectable in the bowel.

> **Inflammatory bowel disease (IBD) is very different from irritable bowel syndrome (IBS).** Constitutional symptoms, such as fever and weight loss, and evidence of GI bleeding effectively rule out a diagnosis of IBS; it is a diagnosis of exclusion.

> Remember the causes of acute pancreatitis by using the mnemonic **I GET SMASHED**. Ethanol and gallstones are by far the most common.
> ■ **I**diopathic
> ■ **G**allstones
> ■ **E**thanol (alcohol excess)
> ■ **T**rauma
> ■ **S**teroid use
> ■ **M**umps
> ■ **A**utoimmune
> ■ **S**corpion venom
> ■ **H**yperlipidaemia / hypercalcaemia
> ■ **E**ndoscopic retrograde cholangiopancreatography
> ■ **D**rugs, including azathioprine

Table 6.9 *Comparing ulcerative colitis and Crohn's disease*

	UC	Crohn's disease
Affected sites	Colon and rectum only	Any part of the GI tract, including mouth, oesophagus and rectum
Macroscopic appearance	One continuous section of bowel affected	Areas of normal bowel in between affected areas ('skip' lesions)
Nature of flares	Systemic signs of inflammation: ■ fever ■ tachycardia ■ raised WCC ■ abdominal pain ■ diarrhoea and increased stool frequency ■ bloody diarrhoea more common in UC	
Pain	Usually left iliac fossa	Depending on site of affected bowel
Extra-intestinal features	Pyoderma gangrenosum: deep necrotic ulcers on the shins Erythema nodosum: tender nodules on shins Iritis / uveitis: inflammation of anterior eye Primary sclerosing cholangitis Joint inflammation and pain (enteropathic arthropathy)	
Surgical complications	Fistulae and strictures more common, requiring numerous surgeries	May require colectomy and colostomy formation

Pancreatitis

Pancreatitis presents as excruciating stabbing epigastric pain that radiates to the back. It is associated with profound nausea and vomiting.

6.3.3 Change in bowel habit

Stool frequency of between three times per day and three times per week is normal.

Diarrhoea

Increased volume of loose stool is commonly called 'diarrhoea' by patients (see *Starter question 5*).

Intestinal causes

IBD. Increasing bowel frequency is one of the hallmarks of an acute flare of IBD. Acute flares of both UC and Crohn's disease cause:
■ increased stool frequency (more than five per day)

■ loose stool, often with mucus or 'slime'
■ fresh rectal bleeding
■ abdominal pain
■ systemic features of inflammation.

Malignancy. Cancer of the colon impairs its ability to absorb water from the bowel. This causes watery stool.

Small bowel disease. Small bowel diseases cause malabsorption: a partial failure to absorb nutrients. This leads to diarrhoea. Common causes of malabsorption are:
■ small bowel bacterial overgrowth
■ untreated coeliac disease
■ infection, such as Whipple's disease, giardiasis, and human immunodeficiency virus (HIV)
■ lactose intolerance
■ radiation enteritis due to previous radiotherapy
■ small bowel Crohn's disease
■ bile salt malabsorption in the ileum.

Endocrine

Diarrhoea is a feature of hyperthyroidism and hypercortisolism.

Chronic pancreatitis

This leads to impaired exocrine secretion of digestive fluid and enzymes, causing malabsorption. It causes steatorrhoea.

> **Steatorrhoea is the presence of fat in the stools.** It manifests as pale or creamy diarrhoea, which is difficult to flush. It is caused by processes that lead to fat malabsorption:
> - Chronic pancreatitis
> - Cystic fibrosis
> - Pancreatic tumours
> - Coeliac disease
> - Bile duct obstruction
> - Weight loss medications that prevent fat absorption, such as orlistat.

Constipation

This is either an inability to evacuate the bowels satisfactorily, or a lack of urge to open the bowels.

Intestinal causes

Malignancy. Tumours of the distal colon or rectum cause obstruction to the normal passage of faeces. These tumours are often associated with tenesmus: the sensation that one has not properly emptied the rectum after defecation.

Inflammatory bowel disease. Ulcerative colitis and Crohn's disease often affect the distal colon and rectum. If the disease is severe enough, an inflammatory mass develops, which obstructs proper evacuation of the bowels.

Drugs. Some prescribed medications cause constipation as a side-effect, including:
- opiates: either prescribed (e.g. morphine) or drugs of abuse (e.g. heroin)
- CCBs, e.g. nifedipine
- ondansetron (an anti-emetic)
- drugs with anticholinergic effects, e.g. amitriptyline.

Endocrine disorders

Constipation is a feature of:
- hypothyroidism

- hyperparathyroidism (due to high calcium levels).

Diverticulosis

This is the development of small pockets of large intestine (diverticula) which pouch out through weaknesses in the colonic smooth muscle. Patients develop abdominal pain alongside alternating bowel habit. If a diverticulum becomes infected, diverticulitis develops.

6.3.4 Swallowing difficulty

This is called dysphagia. Causes of dysphagia are physical obstruction or neurological disease (**Table 6.10**).

Severe dysphagia is associated with aspiration, where food and fluid passes into the trachea, causing choking. Patients often describe this as 'food going down the wrong way'. Aspiration is a risk factor for aspiration pneumonia.

If the patient has a physical obstruction, they notice dysphagia to solids before liquids. In cases of neurological disease, they notice dysphagia to liquids before solids, or both at the same time.

> **Avoid using the words 'oesophagus' and 'trachea', which are unlikely to be understood by patients.** The terms 'food pipe' and 'windpipe' are more helpful when discussing symptoms.

6.3.5 Vomiting

Vomiting is the expulsion of partially digested food and stomach acid.

The commonest cause of acute vomiting is an infection (gastroenteritis). These infections are usually viral and resolve in 24–48 hours without treatment. Vomiting is strongly associated with nausea.

There are many causes of chronic vomiting (**Table 6.11**). Chronic vomiting causes several secondary problems, including:
- loss of electrolytes from gastric juice, especially potassium and sodium
- oesophageal inflammation and ulceration
- loss of tooth enamel.

Table 6.10 *Causes of dysphagia*

Symptom	Reason	Causative conditions
Choking	Aspiration – swallowed material moving into the trachea due to dyscoordinated swallow reflex	Neurological impairment of swallow reflex: ▪ motor neurone disease ▪ Parkinson's disease ▪ stroke ▪ myasthenia gravis
Food 'getting stuck'		
In posterior pharynx	Mechanical obstruction	Pharyngeal tumour Large thyroid goitre
In mid-oesophagus	Mechanical obstruction	Oesophageal tumour Obstructing food bolus, e.g. unchewed meat Oesophageal web – a thin membrane across the oesophagus due to chronic iron-deficiency anaemia Oesophageal stricture due to scarring
Distal oesophagus / retrosternally	Mechanical obstruction	Tumour Stricture Large ulcer
	Failure of lower sphincter to relax	Achalasia
Painful swallow (odynophagia)	Inflammation of oesophagus	Oesophagitis / Barrett's oesophagus Oesophageal candida Oesophageal Crohn's disease

6.3.6 Regurgitation

Regurgitation is the immediate bringing-up of undigested food, and is due to obstruction of the oesophagus or stomach. Common causes of regurgitation are:
▪ intrinsic obstruction of the oesophagus, due to tumour, ulcer or severe GORD
▪ extrinsic obstruction of the oesophagus, e.g. due to mediastinal tumour
▪ achalasia
▪ small stomach size following bariatric surgery
▪ gastric outlet obstruction
▪ rumination syndrome, a functional disorder.

6.3.7 Fatigue

This may be due to inflammation or anaemia.

Inflammation

Chronic inflammation in the body is associated with tiredness, likely due to the inflammatory mediators of the immune system dysregulating the release of pituitary hormones, and interacting with the central nervous system (CNS). Diseases associated with chronic inflammation include inflammatory bowel disease and cirrhosis.

Anaemia

Anaemia causes fatigue due to the decreased delivery of oxygen to tissues.

Iron-deficiency anaemia

Chronic iron deficiency results in small, pale red blood cells (microcytosis) with reduced oxygen-binding ability. Causes of iron deficiency are either poor dietary intake, poor absorption from the GI tract, or iron loss.

Table 6.11 *Causes of nausea and vomiting*

Trigger for nausea / vomiting	Typical causes	Associated features
Gastric outlet obstruction	Pyloric tumour Pyloric ulcer	Succussion splash Abdominal pain
Gastroparesis	Autonomic failure – usually due to diabetes mellitus Long term opiates	Severe abdominal pain Opiate use / abuse
Small bowel obstruction	Paralytic ileus – recent abdominal surgery, severe sepsis	Abdominal distension
Large bowel obstruction	Colonic mass Severe constipation	Chronic anaemia Bowels not opening
Centrally mediated	Drugs Electrolyte derangement Raised intracranial pressure	Prescription of chemotherapy, morphine Neurological impairment Visual changes, headache
Infection	Viral gastroenteritis	Abdominal pain, diarrhoea, fever
Pancreatitis	Alcohol Gallstones	Steatorrhoea, epigastric pain, anorexia
Psychological	Bulimia nervosa	Anorexia nervosa, anxiety, depression
Other	Migraine	Headache

Reduced iron absorption. Iron absorption is affected by:

- achlorhydria (poor gastric acid secretion), as acidic pH is required for iron absorption; achlorhydria is caused by autoimmune gastritis (**Table 6.1**)
- coeliac disease, which causes villous atrophy and poor iron absorption in the duodenum.

Iron loss. The only cause of iron loss is chronic bleeding. Bleeding into the GI tract often goes unnoticed by patients, so presentation to a doctor is delayed until they begin to feel symptoms of anaemia. Chronic GI bleeding is due to:

- colorectal cancer
- IBD
- angiodysplasia.

B12 deficiency anaemia

Lack of vitamin B12 disrupts normal red blood cell cleavage. This leads to a macrocytic anaemia – the red blood cells are large. Due to a deficiency of intrinsic factor, vitamin B12 cannot be absorbed in the ileum. It is usually due to autoimmune gastritis or surgical resection of the ileum.

Folate-deficiency anaemia

This also causes a macrocytosis. Mild folate deficiency is common in pregnancy, so all pregnant women are recommended to take folate supplements. Folate deficiency is a common sequela of malabsorption syndromes (**Table 6.1**).

6.3.8 Gastrointestinal bleeding

Bleeding within the GI tract occurs at any point of its course.

- From the oesophagus, stomach and duodenum – termed 'upper GI bleeds'
- From the jejunum, ileum, colon and rectum – termed 'lower GI bleeds'.

The severity of an upper GI bleed is assessed using the Glasgow-Blatchford score (**Table 6.12**). This

Table 6.12 *The Glasgow-Blatchford score for assessing severity of an upper GI bleed.*	
Feature	**Score**
Blood urea (mmol/L)	
6.5–7.9	2
8.0–9.9	3
10–24.9	4
>25	6
Haemoglobin for men (g/L)	
12–13	1
10–11.9	3
<10	6
Haemoglobin for women (g/L)	
10–12	1
<10	6
Systolic blood pressure	
100–110mmHg	1
90–99mmHg	2
<90	3
Pulse rate >100bpm	1
Melaena	1
Syncope	2
Known liver disease	2
Known cardiac failure	2

The Glasgow-Blatchford score assesses the risk of a patient requiring intervention such as a blood transfusion or endoscopy. A score of 0 confers an extremely low risk of morbidity / mortality, and the patient can be investigated as an outpatient.

tool helps you decide whether the patient needs emergency, urgent or routine endoscopy to identify and control the source of bleeding.

Haematemesis

This means vomiting blood. Haematemesis is due to an upper GI bleed. If the blood is vomited immediately it appears red. If the blood has lain for a while in the stomach or small intestine it becomes partially digested. Partially digested blood, when vomited, has the appearance of ground coffee, and is therefore called 'coffee ground vomit'.

Oesophageal bleeding

Mallory–Weiss tear. A Mallory–Weiss tear is a longitudinal break in the oesophageal mucosa, usually as a consequence of protracted vomiting. The typical history is that of repeated vomiting for many hours, with a small amount of red blood mixed in with subsequent vomits. The bleeding is mild, and treatment is supportive.

Inflammation / ulceration. Chronic acid regurgitation into the oesophagus is the causative mechanism behind gastro-oesophageal reflux disease (GORD). Patients with GORD experience retrosternal burning and pain. The inflamed oesophagus (oesophagitis) bleeds easily. Ulceration of the oesophagus is rare.

Varices. These are dilated blood vessels within the walls of the oesophagus and stomach. Chronic liver disease causes portal hypertension: high back-pressure within the blood vessels that flow into the liver. In response to this, oesophageal and stomach blood vessels expand and experience high pressures. If varices start bleeding, they cause devastating haemorrhage, manifesting as profound fresh upper GI bleeding and melaena.

Cancer. Some patients with oesophageal cancer experience some bleeding from the tumour, but a more common symptom is regurgitation.

Stomach bleeding

Peptic ulcer disease. Gastritis is inflammation of the stomach lining. Severe inflammation, or *Helicobacter pylori* infection, causes ulceration. Both gastritis and gastric ulcers cause gastric bleeding. Bleeding from an ulcer can be a mild ooze or a profound haemorrhage, in accordance with the size and depth of the ulcer.

Cancer. Some tumours of the stomach distort mucosal blood vessels and cause bleeding. More common symptoms of gastric cancer are early satiety, weight loss, regurgitation or vomiting.

Duodenal bleeding

PUD. Duodenal ulcers are the commonest cause of duodenal bleeding.

Crohn's disease. This affects any part of the GI tract. However, duodenal Crohn's is extremely rare.

Per rectum bleeding

This is usually called 'PR bleeding', and is due to either an upper or a lower GI bleed.

Melaena

This is due to PR bleeding from an upper GI source. Melaena is blood that has been fully digested. It has the appearance of thick liquid black tar, and has a distinctive and very offensive odour.

PR bleeding from a lower GI source is undigested and therefore bright red.

> **Rarely, if a patient has rapid bowel transit, upper GI bleeding appears as fresh red PR blood**, as there has not been adequate time to digest it into melaena.

Colorectal bleeding

Inflammatory bowel disease. Both Crohn's and ulcerative colitis cause bleeding as part of their constellation of intestinal symptoms. The bleeding worsens when the patient is having an acute 'flare up' of their condition. Six or more bloody stools per day in association with signs of generalised inflammation is a sign of a severe IBD flare, and requires specialist review, as the patient often needs treatment with IV fluid and steroids. Signs of generalised inflammation are:

- fever
- tachycardia
- elevated WCC.

Cancer. Colorectal cancers damage the vascular supply to the gut mucosa. This results in chronic and often unnoticed loss of blood into the GI tract, resulting in an iron-deficiency anaemia. It is rare for a colorectal tumour to cause noticeable PR bleeding.

Angiodysplasia. Dysplastic blood vessels have an abnormal development and structure, and bleed easily, causing fresh PR bleeding. They rarely result in severe haemorrhage. They are painless. The use of any drugs that affect coagulation, including anticoagulants and NSAIDs, increases the risk of bleeding from angiodysplastic vessels.

Rectal bleeding

Haemorrhoids. Haemorrhoids are dilated vessels, which are either external to the anus or within the rectum or anal canal. They are very common. Internal haemorrhoids are usually painless, and cause bright red PR bleeding. External haemorrhoids are painful, especially during defecation. The patient often notices swelling around the anus on palpation. They are also associated with 'pruritus ani': anal itching.

Anal fissures. These are small tears in the superficial mucosa of the anal canal. They are a sequela of passing hard or impacted stool. They are a very common and trivial cause of PR bleeding, despite being painful during defecation. They heal without the need for treatment.

> **If a patient experiences fresh PR bleeding, ask them whether the blood is usually on the toilet paper when they wipe, or mixed in with the stool in the toilet bowel**. Haemorrhoids generally cause the former, whilst angiodysplasia causes the latter.

6.3.9 Unintentional weight loss

Unintentional weight loss has many potential causes (**Table 6.13**). Weight loss with a normal or increased appetite is usually due to hyperthyroidism. Weight loss is more commonly associated with loss of appetite (anorexia – not to be confused with anorexia nervosa).

Weight loss with anorexia is often a presenting symptom of malignancy of any cause, not just the GI tract.

> **Patients often underestimate or underplay their own weight loss.** Try to quantify it in terms of kilograms over a certain time period. If they do not regularly weigh themselves, ask them if their clothes have become too loose, or if they have had to change belt notches.

Table 6.13 *Causes of unintentional weight loss*	
Cause	**Process**
Hyperthyroidism	Increased metabolic rate
Malignancy	Cancer affects appetite and nutritional status via many pathways, including chronic nausea, chronic pain, constipation and psychological changes
Adrenal insufficiency	Chronic fatigue and nausea lead to poor appetite
Psychological	Depression is often associated with poor appetite and weight loss
Undiagnosed type 1 diabetes	Inability to metabolise glucose leads to profound weight loss
Malabsorption syndromes	Inability to absorb nutrients from gut
Dysphagia	Inability to ingest nutrients
Chronic infection	Chronic TB symptoms often mimic those of malignancy

6.3.10 Abdominal swellings

Discrete masses in the abdomen are due to enlarged abdominal organs, tumours or hernias.

Organomegaly

Hepatomegaly presents as right upper quadrant swelling, and splenomegaly presents as left upper quadrant swelling. Splenomegaly is usually due to chronic liver disease, due to their shared blood supply (the portal system). Chronic liver disease causes increased back pressure to the spleen, causing it to enlarge.

Tumours

Liver tumours cause organomegaly. Ovarian tumours are a more diffuse swelling that are often misinterpreted as abdominal bloating by the patient (see *Section 8.5.1*). Uterine tumours are usually detected due to vaginal bleeding long before they cause a noticeable abdominal swelling.

Hernias

Hernias are caused by abdominal contents extruding through a weak area of musculature or connective tissue. The commonest types are inguinal and femoral hernias. These terms refer to their anatomical origin – however, they both present as swellings in the right or left groin.

Reducible hernias cause a groin swelling that the patient manually pushes back inside, and become more prominent on standing up, due to gravity. They are usually painless. Irreducible hernias are permanent swellings that cannot be pushed back, and are usually more painful.

Other abdominal hernias are:

- incisional hernias: the bowel herniates through a previous surgical incision
- umbilical hernias: the bowel herniates through weakness in abdominal muscles under the umbilicus
- hiatus hernia: the stomach herniates up through the diaphragm into the thoracic cavity; it causes GORD.

6.4 The gastrointestinal history

6.4.1 Past medical history

Questions to ask a patient presenting with abdominal complaints include:

"Do you have a diagnosis of inflammatory bowel disease?"

IBD lies dormant for periods of time, then presents as acute flares. These flares have similar clinical appearances to acute GI infections and the diagnostic uncertainty leads to a delay in appropriate treatment. A known diagnosis of IBD means rapid treatment of the flare.

Primary sclerosing cholangitis, an autoimmune disease of the liver, is strongly associated with UC, so this must be suspected in new cases of liver dysfunction in known UC patients.

"Do you have any existing autoimmune diseases?"

There are three autoimmune diseases that affect the liver (**Table 6.6**):

■ primary biliary cholangitis
■ autoimmune hepatitis
■ primary sclerosing cholangitis.

Patients often have more than one autoimmune disease, and these hepatic illnesses often occur alongside other autoimmune conditions, such as vitiligo, thyroid disease, alopecia, rheumatoid arthritis and SLE.

Whilst liver disease of any cause leads to chronic pruritus, **primary biliary cholangitis in particular is associated with intense intractable itching**. It is thought to be due to the presence of excessive bile acids.

"Have you ever had a blood transfusion?"

Hepatitis B and C are rare but important complications of blood transfusions, despite sophisticated screening programmes.

"Have you ever had radiotherapy?"

Radiotherapy of abdominal malignancies causes radiation enteritis: inflammatory damage to the bowel. This causes chronic loose stool and nutritional deficiencies.

"Have you ever suffered with jaundice?"

Gilbert's disease is a benign hereditary hyperbilirubinaemia that causes recurrent jaundice, especially during acute infections. Viral hepatitis causes transient jaundice during the initial infection, which may have been unreported by the patient.

6.4.2 Medications

Many prescribed medications cause gastrointestinal disturbance, change in bowel habit or acute liver dysfunction (**Table 6.14**). Ask whether the symptoms coincided with any new drug treatment, or whether they have started new medications in the last year.

Table 6.14 *Common medications causing GI disease*		
Medication	**Indication for medication**	**Effect**
Flucloxacillin	Antibiotic	Intrahepatic cholestasis
Co-amoxiclav	Antibiotic	
Methotrexate	Immunosuppressant	Hepatotoxicity
Isoniazid	TB treatment	
Amiodarone	Anti-arrhythmic	
NSAIDs	Pain and inflammation	PUD
Steroids	Immunosuppression Severe inflammation	
PPIs	GORD	Microscopic colitis
Bisphosphonates	Osteoporosis	Severe oesophagitis

Ask specifically about OTC medications. These are often forgotten, and generally considered as benign by patients. NSAIDs such as aspirin and ibuprofen cause peptic ulceration and GI bleeding.

Paracetamol overdose, whether intentional or accidental, is the commonest cause of acute liver failure in the UK.

Ask about non-prescribed or alternative medication, because some herbal medicines cause severe idiosyncratic reactions, including liver or kidney failure. It is not known why only some patients are affected.

6.4.3 Social history

Smoking
Tobacco smoking raises the risk of oesophageal and stomach cancer. It also increases the risk of PUD.

Alcohol
Alcohol abuse is the leading cause of liver disease worldwide. Ask about alcohol use, both currently and in the past. Some patients have strong views as to what constitutes 'excessive' alcohol intake, so it must be quantified in units per day or per week.

Illicit drugs
Chronic cannabis use has been linked to cannabinoid hyperemesis syndrome – a condition categorised by hours or days of intractable vomiting and abdominal pain, followed by periods of normality. Patients often take multiple hot showers per day in an attempt to improve their symptoms. The mechanism by which hot showers improve the symptoms of cannabinoid hyperemesis syndrome is not understood.

Ecstasy is extremely hepatotoxic, and causes sudden and profound acute liver failure in some users.

High risk behaviour
These are behaviours that dramatically increase the chances of contracting hepatitis B and C – viral infections that cause chronic liver disease and HIV. These are blood-borne viruses, so are transmitted by:
- IV drug users sharing needles
- unprotected sex
- extensive tattooing or piercing (the virus withstands the suboptimal sterilisation techniques used in many establishments)
- accidental needlestick injuries in healthcare workers.

6.4.4 Family history

Hereditary diseases that present with GI symptoms include:
- IBD
- coeliac disease
- autoimmune liver disorders
- polycystic kidney disease (causes abdominal swelling).

6.4.5 Systems review

A full systems review for digestive disorders is detailed in **Table 6.15**.

6.5 Signs of gastrointestinal disease

The wealth of extra-abdominal signs in gut, liver and pancreas disease means that a diagnosis is often reached before the abdomen is even examined.

6.5.1 Jaundice

Jaundice (icterus) is caused by the abnormal accumulation of bilirubin (the main component of bile) in the blood. It is usually noticeable in the whites of the eyes (the sclera) before there is obvious skin discolouration (**Figure 6.5**).

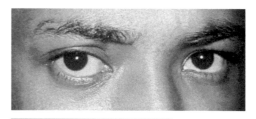

Figure 6.5 Jaundice of the sclera.

It is useful to classify jaundice into prehepatic, intrahepatic and posthepatic causes (**Table 6.16**):

- Prehepatic jaundice is due to excess production of bilirubin.
- Intrahepatic jaundice is due to impaired breakdown of bilirubin.
- Posthepatic jaundice is due to impaired excretion of bilirubin.

Table 6.15 *A full systems review for GI disease*

System	Symptoms	GI causes
Respiratory	Cough	Gastro-oesophageal reflux
	Breathlessness	Left-sided pleural effusion due to severe pancreatitis
		Restriction of the diaphragm due to ascites
Cardiovascular	Chest pain	Gastro-oesophageal reflux
		Oesophageal spasm
	Hypercholesterolaemia	Liver disease
Neurology	Weakness	Anaemia
Endocrine	Diabetes	Severe pancreatic disease

Table 6.16 *The causes of jaundice are divided in prehepatic, intrahepatic, and posthepatic*

	Example	Pathology	Clinical clues
Prehepatic: Excessive haemolysis	Sickle cell disease	Haemolysis of structurally abnormal erythrocyte	Acute attacks of anaemia and jaundice precipitated by infection Patient of Afro-Caribbean descent
	Glucose 6-phosphate dehydrogenase deficiency	Haemolysis due to impaired erythrocyte metabolism	Dark urine
	Malaria	Parasitic destruction of erythrocytes	Recent foreign travel High fever
Hereditary	Gilbert's disease	Disorder of bilirubin metabolism	Mild jaundice during acute illnesses
Intrahepatic	Liver disease of any cause		
Posthepatic: Obstruction of common bile duct	Head of pancreas tumour	Extrinsic compression	Systemic features of malignancy
	Bile duct malignancy (cholangiocarcinoma)	Intrinsic obstruction	
	Acute inflammation	Acute cholecystitis Acute cholangitis	Fever Right upper abdominal pain
	Gallstones	Intrinsic obstruction	Biliary colic

Jaundice is one of many signs of chronic liver disease (**Figure 6.6**).

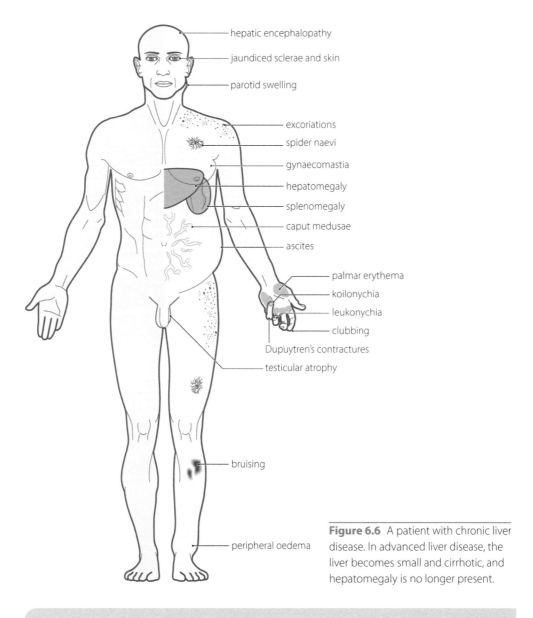

hepatic encephalopathy

jaundiced sclerae and skin

parotid swelling

excoriations

spider naevi

gynaecomastia

hepatomegaly

splenomegaly

caput medusae

ascites

palmar erythema

koilonychia

leukonychia

clubbing

Dupuytren's contractures

testicular atrophy

bruising

peripheral oedema

Figure 6.6 A patient with chronic liver disease. In advanced liver disease, the liver becomes small and cirrhotic, and hepatomegaly is no longer present.

New onset jaundice in the absence of abdominal pain ('painless jaundice') is characteristic of malignant obstruction of the bile duct. This is due to cancer of the bile duct (cholangiocarcinoma) or the head of the pancreas. Ask about other constitutional (non-specific and body-wide) symptoms of malignancy to further assess this, such as weight loss, anorexia and lack of energy.

New onset jaundice associated with right upper quadrant pain and fever is known as Charcot's triad. It is highly suggestive of biliary infection.

6.5.2 Hands and nails

Clubbing

The abdominal causes of nail clubbing are:
- cirrhosis
- IBD.

Palmar erythema

This is reddening of the palmar aspect of the hands (**Figure 6.7**), and indicates elevated circulating oestrogens (it is therefore also a normal sign in pregnancy, where it is also seen). Patients with cirrhosis are unable to break down circulating oestrogen.

Asterixis

Asterixis is a 'flapping' tremor of the hands, best seen with the patient's hands outstretched in front of them. It is often called a 'liver flap' because it is a manifestation of hepatic encephalopathy.

Leukonychia

This is white colouration of the nails, or white patches or flecks in the nails (**Figure 6.8**). It is often present in healthy individuals, but there is an association with cirrhosis and hypoalbuminaemia.

Koilonychia

Koilonychia are concave, 'spoon-shaped' nails. It is a sign of iron-deficiency anaemia.

Dupuytren's contracture

Dupuytren's contracture is a fibrotic thickening of the palmar fascia, leading to fixed flexion of the fingers. It is either idiopathic, or an association of liver dysfunction – particularly alcoholic liver disease.

> **There is a theory that Dupuytren's contracture is related to Viking ancestry** – although unproven, this is a common myth that patients often embrace. There is certainly a genetic susceptibility but other risk factors include alcohol excess or excessive finger flexion (e.g. rock climbers).

6.5.3 Hepatic encephalopathy

Impaired handling of protein metabolism in the diseased liver leads to impaired excretion of nitrogenous waste products from the gut, most notably ammonia. These compounds enter the circulation and cross the blood–brain barrier, where they interfere with the normal function of CNS neurotransmitters. These waste products cause confusion and altered mental states. Hepatic encephalopathy is graded according to severity:
- Grade 1: asterixis, poor concentration
- Grade 2: lethargy, personality change, disorientation
- Grade 3: obtunded
- Grade 4: coma

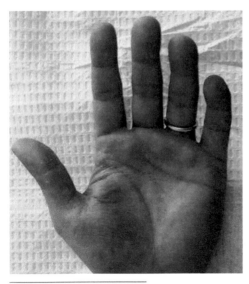

Figure 6.7 Palmar erythema.

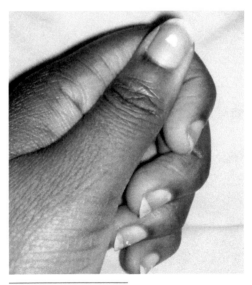

Figure 6.8 Leukonychia.

6.5.4 Skin

Pallor
Bleeding from the GI tract leads to iron-deficiency anaemia. Anaemia manifests as pale skin tone, pale gums and pale conjunctivae.

Jaundice
Elevated levels of circulating bilirubin cause yellow discolouration of the skin and sclerae (**Figure 6.5**).

Scars
Certain abdominal surgeries leave specific scars, making it possible to diagnosis the disorder from the shape of the scar (**Figure 6.9**). IBD – particularly Crohn's disease – often necessitates multiple bowel resections, so if there are numerous scars of indeterminate pattern IBD is a strong likelihood.

Caput medusae
Portal hypertension causes dilated superficial abdominal veins called caput medusae ('Medusa's head') which radiate out from the umbilicus.

Dermatitis herpetiformis
This is an intensely itchy skin eruption, associated with coeliac disease. It consists of small vesicles and erythema.

Excoriations
Liver disease causes generalised itching, probably due to bile salt accumulation. Severe itch ('pruritus') is implied by the presence of multiple skin excoriations (scratch marks) from constant scratching.

Bruising
Chronic liver failure causes a decline in clotting factor production, leading to bruising of the skin and increasing the risk of bleeding briskly from a minor injury. If the cause of liver failure is alcohol excess, the patient will also have low platelets (less than 150×10^9/L), as alcohol suppresses bone marrow manufacture of thrombocytes. Portal hypertension and splenomegaly cause destruction of circulating platelets.

Xanthelasma
These are yellowish-white cholesterol deposits around the eye (derived from the Greek *xanthe*, meaning yellow) due to hypercholesterolaemia. They are particularly associated with primary biliary cholangitis.

Erythema nodosum
This is a rash seen in association with IBD, classically presenting as palpable painful nodules on the shin.

Pyoderma gangrenosum
This is an ulcerated area of necrosis, usually on the lower limbs. It is associated with IBD.

Acanthosis nigricans
This is dark discolouration of the axillae, which is associated with insulin resistance, obesity and GI cancers.

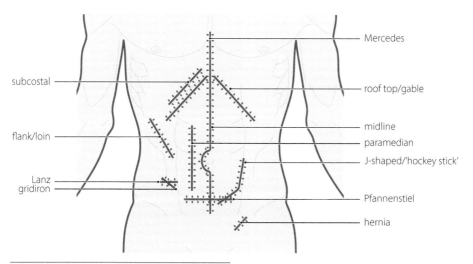

subcostal

flank/loin

Lanz
gridiron

Mercedes

roof top/gable

midline
paramedian
J-shaped/'hockey stick'

Pfannenstiel

hernia

Figure 6.9 Common abdominal surgical scars.

Telangectasia

These are very small dilated capillaries. They are associated with the following conditions:

- Hereditary haemorrhagic telangiectasia: a congenital disorder characterised by numerous telangiectasia on the skin and GI mucosal surfaces. It is a rare cause of GI bleeding.
- Scleroderma – an autoimmune disease affecting connective tissue. The mnemonic **CREST** identifies the key features: **C**alcinosis, **R**aynaud's syndrome, o**E**sophageal dysmotility, **S**clerodactyly, **T**elangiectasia. Scleroderma is a rare cause of dysphagia.

6.5.5 Eyes

Kayser–Fleischer rings are a gold, brown or green discolouration in the iris, as a result of abnormal copper deposition. They are due to Wilson's disease – a rare genetic abnormality of copper metabolism. Copper also accumulates in the liver, causing chronic liver disease and neurological impairment due to cerebral copper deposition.

6.5.6 Mouth

Ulcers

Aphthous ulcers are small painful breaks in the oral mucosa. They are common and self-limiting in most people. Recurrent ulcers are a sign of:

- Crohn's disease
- immunodeficiency
- herpes simplex infection
- Behçet's disease – an autoimmune condition causing oro-genital ulceration.

Parotid swelling

Enlargement of the parotid glands is particularly associated with alcohol-induced liver disease.

6.5.7 Chest

Gynaecomastia

Males with liver cirrhosis develop glandular breast tissue due to elevated oestrogens.

Spider naevi

These are dilated arterioles, usually visible on the chest (**Figure 6.10**), in the distribution of the superior vena cava. They blanch with gentle pressure, then quickly refill from the centre. They are caused by elevated oestrogen. Having fewer than five spider naevi is considered normal.

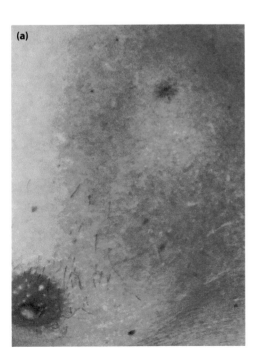

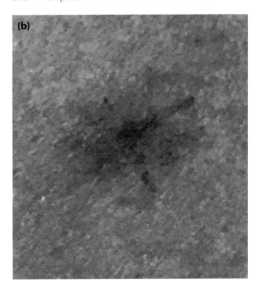

Figure 6.10 Spider naevus, a dilated network of capillaries.

6.5.8 Abdominal swelling

There are several causes of abdominal distension. They are remembered using the 6 Fs (**Table 6.17**).

Organomegaly

Hepatomegaly (enlarged liver) and splenomegaly (enlarged spleen) are detectable on palpation of the abdomen (see *Section 6.6.4*).

Hepatomegaly

Patients with chronic liver disease or cirrhosis have hepatomegaly in the early stages, before developing cirrhosis; a cirrhotic liver is not clinically palpable. Other causes of hepatomegaly include:
- chronic hepatic engorgement with blood due to severe right heart failure
- acute hepatic engorgement due to hepatic vein thrombosis (Budd–Chiari syndrome)
- hepatic tumours.

Splenomegaly

Splenomegaly is usually a consequence of:

- chronic liver disease, leading to portal hypertension and splenic engorgement
- sickle cell disease
- acute inflammation due to Epstein–Barr virus or cytomegalovirus infection
- haematological malignancies, especially chronic myeloid leukaemia and myelofibrosis
- malaria.

Kidney enlargement

Palpable kidneys indicate polycystic kidney disease, an inherited condition that causes massive cyst formation in the renal tissue and chronic renal failure, usually requiring transplantation.

Peripheral oedema

Hypoalbuminaemia in liver disease leads to reduced intravascular oncotic pressure, resulting in fluid moving into the interstitial space. As with cardiac failure, oedema collects in gravity-dependent areas, i.e. the lower limbs and sacrum.

6.6 The abdominal examination

The examination sequence is laid out in **Table 6.18**.

6.6.1 'ID CHECK'

This is detailed in *Section 3.2*.

The patient should be exposed adequately (ideally from nipples to knees, but often in reality from xiphisternum to suprapubic region), whilst trying to maintain patient modesty. The patient must lie flat on their back with one pillow, in order

Table 6.17 *The causes of abdominal distension – the 6 Fs*		
Cause of distension	**Reason**	**Mechanism**
Fluid	Accumulation of ascites	Portal hypertension raises the hydrostatic pressure in the GI circulation, resulting in fluid moving from the vessels into the peritoneal space
Fat	Obesity	Adipocyte hypertrophy and hyperplasia
Faeces	Severe constipation	Delayed or obstructed passage of faeces in large bowel
Flatus	Bowel obstruction	Obstruction of the distal bowel results in accumulation of bowel gas
Foetus	Pregnancy	Developing foetus
Fulminant tumours	Benign or malignant growths of abdominal organs	Insidious growth of ovarian, renal, bowel, hepatic or bladder

Element	Details
General inspection	Appearance: are they pale or jaundiced?
	Environment: are there clues suggesting disease?
	Skin: are there any dermatological signs of bowel or liver disease?
Hands	Are there any nail abnormalities?
	Are there peripheral signs of chronic liver disease?
Face	Is the conjunctiva pale?
	Is the sclera jaundiced?
	Is there any angular stomatitis or mouth ulcers?
	Is there parotid swelling?
Neck	Is there any lymphadenopathy?
Chest	Is there gynaecomastia?
	Are there any spider naevi?
Abdomen	Is there any pain?
	Are there any masses?
	Is there any organomegaly?
	Is there any abdominal distension? If so, is there shifting dullness?
	Are there active bowel sounds?
Legs	Is there any peripheral oedema?

Table 6.18 *The sequence of the abdominal examination*

to fully palpate the abdomen; this is in contrast to most other bedside examinations, where the patient will lie at 45°.

6.6.2 Endobedogram

In a hospital setting, look around the bedside for:

- stoma: this is an opening on the abdominal wall that allows body waste to pass from the bowel or urinary system into an adherent bag (a urostomy drains urine, a colostomy drains colonic contents and an ileostomy drains ileal contents)

- medications, including nutritional supplements and pancreatic enzymes
- any clue as to special nutritional requirements, e.g. a nasogastric or percutaneous feeding tube
- total parenteral nutrition (TPN), 'puréed diet' or 'nil by mouth' sign.

Does the patient appear pale or jaundiced? What is their approximate body habitus and general nutritional state? Are they withdrawing from alcohol or drugs? Are there obvious bruises, superficial abdominal veins or excoriation marks?

Ask the patient to take a deep breath in and out. Check for any scars (**Figure 6.9**), abdominal distension or hernias.

6.6.3 Inspection

Hands
Check hands and nails for the stigmata of chronic liver disease (**Figure 6.6**).

Skin
Examine the skin for any rashes.

Face and eyes
Gently check the lower eyelid for conjunctival pallor. Check for jaundice of the sclera.

Neck
Palpate for enlarged cervical lymph nodes, and check for a left supraclavicular node enlargement (Virchow's node), which is associated with stomach cancer.

Chest
Look for spider naevi and gynaecomastia.

Abdomen
Look for old scars or any abdominal distension. Examine for caput medusae.

Lower limbs
Look for any peripheral oedema.

6.6.4 Palpation

General palpation
Use light, gentle palpation in each of the nine areas of the abdomen (**Figure 6.4**), checking for any obvious masses or tenderness. Then, use deep firmer palpation in each area to check

for any masses or enlarged organs. Note the consistency of the abdomen – it should be soft and compressible. Patients with pain exhibit involuntary 'guarding' – contraction of the abdominal muscle over a tender or inflamed area.

> **Always watch the patient's face whilst palpating the abdomen.** Politeness or timidity mean that patients often don't tell you when you are hurting them, but they usually grimace if in pain.

If you suspect a gastric outlet obstruction or gastroparesis, place your hands on either side of the abdomen and gently shake it from side to side. If there is a splashing sound (a succussion splash), it indicates a distended, fluid-filled stomach.

Place your hands over both groins (midway between the hip and the pubis symphysis) and ask the patient to cough. If the patient has a hernia you will feel the area expand. Also, consider asking the patient to stand up, to see whether a reducible hernia becomes apparent.

Assess for organomegaly

It is rarely possible to identify organomegaly by inspection alone; therefore you palpate and percuss.

Liver

Palpation. Palpate the abdomen to feel for hepatomegaly. Start in the right iliac fossa (RIF). Ask the patient to take a deep breath in, and as they do, press firmly down and upwards with your fingers (**Figure 6.11**). In hepatomegaly, you will feel the liver edge pressing down to meet your fingers as the patient inhales. Gradually move up the abdomen towards the right costal margin, always pressing deeply during the in-breath.

Percussion. Start percussion in the RIF and move up to the right lower ribs, listening for the resonant abdominal percussion note changing to the dull hepatic percussion note, to ascertain the position of the lower liver border. A normal liver does not extend below the right costal margin.

> **Hyperexpansion of the lungs, e.g. due to COPD, displaces the liver downwards and gives a false impression of hepatomegaly.** If this is suspected, percuss above the liver over the right thorax to detect the upper edge, to verify whether the liver is indeed enlarged.

Spleen

Palpation. Palpate the abdomen, feeling for a splenic edge. Starting in the RIF, use the method of pressing firmly during deep inspiration, and work up towards the left costal margin to detect the downward displacement of an enlarged spleen.

Percussion. Start in the RIF once more (both hepatomegaly and splenomegaly enlarge in the direction of the RIF). Work diagonally upwards towards the left costal margin, listening for the dull percussion note over the spleen. A normal spleen does not extend below the left costal margin.

Kidneys

The kidneys are not normally palpable in the abdomen. Assess for renal masses and swelling by balloting the kidney between both hands. Push upwards with your right hand on the posterior aspect of the abdomen and feel for an enlarged kidney pressing against your anterior left hand (**Figure 6.12**).

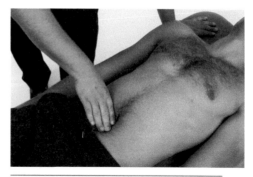

Figure 6.11 As the patient breathes in, press firmly into the abdomen, feeling for the inferior border of an enlarged liver pushing against your fingers.

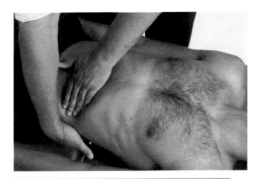

Figure 6.12 Balloting the kidney. As you push upwards with your right hand, press down firmly on the abdomen with your left, to feel the kidney push up towards you.

Check the iliac fossae for transplanted kidneys. These are large, soft masses with an overlying scar.

Aorta

If you detected a pulsatile mass of an aortic aneurysm in the central abdomen, attempt to quantify its size by palpating the lateral edges.

Bladder

Assess for a palpable bladder in the suprapubic region. The bladder should not normally be palpable. If a bladder is detected, it implies urinary retention, and the patient will require a urinary catheter to drain the bladder.

Assess for ascites

If the abdomen is distended, decide whether the cause is ascites. In ascites, the percussion note over the umbilicus is resonant, but becomes stony dull as you gradually percuss laterally down to the flank. In this case, ask the patient to roll onto their left side (away from you). After 30 seconds, gravity pulls the fluid away from the flank to the centre of the abdomen, causing a resonant note in the flank and stony dull note in the umbilical region (**Figure 6.13**). This is termed 'shifting dullness'.

6.6.5 Auscultation

Place the diaphragm of the stethoscope on either side of the umbilicus for 10–20 seconds each. Bowel sounds occur at least every 10 seconds.

■ An absence of bowel sounds indicates paralysis of the digestive tract (paralytic ileus) which is a common complication following abdominal surgery, or in intra-abdominal inflammation, such as acute pancreatitis or peritonitis

■ High-pitched 'tinkling' bowel sounds indicate that the bowel is trying to overcome a total or sub-total obstructive lesion.

Renal arterial bruits are due to stenosis of the renal arteries (see *Section 4.6.5*). Renal artery stenosis is a rare cause of chronic renal failure. Patients with severe peripheral arterial disease have bruits over the femoral arteries.

6.6.6 Finishing off

A digital rectal examination (DRE) is a crucial part of the abdominal examination in cases of PR bleeding and altered bowel habit. The presence of melaena or fresh red blood on DRE confirms the diagnosis of an upper or lower GI bleed. DRE also detects large rectal tumours, prostatic enlargement and external haemorrhoids.

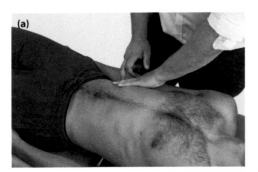
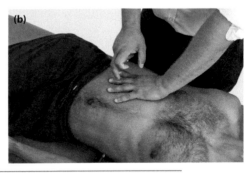

Figure 6.13 If you (a) elicit a stony dull percussion note in the flank, (b) roll the patient away from you and see whether it has moved to the umbilical area, indicating shifting ascitic fluid.

6.7 Further investigations

GI investigations (**Table 6.19**) are either:
- imaging modalities
- endoscopic
- functional studies.

6.7.1 Imaging

Ultrasound

Ultrasound (US) is used to assess the soft tissue organs of the abdomen and detects peritoneal fluid collections, including ascites and inflammatory collections. The pancreas is poorly imaged due to overlying bowel.

X-ray

Plain abdominal X-rays detect constipation and retained foreign bodies, or flatus within the peritoneal cavity due to intestinal perforation.

Radiopaque contrast (usually barium) reveals any narrowing of the GI tract. A 'barium swallow X-ray' reveals oesophageal narrowing, whereas a 'barium enema X-ray' delineates the distal bowel lumen.

Computed tomography

CT scanning is used to diagnose acute abdominal disorders, such as masses, perforation and abscesses. CT angiogram detects the bleeding point in abdominal haemorrhage.

6.7.2 Endoscopy

Endoscopy is the use of flexible fibreoptic scopes to directly image the GI tract. The endoscopist takes biopsies of any abnormal findings, and gives haemostatic treatments to bleeding ulcers and varices.

Table 6.19 *Choosing investigations in GI medicine*

Investigation	Indication	Benefits	Limitations
Abdominal X-ray	To assess for free air in the peritoneal cavity	Quick, easy to do	Does not show soft tissue organs Small dose of ionising radiation
US	To assess the soft tissue organs of the abdomen	Excellent modality for detecting soft tissue abnormalities	Does not visualise pancreas Limited usefulness in obese patients
CT scan	Detailed imaging of abdominal contents	Cross-sectional imaging of abdomen, providing detailed and accurate information Detects bowel perforation Quantifies ascites	Requires ionising radiation Requires administration of IV contrast (contraindicated in renal failure) Inferior to US in examining soft tissue masses
Endoscopy	To visualise the GI tract To administer treatment to bleeding GI tract lesions	Direct visual inspection of GI tract diseases Obtains biopsies and administers treatments without the need for open abdominal surgery	Invasive Requires sedation of the patient Poorly tolerated in patients with significant co-morbidities
Functional studies	To assess movement and function	Provides information on the GI system 'in action' Identifies obstructing lesions or motility problems	Ionising radiation involved

In upper endoscopy (oesophago-gastroduodenoscopy; OGD), the endoscope is inserted via the mouth. In lower endoscopy (colonoscopy or sigmoidoscopy), the endoscope is inserted via the anus.

Capsule endoscopy, where the patient swallows a small camera the size of a pill, allows visualisation of the small bowel.

6.7.3 Functional studies

Nuclear medicine scans assess the functional movement of the GI tract. A gastric emptying study helps diagnose gastroparesis.

6.8 Answers to starter questions

1. Diseases of malnutrition such as scurvy and rickets are now considered to be historical. However, increased movement of people from developing to developed countries has brought nutritional diseases back into focus. Additionally, the prevalence of alcohol and drug abuse in the UK plays a role. Habitual alcohol and drug users often have poor self-care and nutritional states. Thiamine (vitamin B1) deficiency is common in chronic alcoholism.

   Patients who have significant bowel resection develop malabsorption disorders, due to a functionally short bowel. Chronic malabsorption is also a recognised side-effect of bariatric surgery due to obesity.

2. General fatigue is the commonest symptom of iron-deficiency anaemia. The commonest cause of iron deficiency in men and post-menopausal women is GI malignancy. Chronic bleeding into the GI tract often goes unnoticed by patients, and is often the presenting feature of GI malignancy. Whilst many GI malignancies are surgically resected with an internal anastomosis, some require the formation of a stoma.

3. Although alcohol is a major cause of liver disease in the western world, there are many other causes. Patients with non-alcohol-related liver disease often worry that they will be assumed to be 'heavy drinkers', which is perceived as carrying a social stigma, so be mindful of other aetiologies. The commonest cause of liver disease worldwide is NAFLD, which is fatty infiltration of liver tissue, and the incidence is rising along with obesity levels. The most severe form is non-alcoholic steatohepatitis (NASH), which eventually leads to fibrosis and scarring of the liver (cirrhosis).

4. It is a good idea to have a chaperone present when performing all clinical examinations, as they often require various states of undress for the patient. A chaperone reassures the patient, and protects the doctor from any spurious allegations. The abdominal examination is perceived as more intimate than others, and a chaperone is imperative when examining the genitalia and performing a DRE.

5. There is no universally accepted definition of diarrhoea. Many authorities state that it is more than 300g of loose stool per day, although this is challenging to quantify. To some, it is a matter of stool consistency: the stools are soft or liquid. To others, it pertains to volume or frequency: the patient is opening their bowels more than three times per day. Some perceive it as abnormal stool colour. When a patient reports diarrhoea, their meaning needs to be defined. Mostly, they are telling you that something has changed in comparison to their normal bowel habit.

Chapter 7
Genitourinary system

Starter questions

1. Why do some patients with end-stage renal disease not receive haemodialysis?
2. Why do patients with end-stage renal disease need to be careful when ordering at a restaurant?
3. Why is HIV treated outside of the genitourinary medicine clinic?
4. How does genital syphilis infection cause heart failure?

Answers to questions are to be found in *Section 7.9*.

7.1 Introduction

The genitourinary system comprises five separate organs and the tubes that join them. It is responsible for the maintenance of blood electrolyte and pH balance, the filtering of waste products from blood and the production of urine, the production and ejaculation of semen, and the production of hormones leading to sexual maturation.

Diseases of the genitourinary system carry a high burden of stigma and patients often put off presenting due to this. A good knowledge base of the system and a frank and open approach to these disorders is key to providing treatment and relief to patients.

Whilst the urinary system is almost identical between the sexes, the genitals are vastly different. This chapter will focus on the male reproductive system, with the female system being discussed in *Chapter 8*.

Case 7.1 Dysuria

Presentation

Mr Jones is 77 years old. He presents to the Emergency Department feeling unwell, with burning pain on passing urine.

Initial interpretation

Dysuria (the sensation of pain when passing urine) indicates urethral irritation which could be related to stones or infection.

He is of an age where an enlarged prostate causing micturition difficulty is relatively common, but we need more information.

History

Mr Jones reports feeling unwell for the last week with lethargy and intermittent fevers. He has had burning pain on urinating for three days and has noticed his urine has become darker and has sometimes had some blood in it. He reports he has aching in the left side of his back.

Interpretation of history

He is constitutionally unwell with lethargy, dark urine and fevers. This indicates sepsis – an overwhelming infection and medical emergency.

A large stone may be impacted within a ureter, causing urine to back up behind it. This results in hydronephrosis (a blockage of urine flow from the kidney causing dilation) which would account for his back pain. This stagnant urine becomes easily infected. Serious infections damage and scar the renal tract epithelium, causing bleeding.

Further history

Mr Jones has never had a urine infection or difficulty urinating. He has no other medical history and takes no regular medication.

Examination

On examination, he is unwell. His heart rate is 110bpm, blood pressure is 98/64mmHg and temperature is 38.2°C. His hands are cool and his pulse thready. His abdomen is soft but tender in the left flank. There are no palpable masses and bowel sounds are normal. External genital examination and digital rectal examination are normal.

Interpretation of findings

Mr Jones has sepsis and requires urgent resuscitation with fluids and antibiotics. Coupled with his left flank tenderness, it raises the concern of infection within the kidney (pyelonephritis).

Investigations

Serum blood tests reveal white blood cells of 17.2×10^9/L with a neutrophilia and a C-reactive protein of 219mg/L. His urea and creatinine are both raised, at 14.2mmol/L and 151µmol/L, respectively. Haemoglobin, sodium and potassium are within normal limits. When catheterised, he has a residual volume of 20ml turbid urine. The urine dipstick shows protein 3+ and blood 3+ (indicating either glomerular or epithelial damage), and leukocytes 4+ and nitrites positive (reflecting infection). A bedside ultrasound shows a dilated left ureter of 7mm with hydronephrosis.

Diagnosis

Mr Jones has an acute kidney injury and sepsis due to pyelonephritis and a left-sided ureteric obstruction. He requires intravenous fluids and antibiotics and a non-contrast CT of his renal tract to characterise this obstruction and guide further intervention.

7.2 System overview

The genitourinary system encompasses the kidneys, bladder, prostate, penis, testes and tubes that connect them (**Figure 7.1**).

7.2.1 Kidneys

The kidney comprises an outer cortex and inner medulla (**Figure 7.2**). Nephrons are the functional unit of the kidney. They span both regions and drain into a central collecting duct. Ducts empty into larger chambers called calyces which converge at the renal pelvis.

Blood from renal arteries perfuses the glomeruli which comprise a network of single cell-walled tubes that filter water, electrolytes, proteins and waste products into the nephron.

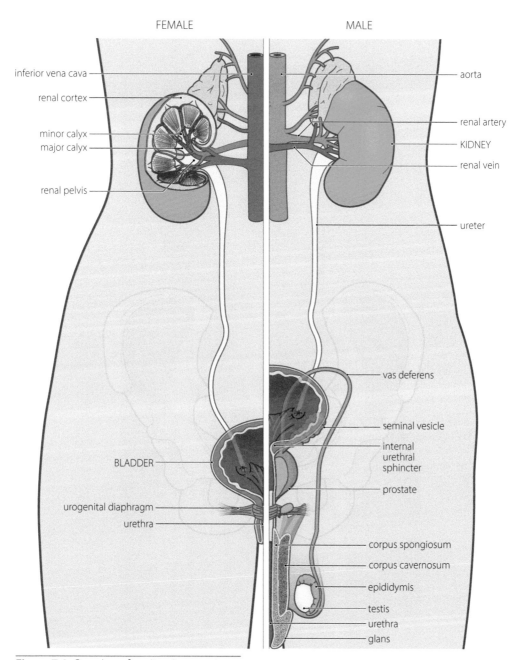

FEMALE

MALE

inferior vena cava

aorta

renal cortex

minor calyx

major calyx

renal artery

KIDNEY

renal vein

renal pelvis

ureter

vas deferens

seminal vesicle

internal urethral sphincter

BLADDER

prostate

urogenital diaphragm

urethra

corpus spongiosum

corpus cavernosum

epididymis

testis

urethra

glans

Figure 7.1 Overview of genitourinary anatomy.

As this solution passes through the nephron, the kidneys:

■ reabsorb water
■ reabsorb nutrients (albumin, glucose)
■ maintain acid–base balance (adapting ion reabsorption)

■ regulate electrolyte balance.

The kidneys also produce hormones such as erythropoietin (stimulates erythrocyte production), calcitriol (activated vitamin D involved in calcium homeostasis) and renin (involved in blood pressure control).

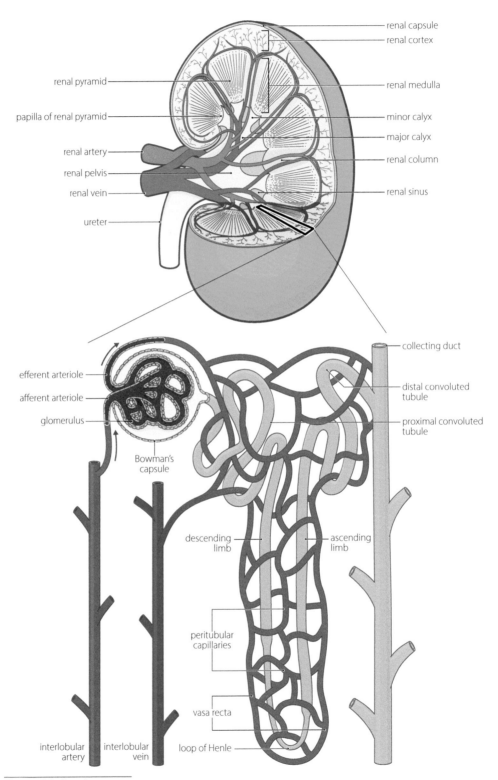

Figure 7.2 Renal anatomy.

A deterioration in kidney function is either acute (acute kidney injury; AKI) or chronic (chronic kidney disease; CKD). AKI is reversible if recognised and treated early. There are three types:

- Prerenal: reduced circulating volume impairing renal perfusion (e.g. dehydration, medications, sepsis, renal artery disease)
- Renal: primary nephron disorders (e.g. nephrotoxic medications, acute glomerulonephritis)
- Postrenal: disrupted urinary drainage causing back-pressure (e.g. obstructing ureteric stones, extrinsic ureteric compression, urinary retention).

The glomerulonephritides are a group of disorders causing damage to the glomerulus (**Table 7.1**). They present in two ways:

- Nephrotic syndrome: glomerular wall changes, allowing larger molecules to enter the nephron. This causes massive proteinuria, hypoalbuminaemia and oedema.
- Nephritic syndrome: inflammation, proliferation and damage to glomeruli cause haematuria, oliguria, proteinuria and hypertension. Hypertension is in response to the increased vascular resistance of damaged vessels.

CKD is an irreversible decline in renal function. It progresses if the cause remains untreated. The commonest causes are:

- poorly controlled diabetes mellitus
- poorly controlled hypertension
- polycystic kidney disease (autosomal dominant disorder causing multiple renal cysts)
- glomerulonephritides.

Impaired renal function causes:

- uraemia – toxic accumulation of urea causing encephalitis and pericarditis

Table 7.1 *Overview of the glomerulonephritides*

	Type	Cause	Prognosis	Associations
NEPHROTIC	Minimal change disease	Unclear	Good	Usually affects children
	Focal segmental glomerulosclerosis	Unclear	Poor	HIV infection. Heroin abuse
	Membranous nephropathy	Immune complex deposition	Good	
	Membranoproliferative glomerulonephritis	Thickened glomerular basement membrane	Poor	Hepatitis C virus infection. Cryoglobulinaemia
NEPHRITIC	Post-streptococcal glomerulonephritis	Antigen-antibody deposition	Good (in children)	Post-group A *Streptococcus* infection
	IgA nephropathy	Increased IgA following upper respiratory tract infection	Good	Post-upper respiratory tract infection
	Hereditary nephritis	Basement membrane protein mutations	Poor	Mostly X-linked mutations (e.g. Alport's syndrome)
	Rapidly progressive glomerulonephritis	Immune mediated or vasculitic-related	Poor	Linked to vasculitides

- fluid overload due to poor excess water excretion and nephrotic syndrome
- acidaemia
- hyperkalaemia
- reduced hormone production causing anaemia, hypocalcaemia and hypertension.

Symptoms of kidney disease worsen as renal function declines, leading to total failure (end-stage renal disease; ESRD). The only treatment for ESRD is renal replacement therapy (**Table 7.2**).

7.2.2 Ureters

The ureters are 3–4mm diameter tubes containing smooth muscle, that transport urine from the renal pelvis to the bladder.

7.2.3 Bladder

The bladder receives urine from the ureters and stores it until urination. The wall contains a smooth muscle layer called the detrusor muscle. This contracts downwards, collapsing the bladder and expelling urine. Two sphincters at the bladder outlet, one under autonomic and one voluntary control, open in coordination with detrusor contraction to allow voiding.

7.2.4 Urethra

The urethra originates at the bladder outlet and carries urine to the urethral meatus. In men, the urethra also carries semen during ejaculation.

7.2.5 Prostate

The prostate is a muscular exocrine gland that surrounds the urethra at the bladder outlet in males. It produces alkaline fluid which is mixed with spermatozoa from the vas deferens and semen from the seminal vesicles. This is passed into the urethra via the ejaculatory duct during ejaculation (**Figure 7.3**). The smooth muscle within the prostate ensures that ejaculate is expelled away from the body and does not mix with urine.

Table 7.2 *Methods of renal replacement therapy*

	Indications	Method	Limitations
Haemodialysis	Renal failure with: - fluid overload - hyperkalaemia - hypercalcaemia - metabolic acidosis - pericarditis - uraemia	Blood removed via arteriovenous fistula, filtered through dialysis machine and reinfused	Not suitable for haemodynamically unstable patients Requires fistula formation prior to initiation
Peritoneal dialysis	As above in those who prefer self-therapy or do not have vascular access	Infusion and removal of dialysate into peritoneal cavity	High infection risk Unsuitable with many bowel conditions (inflammatory bowel disease, diverticulosis)
Haemofiltration	As for haemodialysis	Blood removed via venous line, filtered through dialysis machine and reinfused	Not suitable for haemodynamically unstable patients (to a lesser extent than haemodialysis)
Renal transplant	As for haemodialysis in patients with a matched organ	Surgical implantation and medical immunosuppression	Patient needs to be fit for surgery Needs allogenic-matched organ Long waiting list

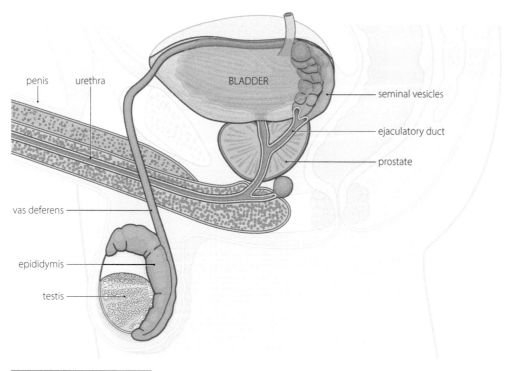

Figure 7.3 Prostate anatomy.

7.2.6 Penis

The penis contains two sponge-like corpora cavernosa which fill with blood during sexual arousal to give an erection. The central corpus spongiosum carries the urethra. At the tip, the glans penis transmits the urethra to the urethral meatus.

7.2.7 Scrotum and testes

The scrotum contains the testes – exocrine and endocrine glands producing:

- germ cells (spermatozoa) produced in Sertoli cells
- testosterone and other androgens produced in Leydig cells.

Spermatozoa are transported to and stored in the epididymes then travel through the vas deferens to the prostate.

The wall of the scrotum contains the cremaster muscle which relaxes and contracts to help regulate scrotal temperature.

7.3 Symptoms of genitourinary disease

History and examination assess for the features of the main genitourinary diseases (**Table 7.3**) and their impact on quality of life. These are often embarrassing to talk about and some patients may not openly discuss them.

7.3.1 Abdominal pain

Causes outside the urinary system are explored in *Section 6.3.2*.

Renal capsule stretch

Each kidney is surrounded by a highly innervated capsule, causing pain when the kidney is enlarged. This is exacerbated by movement and patients prefer to lie still. Causes include:

- infection (e.g. pyelonephritis)
- bleeding (e.g. traumatic or ruptured cyst)
- masses (e.g. tumours or large / multiple cysts).

Table 7.3 *The main features of genitourinary disease*

Disease	Symptoms	Signs
ESRD	Lethargy Itch Breathlessness Weight gain	Leukonychia Oligouria / anuria Oedema and ascites
Upper UTI	Fevers +/− rigors Abdominal pain (typically dull ache)	Febrile Features of sepsis if severe Tenderness in affected renal angle Pyuria
Lower UTI	Dysuria Haematuria	Febrile Features of sepsis if severe Pyuria Urethral discharge
Renal colic	Abdominal pain (typically sharp, radiating from loin to groin)	Haematuria Features of upper UTI if infection present
Urinary retention	Inability to pass urine Lower abdominal pain	Anuria Palpable bladder Possible prostatic enlargement
Prostatic enlargement	Progressive micturition difficulty Possible haematuria	Prostatic enlargement
Epididymo-orchitis	Fevers Dysuria Testicular pain Testicular swelling	Febrile Swollen, warm, tender testicle Haematospermia +/− urethral discharge

Ureteric colic

This is typically an intermittent, sharp pain that radiates from "loin (posterior area between ribs and pelvis) to groin" caused by a calculus within the ureter. Patients find it difficult to find a comfortable position.

Urinary retention

This is an inability to pass urine associated with progressively worsening suprapubic pain. Causes are explored below.

7.3.2 Difficulty and discomfort passing urine

Lower urinary tract symptoms (LUTS) is an umbrella term related to micturition difficulty.

They are split into two groups (**Table 7.4**) but have a variety of causes.

Obstructive

Obstruction of the bladder outlet or urethra impedes urine flow. Causes include:

- prostatic enlargement (either benign or malignant)
- urethral stricture (a narrowing of the urethra caused by scar tissue, usually from an injury or infection)
- urethral stone.

Detrusor atony

Chronic retention causes the detrusor muscle to overstretch and lose its ability to contract efficiently during voiding.

Table 7.4 *LUTS symptoms*	
LUTS group	**Symptoms**
Filling and irritative symptoms	Urinary frequency
	Urinary urgency
	Painful urination
	Nocturia
Voiding and obstructive symptoms	Poor stream
	Hesitancy
	Terminal dribbling
	Incomplete voiding
	Overflow incontinence
	Retention

Table 7.5 *Pharmacological causes of urinary retention*	
Class	**Examples**
Alpha-receptor agonists	Ephedrine
	Pseudoephedrine
Anticholinergics	Atropine
	Glycopyrrolate
	Oxybutynin
Antidepressants	Amitriptyline
	Imipramine
	Nortriptyline
Antihistamines	Chlorpheniramine
	Hydroxyzine
Antihypertensives	Hydralazine
	Nifedipine
Antiparkinsonian medication	Amantadine
	Bromocriptine
	Levodopa
Antipsychotics	Chlorpromazine
	Haloperidol
	Prochlorperazine
Beta-receptor agonists	Terbutaline
Hormonal treatments	Oestrogen
	Progesterone
	Testosterone
Muscle relaxants	Baclofen
	Diazepam
Other	Carbamazepine
	Dopamine
	NSAIDs
	Opioid analgesics

Neurological

Impaired bladder innervation disrupts the sensation of bladder fullness and the stimulation of bladder contraction. Damage to the nervous supply can occur at:

- peripheral nerves (e.g. nerve trauma typically during abdominal surgery or poorly controlled diabetes mellitus)
- spinal cord (e.g. cord compression, cauda equina).

Infection

Inflammation and pus from urinary tract infections (UTIs) cause LUTS.

Pharmacological

See **Table 7.5** for pharmacological causes of urinary retention.

7.3.3 Urinary incontinence

Urinary incontinence is the involuntary leaking of urine, which can be highly embarrassing. There are four main types:

Urge incontinence

Detrusor muscle overstimulation and activity causes sudden and frequent voiding. Patients with urge incontinence tend to get little warning that they are about to pass urine and are unable to reach the bathroom in time.

Stress incontinence

Weakness of the sphincters controlling the bladder outlet allows urine to leak from the bladder. The commonest cause for this is damage after pregnancy and childbirth. Patients with stress incontinence tend to accidentally pass urine during manoeuvres where the intra-abdominal pressure is raised (e.g. heavy lifting, sneezing, laughing).

Overflow incontinence

When the bladder is over-full, such as with chronic urinary retention, the detrusor muscle contracts involuntarily, causing the patient to urinate. Patients with overflow incontinence tend to have accompanying LUTS.

Functional incontinence

Functional incontinence is not a disorder of the urinary tract but a reflection of an inability to reach the bathroom in time (such as for patients with poor mobility).

7.3.4 Haematuria

Blood in the urine is always abnormal and should be thoroughly investigated for sinister causes. It is either macroscopic (visible) or microscopic (detected on urinalysis).

Renal

Damage to the glomerulus allows blood to leak into the renal tract, causing a microscopic haematuria. Causes include the glomerulonephritides (**Table 7.1**) or trauma.

Ureteric

Stones damaging the ureteric epithelium cause both macroscopic and microscopic haematuria.

Infection

Severe infections invade and damage the urinary tract epithelium, leading to microscopic or macroscopic haematuria.

Malignancy

Malignancy in any part of the renal tract often presents with haematuria and is accompanied by other constitutional symptoms such as fatigue, weight loss and loss of appetite.

7.3.5 Erectile dysfunction

Cardiovascular

Damage to blood vessels by atherosclerosis, poorly controlled hypertension and diabetes mellitus impedes blood flow to the penis.

Neurological

The nerve supply to the penis may be interrupted by:
- poorly controlled diabetes mellitus
- multiple sclerosis
- nerve damage (e.g. during pelvic surgery).

Pharmacological

See **Table 7.6** for pharmacological causes of erectile dysfunction.

Psychological

Depression and anxiety cause psychogenic impotence. This may be associated with a decreased libido.

Table 7.6 *Pharmacological causes of erectile dysfunction*	
Class	**Examples**
Antihypertensives	Enalapril
	Hydralazine
	Nifedipine
	Verapamil
	Atenolol
	Bisoprolol
Antidepressants	Amitriptyline
	Fluoxetine
	Sertraline
Antihistamines	Hydroxyzine
Antiparkinsonian medication	Bromocriptine
	Levodopa
Diuretics	Bendroflumethiazide
	Furosemide
	Spironolactone
Muscle relaxants	Diazepam
	Chlordiazepoxide
Other	Carbamazepine
	Dopamine
	Histamine H_2-receptor antagonists
	NSAIDs
	Opioid analgesics

7.3.6 Urethral discharge

Both structural and infective disorders cause urethral discharge. Note that not all are sexually transmitted (**Table 7.7**).

7.3.7 Testicular pain or swelling

Testicular pain and swelling are common and distressing (**Table 7.8**).

7.3.8 Generalised swelling

There are two main causes for generalised swelling in renal disease:
- nephrotic syndrome
- inability to excrete excess water in ESRD, leading to fluid overload.

7.4 The genitourinary history

7.4.1 Past medical history

For patients with established genitourinary disease, explore previous interventions including:
- methods of or plans for future renal replacement therapies (including any associated adverse events)
- previous instrumentation (urinary catheterisation, urethral dilatation)
- surgical interventions (e.g. renal transplants, ureteric stenting, prostatic surgery).

Renal disease is caused by and then greatly affected by many systemic diseases. Always ask about:

Table 7.7 *Causes of urethral discharge*

Cause	Sexual transmission	Treatment
Neisseria gonorrhoeae	Yes	Cephalosporin Azithromycin
Chlamydia trachomatis	Yes	Doxycycline Azithromycin
Treponema pallidum (syphilis)	Yes	Benzyl-penicillin Doxycycline
Trichomonas vaginalis	Yes	Metronidazole Tinidazole
Escherichia coli	No	Penicillin-based antibiotics (co-amoxiclav)
Herpes simplex virus	Yes	Aciclovir, famciclovir or valaciclovir
Prostatitis	Both	Sexually transmitted: cephalosporin + doxycycline Non-sexually transmitted: ciprofloxacin
Epididymo-orchitis	Both	Sexually transmitted: cephalosporin + doxycycline Non-sexually transmitted: ciprofloxacin
Urethral stricture	No	Correction of stricture
Renal calculi	No	Passage or removal of stone

Table 7.8 *Causes of testicular pain and swelling*

Cause	Pathology	Painful	Swelling	Notes
Epididymo-orchitis	Infection within testis or epididymis	Very	Mild	Usually due to an STI
Testicular torsion	Occlusion of blood flow to testis caused by twisting of vasculature	Extremely	None	Surgical emergency
Hydrocele	Excessive production or impaired absorption of fluid within a remnant piece of peritoneum wrapped around a testis	Mild	Yes	Transilluminates brilliantly
Varicocele	Abnormal enlargement of veins draining a testis	Mild	Yes	Feels like a bag of worms
Malignancy	Primary tumour of testicular cells	Depends on size	Depends on size	
Inguinal hernia	Protrusion of abdominal contents through inguinal canal and into the scrotum	If hernia becomes strangulated	Yes	
Scrotal oedema	Collection of fluid within scrotum, usually from ascites draining through the inguinal canal	Yes	Yes	

- diabetes mellitus: this is the leading cause of ESRD worldwide; many oral antidiabetic medications are contraindicated with poor renal function thus complicating management.
- hypertension: ESRD is complicated by fluid overload causing increased blood pressure; many antihypertensives and diuretics worsen renal function or are less effective in ESRD
- ischaemic heart disease: CKD is an independent risk factor for developing ischaemic heart disease; additionally, these patients have worse outcomes following cardiac events.

Recurrent UTIs are often related to structural abnormalities so ask about previous infections or surgeries, especially during childhood.

Ask about previous abdominal surgery including previous caesarian section which may contribute to neurological and structural damage or the presence of adhesions.

In men with testicular problems, ask about whether they had undescended testes as a newborn, as this is a risk factor for developing testicular cancer.

7.4.2 Medications

A vast range of medications are nephrotoxic (**Table 7.9**). Water-soluble drugs are excreted via the kidneys so their doses often need changing in periods of renal dysfunction. With recurrent infections, ask about previous antibiotic usage including route of administration and duration.

7.4.3 Social history

This focuses on establishing the presence of modifiable risk factors and how the patient's health is impacting on their life.

Sexual history

A detailed sexual history is imperative for the

Table 7.9 *Common nephrotoxic drugs*

Nephrotoxic effect	Class	Example
Interstitial nephritis	NSAIDs	Ibuprofen, indomethacin, naproxen
	Antibiotics	Aminoglycosides, rifampicin, tetracyclines
Acute tubular necrosis	Antipsychotics	Lithium
	IV contrast media	
	Antibiotics	Aminoglycosides
Precipitating renal artery stenosis	ACE inhibitors	Ramipril, verapamil
Glomerular damage	NSAIDs	Ibuprofen, indomethacin, naproxen
	Disease-modifying antirheumatic drugs (DMARDs)	Gold, penicillamine, methotrexate

genitourinary system. Particular detail should be paid to the type of encounter (insertive or receptive), the orifice (vagina, mouth or anus) and whether protection was used. Always ask about high risk sexual encounters where blood-to-blood transmission is more likely (chemsex, BDSM). Consider also the impact of any condition on a patient's ability to pursue and enjoy sexual intercourse.

Smoking

Tobacco smoking is an important risk factor for the development of cancer and renovascular disease. Smoking is attributable to 40% of erectile dysfunction, due to a combination of vascular disease and the vasoconstricting effect of nicotine.

Alcohol

High alcohol intake is a risk factor for renovascular disease in the same way as in cardiovascular disease (both as a CNS depressant in binges and as a risk factor for peripheral neuropathy in chronic use).

Illicit drugs

Intravenous drug injection is a risk factor for developing HIV which, if untreated, lowers immunity and increases the risk of acquired infections.

Employment

Patients with urinary incontinence or chronic urinary retention requiring intermittent self-catheterisation (where the patient inserts a urethral catheter to allow bladder emptying, then removes it) may struggle if working in busy jobs that do not allow for regular comfort breaks.

Physical activity

Enquire whether the patient is active in their daily life, and whether they take any exercise. The vascular supply to the kidneys is prone to the same problems that affect the heart's coronary arteries. A sedentary lifestyle greatly affects cardiovascular and hence renal health.

Social circumstances

Psychological stresses of any type can manifest with problems such as erectile dysfunction. Urine management systems (such as catheters) impact on patients' confidence and self-image as well as their sexuality. STIs carry stigma and negatively impact intimacy.

Functional capacity

Establish functional capacity and how this might affect the management of genitourinary disease:

■ Patients with poor mobility and incontinence sometimes require long-term catheterisation for comfort and to prevent skin damage.
■ Aggressive treatment plans (e.g. haemodialysis for ESRD or chemotherapy for renal cell carcinoma) are often not appropriate for patients with a poor physical baseline.

7.4.4 Family history

Ask about:
■ diabetes
■ cardiovascular disease
■ polycystic kidney disease.

7.4.5 Systems review

Ensure to ask about other symptoms patients have, as they might be associated with genitourinary disease (**Table 7.10**).

Table 7.10 *Genitourinary manifestations of systemic diseases*	
Disease	**Manifestation**
Cryoglobulinaemia	Membranoproliferative glomerulonephritis
Diabetes mellitus	Nephrotic syndrome
	Nephropathy
	Polyuria
	Erectile dysfunction
	Recurrent UTI
Dupuytren's contracture	Peyronie's disease (fibrous tissue in penis causing curved, painful erection)
Haemolytic uraemic syndrome	Renal microangiopathy
Hypertension	Nephropathy
	Nephrosclerosis
Immunosuppressive states	Recurrent infection
	Glomerulonephritis (HIV)
Multiple myeloma	Light chain deposition
	Amyloidosis
	Cast nephropathy
Progressive systemic sclerosis	Renal microangiopathy
Sickle cell disease	Polyuria
	Nocturia
	Priapism (painful erection)
Sjögren's syndrome	Renal tubular dysfunction
SLE	Nephrotic syndrome
Vasculitides	Glomerulonephritis

7.5 Signs of genitourinary disease

7.5.1 Hand and nail changes

Capillary refill time
This is prolonged in severe infections and kidney failure.

Leukonychia
White discolouration of the nails is a sign of hypoalbuminaemia, a cause of which is protein loss in kidney failure (**Figure 6.8**).

7.5.2 Pulse

A 'bounding', high volume pulse is felt in fluid overloaded states. A weak and thready pulse is associated with low volume states such as dehydration or overwhelming infection.

7.5.3 Blood pressure

A low BP represents shock caused by a severe dehydration and sepsis. High BP is a key cause of renal disease and also a manifestation of existing renal disease, reflecting fluid overload.

7.5.4 Eyes

Conjunctival pallor
A pale appearance of the conjunctiva associated with renal disease is caused by anaemia secondary to reduced erythropoietin production.

Periorbital swelling
Oedema of the skin and soft tissues around the eyes is seen in nephrotic syndrome (a sequela of some forms of renal disease typified by a triad of proteinuria, hypoalbuminaemia and oedema).

7.5.5 Raised jugular venous pressure

A raised jugular venous pressure is a sign of fluid overload in ESRD.

7.5.6 Evidence of renal replacement therapy

There are several different forms of renal replacement therapy (**Figure 7.4**). Lines and scars give clues as to what forms have been attempted.

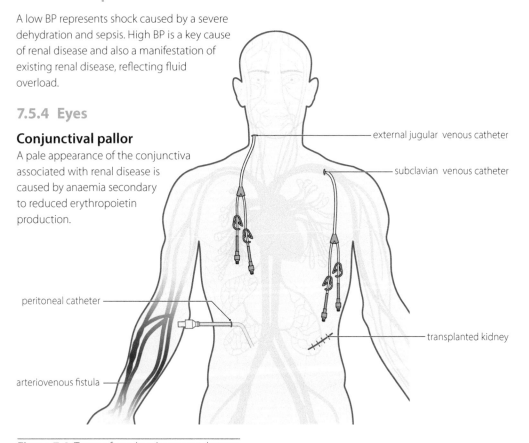

external jugular venous catheter

subclavian venous catheter

peritoneal catheter

transplanted kidney

arteriovenous fistula

Figure 7.4 Types of renal replacement therapy.

7.5.7 Abdominal masses

Kidneys

Enlarged kidneys are due to:

■ polycystic kidney disease – the kidneys will be irregular in shape; this is usually, but not always, bilateral
■ renal cell carcinoma
■ renal metastases (these are rare).

Transplanted kidneys are usually sited in the iliac fossae. Note that native kidneys are not always removed.

Bladder

An enlarged bladder is due to:

■ urinary retention
■ bladder tumours.

Uterine fibroids

These are discussed in *Chapter 8*.

7.5.8 Ascites

This is due to fluid overload, hypoalbuminaemia, or secondary to peritoneal dialysis. Other causes of ascites are discussed in *Chapter 6*.

7.5.9 Urethral discharge

See **Table 7.7**.

7.5.10 Genital skin lesions

Ulcers

There are many causes for genital ulceration which have different appearances (**Table 7.11**).

Ulcers also appear as part of multi-systemic diseases (Behçet's disease, lupus, rheumatoid arthritis).

Lumps

Abnormal growths are:

■ due to infection (genital warts with HPV)
■ malignant
■ benign (pearly penile papules).

Plaques

Genital plaques are:

■ infective (*Candida* spp.)
■ non-infective (lichen sclerosus).

7.5.11 Scrotal masses

Testicular

Tumours and cysts arising from the testicle or epididymis are indistinguishable from the testicle itself. Infections are usually warm, red and tender whilst tumours tend to be non-tender.

> **Testicular torsion is a urological emergency** whereby the testicle twists on its blood supply, causing ischaemia. This presents as an acutely swollen and tender testicle that sits high within the scrotum. It requires urgent surgical correction to prevent testicular loss.

Hydrocele

This is a fluid-filled sac that is distinct from the testicle and should transilluminate.

Table 7.11 *Summary of genital ulcers*				
	Pathogen	**Onset after exposure**	**Lesion**	**Painful?**
Herpes	Herpes simplex virus	4–7 days	Inflamed papule and vesicle clusters	Yes
Syphilis	*Treponema pallidum*	3 weeks to 3 months	Single, firm ulcer (chancre)	No
Chancroid	*Haemophilus ducreyi*	4–7 days	Grey-yellow ulcer that bleeds easily	Yes
TB	*Mycobacterium* spp.	Insidious	Single ulcer	Yes
Malignancy	n/a – may be related to HPV	n/a	Non-healing, spreading ulcer	Either

Herniae

Herniae are either small or large and may be reducible. As they arise from the inguinal ring, it should not be possible to palpate above a hernia.

Varicocele

This is a non-tender, twisted mass along the spermatic cord that feels like a bag of worms. It is not always obvious when the patient is reclined, due to the effects of gravity.

7.5.12 Inguinal lymphadenopathy

Enlarged inguinal lymph nodes are palpated with infections and cancers of the genital tract.

7.5.13 Enlarged prostate

An enlarged prostate can be benign or as a result of infection or cancer.

7.6 The genitourinary examination

As with all examinations, a consistent and thorough approach is required (**Table 7.12**).

7.6.1 'ID CHECK'

This is detailed in *Section 3.2*.

For the abdominal examination the patient should be topless and have their legs exposed. For the genital examination, the patient should remove their underwear. Ensure that patient dignity and privacy are maintained at all times. Your patient should be lying at 45°.

Table 7.12 *Approach to genitourinary examination*

Genitourinary examination

Element	Details
General inspection	Appearance: does the patient look systemically well or unwell?
	Environment: are there any clues suggesting disease?
Hands	Are there any nail abnormalities?
Wrist	What is the pulse rate and volume?
Arm	What is the blood pressure?
	Is there evidence of renal replacement therapy?
Face	Is there conjunctival pallor?
	Is there evidence of fluid retention?
Neck	Is the jugular venous pressure elevated?
Abdomen	Is there any tenderness?
	Are there any masses?
	Are the kidneys ballotable?
	Is the bladder percussable?
	Is there peritoneal fluid?
Genitals	Are there any lesions?
	Are the testes normal?
Prostate	Is the prostate normal?
Legs	Is there any peripheral oedema?

Always offer a chaperone for genital examinations.

7.6.2 Endobedogram

Have a good look at the patient:
- Are they uncomfortable?
- Around the bedside, are there medications?
- Are there abdominal scars (**Figure 7.5**)?
- Are there any catheter bags next to the bed?

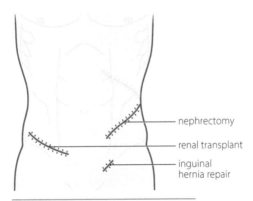

nephrectomy

renal transplant

inguinal hernia repair

Figure 7.5 Abdominal scars relating to genitourinary disease.

7.6.3 Abdominal examination

Inspection

Hands
Ask the patient to hold out their hands.
- Look for nail changes such as leukonychia.
- Note the perfusion of the hand and fingers.
- Is there evidence of capillary blood glucose monitoring, indicating diabetes mellitus?

Radial pulse
Assess the radial pulse rate and volume.

Blood pressure
Measure the blood pressure (see *Section 3.4.2*).

Face and eyes
Inspect the face and around the eyes for:
- periorbital swelling
- conjunctival pallor.

Neck
Examine the JVP. A raised JVP suggests the patient is fluid overloaded.

Evidence of renal replacement therapy
Take a second look at and feel the arms, neck and chest for evidence of previous or current renal replacement therapy (**Figure 7.5**). A fistula will have a continuous vibrating feel from turbulent blood flow.

Legs
Note the presence and extent of any peripheral oedema.

Palpation

Kidneys
Ballot both kidneys, noting the size, nodularity and tenderness of any masses felt (**Figure 7.6**). Palpate the lower abdomen for a transplanted kidney.

Bladder
Palpate for the bladder and note any discomfort.

Percussion
Percuss from the umbilicus to the pubis for a full bladder; then for shifting dullness associated with ascites and peritoneal dialysis.

Auscultation
Use the bell of the stethoscope 5cm superior and lateral to the umbilicus for bruits associated with renovascular disease.

7.6.4 Genital examination

This is performed with the patient lying on the bed or standing up whilst you sit in a chair in front of them. Ensure the examination area is private and always wear gloves.

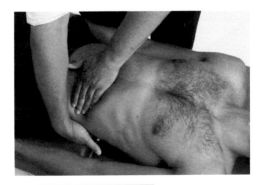

Figure 7.6 Balloting kidneys.

Penis

Are there any abnormal skin lesions? Ask the patient to retract their foreskin to assess the glans. Is the urethral meatus in the correct position? Is there any discharge? If so, note the colour, consistency, the presence of blood and any smell.

Testes

Are there any skin lesions on the scrotum? Ensure to look underneath also. With one finger and thumb, gently feel the outline of one testicle (**Figure 7.7**). Note the size, shape, texture and any tenderness. Palpate the epididymis for any irregularity. Repeat on the opposite side. Examine for testicular herniae (see *Section 6.3.10*).

> **Top tip: shine a light through any scrotal mass.** If the light transmits, this is called transillumination and indicates a fluid-filled collection, usually a hydrocele.

Inguinal lymph nodes

Palpate the inguinal and suprapubic regions for lymphadenopathy. Is it large or small, unilateral or bilateral?

Prostate examination

Ask permission to perform a DRE to examine the prostate (**Table 7.13**). Change your gloves, ask the patient to roll away from you on the couch, drawing their knees to their chest. Insert a single lubricated index finger rectally and palpate the prostate for:

- texture
- enlargement: is this unilateral or bilateral?
- tenderness.

Also consider whether the examination stimulates urethral discharge (this occurs in prostatitis).

7.6.5 Finishing off

Offer the patient some tissue and allow them to dress in privacy.

> "To complete my examination, I would like to perform urinalysis, perform a bladder scan and offer a sexual health screen."

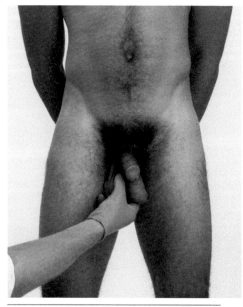

Figure 7.7 Testicular examination technique.

Table 7.13 *Prostate examination findings*				
	Normal	**Benign prostatic hypertrophy**	**Prostatitis**	**Prostate malignancy**
Size	Walnut-sized	Enlarged	Enlarged	Enlarged
Shape	Bilobar	Bilobar	Bilobar	Irregular
Texture	Soft	Firm	Hard	Hard
Surface	Smooth	Smooth	Smooth	Craggy
Tenderness	None	None	Extreme	Possible

7.7 Common investigations

There are many tests used in investigation, diagnosis and monitoring of genitourinary disease (**Table 7.14**). Imaging is the mainstay of assessing structural disease, whilst urinalysis and blood tests monitor disease progression and recovery.

7.7.1 Urinalysis

Urinalysis assesses for blood and protein associated with urinary disease and leukocytes and nitrites associated with UTIs. Note whether this is a 'clean catch' (urinated directly into the bottle) or catheter sample. Sometimes, catheters become colonised with bacteria without causing infection.

7.7.2 Ultrasound

Ultrasound allows easy assessment of the size of the kidneys, bladder and prostate and for the presence of hydronephrosis. Testicular US aids identification and characterisation of any lumps.

7.7.3 Computed tomography

A non-contrast scan gives a cross-sectional image of the kidneys, locates and measures any calculi within the urinary tract and identifies hydronephrosis. Fat stranding around the kidneys is a sign of pyelonephritis.

7.7.4 Magnetic resonance imaging

This is used to assess the prostate and perineum. The addition of IV contrast allows assessment of the renal vascular supply.

7.7.5 Urodynamics

This allows direct assessment of urine flow and bladder emptying during micturition.

7.7.6 Blood tests

Serum blood testing is used to diagnose:
- anaemia
- impaired renal function
- infection (including blood-borne infections such as HIV and hepatitis B and C)
- hypoalbuminaemia
- serum markers of renal, prostate and testicular cancer.

Table 7.14 *Summary of genitourinary investigations*

	Indications	Benefits	Limitations
Urinalysis	Look for evidence of glomerular dysfunction and urinary infection	Quick Easy to perform	Non-specific
Ultrasound	Assess for urinary tract obstruction	Quick Non-invasive	Operator-dependent
CT	Assess for urinary tract obstruction and cause	Quick Diagnostic Non-contrast	Radiation dose (small)
MRI	Assess for renal vasculature and prostatic abnormalities	Reliable Diagnostic	Limited availability Slow
Sexual health screening	Identify or exclude organisms for infection	Limited invasiveness Diagnostic	Stigma of diagnosis Poor uptake of testing

7.7.7 Venous blood gas

Acidaemia and low serum bicarbonate are found in advanced renal disease.

7.7.8 Sexual health screening

This should be performed in a sexual health clinic and offered to all sexually active patients. It includes blood tests, swabs of the oropharynx, penis and rectum and urine tests.

7.7.9 Cystoscopy

This is a procedure whereby a camera is inserted into the bladder via the urethra. Much like OGD in the upper gastrointestinal tract, it allows the clinician to have a direct look at the lining of the bladder, take biopsy samples and perform minor interventions.

7.7.10 Renal biopsy

Sometimes, especially when a primary renal disease is suspected, it is necessary to take a sample of kidney tissue. This allows the sample to be looked at under a microscope. When particular stains are used they characterise the changes which are associated with particular diseases. This procedure requires specialist training.

7.8 System summary

The genitourinary system is complex and involves many organs. Symptoms can be embarrassing and have an extremely negative impact on a patient's quality of life. Understanding the basics of genitourinary disease is key to appreciating the problem as a whole, allowing one to explain the cause of the problem and guide the patient through their investigations towards treatment. Diseases such as ESRD are life-changing. Understanding the risks, symptoms and signs leading to renal failure is key in preventing it from reaching such a point.

7.9 Answers to starter questions

1. There is more than one form of dialysis. Haemodialysis is usually performed three times a week and is only provided in specialist centres. This requires a large amount of time and restricts patients' ability to leave their local areas. The procedure involves the removal, filtering and re-infusion of blood, which results in large changes in circulating volume. It is not suitable for frail patients. Alternative methods include peritoneal dialysis which can be performed and set up at home, usually overnight. Some patients do not want renal replacement therapy and refuse it.

2. In ESRD, the kidneys are unable to filter electrolytes and fluid from the blood. Foods high in sodium and potassium lead to toxic serum levels which affect neurological, cognitive and cardiac function. Patients must be hyper-aware of not only the salt in their food but also the salt their food is cooked in (e.g. salted water when boiling pasta). Most patients with ESRD are restricted to one litre of fluid per day.

3. HIV is a complicated infection that affects multiple organs and risks the development of severe opportunistic infections. The psychosocial impact of HIV is vast and as such, these patients require a coordinated care plan involving many members of the multidisciplinary team. This care is better provided through specialised HIV services with doctors, nurses, therapists, counsellors and social workers all working together.

4. The primary syphilis infection causes a chancre which clears over 6–8 weeks without treatment. These sometimes go unnoticed as they are painless. If untreated, the infection spreads, causing secondary syphilis. This is typified by a maculopapular rash involving the skin and mucous membranes associated with lymphadenopathy. Secondary syphilis also involves the liver, joints and nerves. If still untreated, tertiary syphilis occurs (3–15 years after the primary infection). This causes gummatous syphilis (where benign tumour-like growths develop anywhere in the body), neurosyphilis and syphilitic aortitis. Without intervention, prolonged aortitis leads to the development of left-sided heart failure.

Chapter 8
Female reproductive system

Starter questions

1. Why do we screen for breast and cervical cancer, but not uterine or ovarian cancer?
2. Why might a woman want to control her periods?
3. Why are diabetic mothers followed up so closely during their pregnancy and delivery?
4. Can a pregnant woman celebrate with a glass of champagne?
5. Can you tell if a woman has a high risk of a complicated pregnancy from examination alone?
6. Why do we weigh patients in the gynaecology outpatients clinic?

Answers to questions are to be found in *Section 8.10*.

8.1 Introduction

Women's health is the specialty concerned with female reproductive health. The organs involved are the breast and pelvic organs, including the ovaries, uterus and vagina. The body regulates and maintains the reproductive system using complex hormonal pathways. Conditions affecting the reproductive system are treated by specialists in obstetrics and gynaecology. Women's health affects all women, whether they have children or not.

Exploring a woman's reproductive or gynaecological history involves asking extremely personal questions. It is essential to develop a rapport and respect a woman's choices and lifestyle. During intimate examinations, a woman must feel safe, and have a female chaperone present.

Women are often profoundly affected by gynaecological diseases. Some feel embarrassment about heavy bleeding or vulval discomfort. Some find sensitive subjects such as abortion, miscarriage and infertility very difficult or painful to talk about. A women's health specialist must therefore maintain an attitude that is sympathetic, non-judgemental and professional.

Case 8.1 Heavy menstrual bleeding

Presentation

Rachael is a 24-year-old female with very heavy periods.

Initial interpretation

Rachael is suffering from menorrhagia. This is defined as heavy menstrual bleeding which is interfering with a woman's physical, social or emotional wellbeing. There are numerous causes of menorrhagia, including diseases of the uterus lining, endocrine disorders, structural problems such as fibroids, clotting disorders or ovarian pathology. Further information is required to narrow down the differential diagnosis.

History

Rachael has always had quite heavy periods since the menarche at age 13. Her menstrual cycle is 30 days, and she bleeds heavily from day 1 to day 7. She often has to use both tampons and sanitary pads to prevent leakage, and she must change these every 2 hours. During the last year, the problem has worsened, and she now describes the bleeding as 'torrential'.

She does not experience any period pain. She has no significant past medical history, except for a tooth extraction when she was 19, which was uneventful. She takes no medication. She is in a long-term relationship, and she and her boyfriend use condoms for contraception. Apart from this menorrhagia, her health is good, although she has been very tired the last few months.

Menorrhagia either coexists with menstrual pain (dysmenorrhoea), or occurs on its own, as in this case. This rules out endometriosis as a cause, as this condition is associated with severe dysmenorrhoea. She is not taking any anticoagulants, and did not suffer severe bleeding after her tooth extraction, so congenital or acquired coagulation disorders are unlikely. Her recent tiredness is likely a sequela of iron-deficiency anaemia, a common complication of menorrhagia. However, hypothyroidism is a potential rare cause of heavy menstrual bleeding and fatigue, and should be investigated.

Uterine hyperplasia and cancer cause menorrhagia, but are usually seen in older women who have completed the menopause. Failure to ovulate (anovulation) causes irregular cycle lengths and unpredictable bleeding patterns. Anovulatory cycles are classically seen at the extremes of reproductive life: around the menarche and the menopause. Considering that Rachael is 24 years old with regular cycle durations, anovulation is not a likely cause.

Fibroids are benign tumours of the womb lining, which cause heavy bleeding and abdominal pain and distension if sufficiently large. They are more common in African-Caribbean patients and women over the age of 40, but remain a possibility in Rachael's case.

If a cause cannot be found, then it is termed idiopathic menorrhagia.

Further history

Rachael has not experienced changes in her weight or appetite, abnormal sleeping patterns, or any other symptoms of hypothyroidism. She has not noticed any abdominal swelling that might indicate a fibroid.

Examination

Rachael is rather pale, and has conjunctival pallor. Her cardiovascular and respiratory examinations are normal. Her abdomen is non-tender, with no masses. There is no goitre. Examination of the vagina and cervix with a speculum is normal. Bimanual palpation of the uterus reveals a small uterus with no masses. There is no cervical excitation or adnexal masses.

Interpretation of findings

The gynaecological examination did not reveal the presence of fibroids or cervical disease, which might explain her symptoms. She has clinical signs of anaemia, which likely reflects iron deficiency due to blood loss.

Investigations

Her full blood count reveals a microcytic anaemia,

with haemoglobin of 80g/L, and a mean cell volume (MCV) of 71fl. Her ferritin is extremely low at 8ng/ml, reflecting poor iron stores. Her thyroid function tests and coagulation tests are normal. Her serum progesterone on day 23 of her cycle is 36, confirming that she has ovulated.

Diagnosis

Rachael has significant menorrhagia in the absence of dysmenorrhoea. Her symptoms are significantly affecting her quality of life. Idiopathic menorrhagia is the diagnosis, as no primary cause has been identified. A serum progesterone

level of >30 taken 7 days before the onset of menstruation (in this case, day 23) confirms the release of an ovum, and therefore rules out an anovulatory cycle.

She requires oral iron therapy and treatment of the menorrhagia. Options for menorrhagia control include:

- the levonorgestrel-releasing intrauterine system
- combined oral contraceptive pill
- tranexamic acid, an anti-fibrinolytic agent that promotes clotting
- mefenamic acid, an NSAID that improves menorrhagia and dysmenorrhoea.

A diagnosis of menorrhagia is not based on a measurement of the actual volume of blood loss.
Traditional texts define menorrhagia as bleeding in excess of 80ml per period, but measuring this is neither accurate nor feasible. It is better to rely on the woman's own judgement of how much blood loss is excessive. Menorrhagia is suggested if she:
- has to wake up and change her tampon / sanitary pad during the night
- finds her sanitary pad is soaked with blood when she changes it
- has to replace her tampon / pad every 2 hours or more frequently.

8.2 System overview

The female reproductive system comprises the breast and the pelvic organs. The pelvic organs are:
- vagina
- cervix
- uterus
- ovaries
- uterine tubes (also called fallopian tubes).

8.2.1 The breast

The breast manufactures and secretes milk. It is a network of lactiferous ducts within adipose tissue, with supportive connective tissue.

The tail of the breast extends into the axilla (**Figure 8.1**). Breast development usually precedes the menarche, occurring between the ages of 9 and 12 years.

Lactation

Lactation is the secretion of breast milk. The hormone prolactin promotes maturation of the lactiferous system and milk production following childbirth.

After birth, suckling of the nipple causes oxytocin release from the pituitary, resulting in ejection of milk via the nipple.

A prolactinoma is a tumour of the pituitary gland which secretes excessive amounts of prolactin in non-pregnant women, resulting in inappropriate lactation. Prolactin also suppresses production of follicle-stimulating hormone (FSH) and luteinising hormone (LH), which leads to subfertility (due to anovulation).

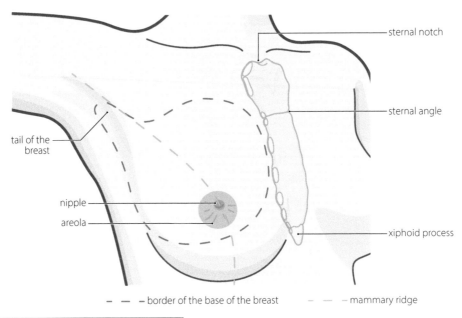

sternal notch

sternal angle

tail of the breast

nipple

areola

xiphoid process

– – – border of the base of the breast   – – – mammary ridge

Figure 8.1 Surface anatomy of the breast.

Lymphatic drainage

Most lymphatic fluid within the breast drains to ipsilateral axillary lymph nodes. Smaller amounts drain to the parasternal nodes and the contralateral breast's lymphatic system.

8.2.2 Vagina

This is a muscular canal extending from the external genitalia (vulva) to the cervix. Both the cervix and vaginal wall secrete lubricating fluid to facilitate sexual intercourse. The vaginal walls have an elastic structure, allowing sufficient dilation for childbirth.

8.2.3 Cervix

The cervix is the channel connecting the vagina to the uterus. It secretes a mucus which changes in consistency during the menstrual cycle. During ovulation the mucus is thin and watery to allow passage of spermatozoa. During the secretory phase, progesterone thickens the cervical mucus so it acts as a barrier to further spermatozoa.

> The main action of the **progesterone-only contraceptive pill** is to thicken the cervical mucus.

8.2.4 The uterus

This is a fist-sized organ in the pelvic cavity. The outer surface is lined with a serous membrane called the perimetrium. The bulk of the uterine walls are smooth muscle fibres, called the myometrium. The myometrium generates the powerful uterine contractions in labour. The inner layer is glandular tissue called the endometrium. The endometrium thickens each month, until it is shed during menstruation.

8.2.5 The ovary

The ovary manufactures ova (gametogenesis) and hormones: oestrogen, progesterone and small amounts of testosterone. Ovaries contain a finite number of immature follicles, and over one monthly menstruation cycle, one of these immature follicles develops into a mature ovum, and is released from the ovary. When the ovaries exhaust their follicular supply, gametogenesis ceases and the ovaries dramatically decrease hormone production, inducing the menopause.

The ovaries are held in place in the pelvis by two ligaments:

- The ovarian ligament anchors the ovaries to the uterus.
- The suspensory ligament of the ovary anchors the ovaries to the pelvic wall.

8.2.6 The uterine tubes

The left and right tubes connect their corresponding ovary to the uterine cavity. They are lined with motile cilia, that 'waft' the ovum released by the ovary during ovulation down towards the uterus.

8.2.7 The menstrual cycle

Menstruation is the normal discharge of blood and endometrial lining through the vagina. The menarche is the onset of menstruation and usually occurs between the ages of 9 and 15 years. It is caused by secretion of gonadotrophin-releasing hormone (GnRH) from the hypothalamus. A normal menstrual cycle is 21–35 days. Menstruation begins on day 1 and ovulation occurs at the mid-point of the cycle (**Figure 8.2**).

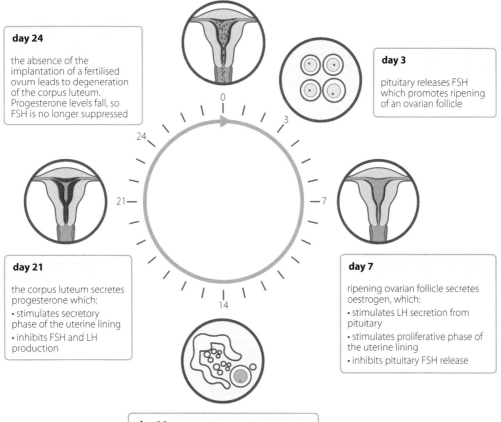

day 0

low levels of progesterone cause endometrial shedding: menstruation begins

day 24

the absence of the implantation of a fertilised ovum leads to degeneration of the corpus luteum. Progesterone levels fall, so FSH is no longer suppressed

day 3

pituitary releases FSH which promotes ripening of an ovarian follicle

day 21

the corpus luteum secretes progesterone which:
• stimulates secretory phase of the uterine lining
• inhibits FSH and LH production

day 7

ripening ovarian follicle secretes oestrogen, which:
• stimulates LH secretion from pituitary
• stimulates proliferative phase of the uterine lining
• inhibits pituitary FSH release

day 14

LH levels become sufficiently high to induce ovulation. The ovum leaves behind the remnant of the ripened follicle, which becomes the corpus luteum

Figure 8.2 Hormonal changes during the menstrual cycle.

Hormonal changes

The menstrual cycle is controlled by the hypothalamic–pituitary–ovarian axis (**Figure 8.3**). The word 'axis' means the entire hormonal pathway. The hypothalamus, pituitary and ovary all secrete hormones that, together, regulate their own production and secretion.

Pituitary hormones

The pituitary hormones FSH and LH are released from the pituitary gland in the brain.
- FSH promotes the ripening of an ovarian follicle into a mature ovum.
- LH stimulates the release of the ovum from the ovary (ovulation).

Ovarian hormones

The ovarian hormones are oestrogen and progesterone.
- Oestrogen is produced by the ripening ovarian follicle. It stimulates the pituitary to secrete LH and promotes the proliferative phase of the uterine lining.
- Progesterone is secreted by the corpus luteum – the remains of the ripened ovarian follicle following ovulation. It promotes the secretory phase of the uterine lining.

Uterine changes

The uterine lining responds to progesterone and oestrogen. The uterus sheds its lining on days 1–7 of the cycle, followed by two further phases:
- Proliferative phase: between days 7 and 14. During this phase the endometrium begins to regenerate in response to oestrogen release from a ripened follicle. It is caused by oestrogen.
- Secretory phase: after ovulation on day 14, the endometrium becomes highly vascular in preparation for implantation of a fertilised ovum. It is caused by progesterone.

Ovarian changes

The ovarian cycle is divided into the follicular and luteal phases:
- Follicular phase: this corresponds to the ripening of an ovarian follicle. It terminates on day 14, when the follicle releases an ovum.
- Luteal phase: the ruptured follicle transforms into the corpus luteum, which secretes progesterone between days 14 and 28. The corpus luteum atrophies over 14 days, until it no longer secretes progesterone; this triggers menstruation.

The hormonal, ovarian and uterine changes evolve together during the menstrual cycle (**Figure 8.4**).

8.2.8 Pregnancy

Pregnancy occurs when a fertilised ovum implants into the highly vascularised endometrial lining during the secretory phase of the menstrual cycle. A normal pregnancy is 40 weeks, measured from the last menstrual period until delivery. There are many physiological changes during pregnancy (**Table 8.1**).

8.2.9 Menopause

This classically occurs at age 50. It occurs due to follicular depletion within the ovaries. In the absence of ovulation, the ovary does not produce oestrogen or progesterone. FSH and LH levels rise due to the loss of negative feedback from the ovarian hormones. Menstruation ceases permanently.

Falling oestrogen and progesterone levels cause the common symptoms of the menopause:

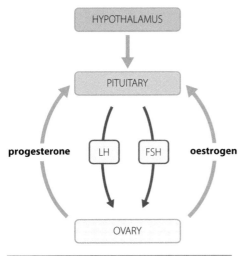

Figure 8.3 The hypothalamic–pituitary–ovarian axis.

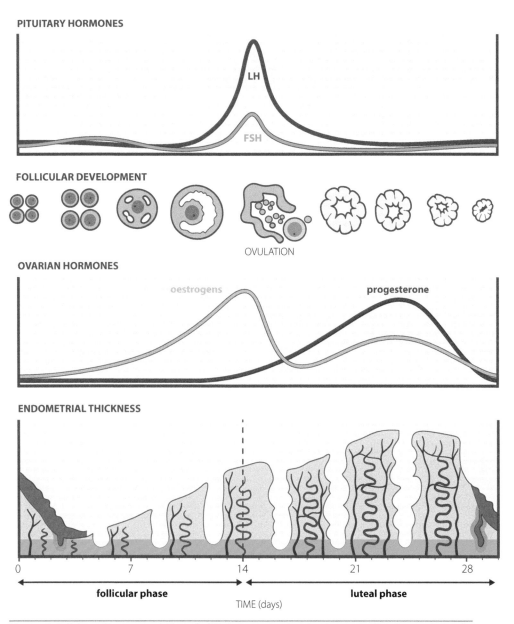

PITUITARY HORMONES

LH

FSH

FOLLICULAR DEVELOPMENT

OVULATION

OVARIAN HORMONES

oestrogens   progesterone

ENDOMETRIAL THICKNESS

0   7   14   21   28

follicular phase   **luteal phase**

TIME (days)

Figure 8.4 Schematic representation of a 28-day menstrual cycle, demonstrating the ovarian cycle, uterine cycle, and key hormonal changes.

- hot flushes, due to vasomotor instability
- vaginal dryness, which often makes sex painful (dyspareunia)
- osteoporosis
- mood changes.

Unbearable vasomotor symptoms are treated with hormone replacement therapy (HRT).

Most of the symptoms of the menopause are caused by oestrogen depletion. However, HRT is a combination therapy with oestrogen and progesterone, as unopposed oestrogen increases the risk of endometrial cancer.

Table 8.1 *Normal physiological changes of pregnancy*		
System affected	**Changes in pregnancy**	**Potential symptoms and signs**
Cardiovascular	Increased stroke volume and heart rate leading to increased cardiac output	Bounding pulse
	Peripheral vasodilation leading to low blood pressure in first two trimesters	Light-headedness, fatigue
Respiratory	Increased tidal volume	Sensation of breathlessness
	Mild respiratory alkalosis	
Haematological	Increased plasma volume in excess of increased red cell mass, resulting in dilutional anaemia	Fatigue
	Increased clotting factors	VTE
Gastroenterological	Morning sickness in early pregnancy	Nausea and vomiting
	Relaxation of GI tract smooth muscle	Gastro-oesophageal reflux Constipation
Genitourinary	Dilation of ureters	Upper urinary tract infections (pyelonephritis)
Musculoskeletal	Pelvic pain	Pubic symphysis dysfunction (very common)

8.3 Breast history

The breast history elicits the symptoms of breast disease and determines the woman's risk for breast cancer. This is for two reasons. Firstly, all breast-related symptoms could be a manifestation of breast cancer. Therefore, no matter what changes there are that a woman notices in her breast tissue, breast cancer must be suspected, investigated and ruled out before any other diagnosis is made. Secondly, breast cancer is very common, and is the only 'breast diagnosis' that results in significant life-altering or life-limiting illness. Therefore, diagnosing a mass, a pain or a nipple discharge as a benign process without first ruling out cancer (either by careful history and examination or by tissue biopsy) is very risky.

8.3.1 Symptoms

The symptoms of breast disease are masses (either in the breast or in the axilla), pain and nipple discharge.

Masses

The main symptom relating to breast disease is the discovery of masses. 'Mass' is a medical term and can be misunderstood by patients as something that is 'massive' in size, so a mass is usually called a lump when talking with patients.

The most common type of breast lump is a fibroadenoma, which is benign. However, all breast lumps are suspected to be cancer until firmly proven otherwise.

The characteristics of different breast masses are explored in **Table 8.2**.

Table 8.2 *Causes of breast masses with associated features*

	Details	Features
Fibroadenoma	Benign tumour of breast connective tissue	Usually mobile within breast Difficult to differentiate from breast cancer without tissue biopsy
Fibrocystic breast changes	Multiple benign masses within the breast tissue	Usually multiple, causing 'lumpy breasts' Causes mild breast pain that worsens just before menstruation Diminishes after the menopause
Breast cyst	Fluid-filled mass	Often tender to palpation Well-defined oval mass, often multiple in each breast
Breast cancer	Neoplastic changes of breast tissue	Irregular, hard, painless lump
Mammary duct ectasia	Widening of the lactiferous ducts in middle age, resulting in ductal discharge	Tender lump around the areola with green nipple discharge
Fat necrosis	Trauma to the adipose tissue of the breast	Hard tender lump following trivial trauma or breast surgery
Breast abscess	Infection and pus collection within the breast	Usually in breastfeeding women Painful red swelling around areola
Galactocele	Milk cyst within the lactating breast	Large, soft, fluctuant lump in lower breast

Breast cancer

Breast cancer affects one in nine women. Most are due to random mutations, whilst 10% are due to inherited mutations of the *BRCA* gene. Breast cancer risk factors are modifiable or non-modifiable (**Table 8.3**).

> **Mutations of the *BRCA1* or *BRCA2* gene confer a lifetime breast cancer risk of 80%, and ovarian cancer risk of 25–50%.** Some women who have these mutations elect to have preventative mastectomies and oophorectomies.

Table 8.3 *Modifiable and non-modifiable risk factors for breast cancer*

Modifiable risk factors	Non-modifiable risk factors
Nulliparity Obesity Alcohol excess HRT Combined oral contraceptive Smoking	Inherited genetic abnormalities, e.g.: ■ *BRCA1* and *BRCA2* mutation ■ p53 mutation ■ early menarche ■ late menopause ■ increasing age

Lymphadenopathy. Most lymphatic fluid within the breast drains to ipsilateral axillary lymph nodes. Therefore cancerous cells from the breast spread to the axillary lymph nodes first in cases of metastatic cancer. This causes firm, non-tender lumps in the axilla.

Pain
Breast pain is a common symptom associated with menstruation (cyclical breast pain), due to high levels of circulating progesterone. This is the same reason many women experience breast pain during pregnancy.

Mastitis is inflammation of the breast tissue, resulting in pain. It occurs in breastfeeding women, and is due to an accumulation of milk (milk stasis). Associated symptoms are cracked nipples, redness of the skin on the breast, and pain on lactation. If infection occurs, the mother experiences fever and general malaise. This is treated with antibiotics.

Many benign breast masses, such as fibroadenoma, breast cysts and fibrocystic changes, often become more tender just before menstruation.

Discharge
Discharge from the nipple is either milk (galactorrhoea), pus or fluid (**Table 8.4**).

8.3.2 Taking a history

The breast history explores the nature of the abnormality, and establishes a time frame. Crucially, it evaluates the woman's individual risk for breast cancer.

Past medical history
Explore the woman's menstrual history, as breast cancer risk is proportional to the number of periods a woman has during her lifetime. Early menarche, late menopause and nulliparity therefore confer a higher risk.

Medications
Ascertain whether they are taking medications that cause galactorrhoea (**Table 8.4**). Ask about HRT if they are postmenopausal, as it increases the risk of breast cancer.

Social history
Both smoking and excessive alcohol have been implicated as causes of breast cancer.

Family history
Ask about a family history of breast or ovarian cancer, which indicates an inherited gene mutation.

Systems review
A full systems review relating to breast disease is in **Table 8.5.**

Table 8.4 *Causes of nipple discharge*		
Discharge	**Causes**	
Galactorrhoea	Physiological	Post-pregnancy
	Prolactin excess	Prolactin-producing tumour of the pituitary gland
	Medication	Methyldopa (antihypertensive)
		Antipsychotics
		Antihistamines
	Idiopathic	
Blood-stained fluid	Ductal papilloma	Benign lesion of breast tissue
	Breast cancer	A rare cause of nipple discharge
Pus	Breast abscess	Infection of breast tissue

System	Symptoms	Breast disease causes
Cardiovascular	Chest pain	Pulmonary embolism due to breast cancer
Respiratory	Breathlessness	Pleural effusion due to breast malignancy
		Lung metastases from breast cancer
		Pulmonary embolism due to breast cancer
Neurological	Headache	Cerebral metastasis from breast cancer
	Focal neurological impairment	

Table 8.5 *Systems review as related to the breast*

8.4 Breast examination

The examination determines the nature and extent of the breast abnormality. In cases of breast pain or nipple discharge, the examination reveals any hitherto unnoticed breast masses. If there is a mass, the examination reveals the size, consistency and any associated features, and determines whether it is in keeping with malignancy. This helps inform decisions about the best investigations to order. If there is a firm mass in keeping with malignancy, mammogram is warranted. If there is evidence of inflamed skin on the breast, and a painful fluctuant lump in keeping with an abscess, then a breast ultrasound is the preferred test.

8.4.1 Signs

Public information programmes have led to a greater awareness particularly of breast cancer, and women are more frequently detecting changes in their breast tissue.

The commonest signs in breast disease are:
- skin changes
- nipple changes
- breast lumps – either as the presenting symptom for the consultation, or a clinical finding detected during a medical examination
- lymphadenopathy.

Skin changes

Peau d'orange
Literally 'orange-peel skin', this is dimpling due to cutaneous lymphatic oedema, seen in inflammatory breast cancer.

Erythema
This is seen in mastitis or overlying a breast abscess. An abscess is localised infection that has developed into a collection of pus.

Scars
Patients who have undergone a mastectomy have a large diagonal scar over the chest wall and an absent breast (**Figure 8.5**). Those who have undergone a lumpectomy have smaller scars and an intact breast.

Skin puckering
This is due to breast cancer becoming tethered to the skin. The skin appears pinched or crumpled,

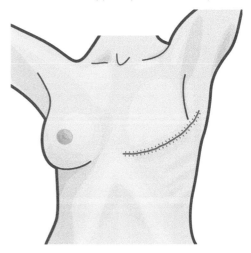

Figure 8.5 Unilateral mastectomy with thoracic scar.

and is pulled in towards the underlying breast lump (to which it is firmly anchored).

Nipple changes

Nipple inversion

An inverted nipple points in toward the breast, rather than out, causing a dimple in the centre of the areola. Congenital nipple inversion is benign, and very common, with an incidence of 10%. New inversion is a sign of breast cancer, and is caused by the skin becoming tethered to the underlying lump.

Paget's disease of the nipple

This is an itching, scaly rash over the nipple and areola. It is a paraneoplastic phenomenon, indicating breast cancer (**Figure 8.6**).

Lymphadenopathy

Lymphadenopathy due to cancer is found in the axilla.

8.4.2 Examination sequence

The examination sequence is detailed in **Table 8.6**.

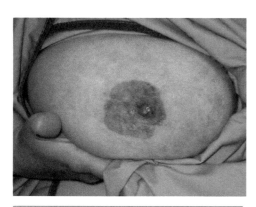

Figure 8.6 Scaling and erythema of the areola in keeping with Paget's disease of the breast.

Table 8.6 *The breast examination sequence*	
Element	**Details**
Inspection	Are there any skin changes?
	Are there any nipple changes?
	Are there any masses?
Palpation	Are there any masses?
	Is there any lymphadenopathy?

'ID CHECK'

This is detailed in *Section 3.2*.

The breast examination is an intimate examination. There must be a female chaperone present, to ensure the woman feels safe and to confirm that the examination was carried out correctly and in a professional manner. Either lock the clinic door to ensure that no other staff member interrupts the examination, or move the woman and chaperone behind a curtain or screen within the room.

> **A chaperone is an impartial observer.** It is usually a nurse or a healthcare assistant. The GMC advises in its *Ethical Guidance for Doctors* that a chaperone must:
> - "be sensitive and respect the patient's dignity and confidentiality
> - reassure the patient if they show signs of distress or discomfort
> - be familiar with the procedures involved in a routine intimate examination
> - stay for the whole examination and be able to see what the doctor is doing, if practical
> - be prepared to raise concerns if they are concerned about the doctor's behaviour or actions."

Endobedogram

Have a good look at the woman. Remember that mild breast asymmetry is normal.
- Has she had any previous breast surgery, or a mastectomy?
- Are there any visible breast masses?
- Are there any abnormalities of the skin or nipples?

Inspection

Asking the woman to move into the following positions may reveal abnormalities.

At rest

Ask her to rest her hands on her thighs whilst seated, and inspect for any visible masses.

Hands on hips

Ask her to place her hands on her hips and push them in (**Figure 8.7a**). This tenses the pectoral muscle and reveals masses tethered to the muscle wall.

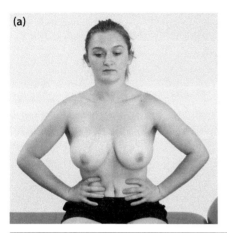
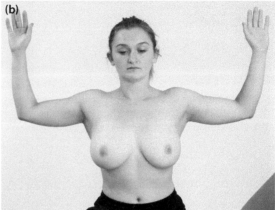

Figure 8.7 (a) Tensing the pectorals and (b) raising the arms may reveal tethered breast masses.

Hands above head

Inspect the under-surface of the breast for skin changes. Elevating the arms (**Figure 8.7b**) reveals any skin puckering.

Palpation

You need to press quite firmly to palpate for deeper masses closer to the chest wall, particularly if the woman has large breasts. Check that your pressure is not causing undue pain.

Breast

Imagining that the breast is a clock face, palpate each 'hour' systematically (**Figure 8.8**). Use the palmar aspect of the fingers to detect any pain or swelling. After each 'hour' has been examined, palpate the breast over the nipple. Finish by palpating the axillary tail of the breast.

If you detect a mass, attempt to clarify:

- location (which 'hour' it is)
- consistency – malignant masses are firm and painless, whereas fibroadenomas are more 'lumpy' and tender
- size in centimetres
- whether it is mobile or tethered to the skin or muscle.

Axilla

Ask the woman to sit on the edge of the bed facing you. Ask her to rest her right hand upon your left shoulder. Use your left hand to palpate all borders of her right axilla, feeling for any lymphadenopathy.

Repeat the process for her left axilla.

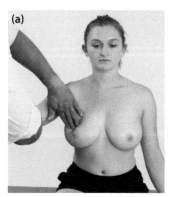
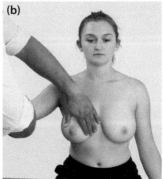
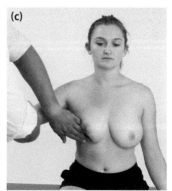

Figure 8.8 Examine the breast using the 'clock-face approach': (a) 11 o'clock; (b) 2 o'clock; (c) 7 o'clock.

8.5 Gynaecology symptoms and history-taking

You are determining the nature and duration of the symptoms and how they affect the woman's life. The history reveals the nature and time course of the gynaecological problem, to make the correct diagnosis. It also investigates how the problem is affecting the woman in her day-to-day life. Determining the severity of the symptoms helps choose the right treatment plan for each patient. For example, if a woman had cyclical pelvic pain (related to menstruation) that was only uncomfortable, painkilling medication would be appropriate. If the pain was too intense to bear, or making her miss work, then she may require more invasive management, such as surgery.

Not all women attending a gynaecology clinic have disease. Some have normal physiological processes that are causing them anguish. A common example is irregular cycle length – the woman does not have an illness, but still requires treatment to help her live a happy life.

8.5.1 Symptoms

The main symptoms are menstrual disturbances, abnormal bleeding, pelvic pain, discharge, abdominal distension and itching.

Heavy periods

This is called menorrhagia. It is either idiopathic or secondary (**Table 8.7**).

Table 8.7 *The causes of menorrhagia*		
Cause	**Mechanism**	**Associated features**
Fibroids	Fibroids are highly vascular and bleed easily	Abdominal distension
Endometriosis	Deposition of endometrial tissue throughout reproductive tract and abdomen	Dysmenorrhoea Dysuria Chronic pelvic pain
Endometrial polyp	Highly vascular benign lesion of the endometrium	May also have cervical polyps causing postcoital bleeding
Anovulation	Follicle is not converted into a corpus luteum, resulting in low progesterone state and endometrial shedding	Occurs with the menarche and menopause Variable menstrual cycle duration
Idiopathic	No cause identified	
Hypothyroidism	Cause unclear; possibly due to failure to ovulate	Lethargy Weight gain Constipation Palpable goitre
Pelvic inflammatory disease (PID)	Chronic inflammation of the pelvic organs due to infection, resulting in vascularised and fragile tissue	Pelvic pain Vaginal discharge Dysuria May be asymptomatic
Intrauterine contraceptive device (IUCD)	The copper IUCD is associated with heavy bleeding for the initial months after insertion	History of device insertion
Clotting disorders	Inability to coagulate blood	Bleeding from other sites

Absent or rare periods

Oligomenorrhoea (infrequent periods) is defined as when a woman has periods less often than every 35 days. Amenorrhoea (absent periods) is either primary or secondary.

Primary amenorrhoea

This is when a woman has never menstruated. It is diagnosed if a woman has not experienced the menarche by age 17. Causes are:

- gonadal dysgenesis, such as in Turner's syndrome
- structural abnormalities of the reproductive tract, such as imperforate hymen.

Secondary amenorrhoea

This is when a woman who experienced menarche has new onset amenorrhoea (**Table 8.8**), defined as missing three periods in a row.

Non-cyclical vaginal bleeding

This is irregular or unexpected bleeding outside the norms of the woman's usual menstrual cycle. This includes:

- intermenstrual bleeding
- postcoital bleeding
- postmenopausal bleeding
- irregular cycle lengths.

Intermenstrual bleeding

Intermenstrual bleeding occurs between periods and could be due to disease in any part of the reproductive tract (**Table 8.9**).

Postcoital bleeding

This is vaginal bleeding in the minutes or hours following intercourse. It is usually very light and often presents as spotting of blood on the underwear. It is caused by diseases of the cervix or vagina, including:

Table 8.8 *The causes of secondary oligo- / amenorrhoea*		
Cause	**Mechanism**	**Associated features**
Pregnancy	High oestrogen and progesterone states preserve the endometrium	Features of pregnancy
Polycystic ovarian syndrome	Elevated androgens and anovulation	Obesity Insulin resistance Hirsutism Subfertility
Low weight	Excessive dieting or exercise inhibits pituitary production of LH and FSH, leading to low oestrogen and progesterone	Subfertility
Excessive prolactin production	Prolactin suppresses LH and FSH levels, disrupting the menstrual cycle	Galactorrhoea Intracranial mass effect of pituitary prolactinoma
Thyrotoxicosis	Suppression of LH and FSH through dopamine and prolactin pathways	Agitation Tachycardia Weight loss Goitre
Cervical stenosis	Usually a consequence of cervical surgery	History of surgery
Early menopause (aka 'premature ovarian failure')	Loss of ovarian function and hormone recreation before 40 years of age; usually idiopathic in aetiology	Usual features of menopause (e.g. vasomotor instability)

Table 8.9 *The causes of intermenstrual bleeding*

	Cause	Associated features
Vaginal causes	Vaginitis	Dyspareunia Postcoital bleeding
	Tumours	Sensation of vaginal mass
Cervical causes	Cervicitis (infective)	Dysuria Pelvic pain Vaginal discharge
	Polyps	Menorrhagia Postcoital bleeding
	Ectropion	Postcoital bleeding Asymptomatic
	Tumour (rare)	Postcoital bleeding
Uterine causes	Fibroids	Abdominal mass Menorrhagia
	Polyps	Menorrhagia
	Cancer	Postmenopausal bleeding
Ovarian	Tumours (rare)	Pelvic masses
Iatrogenic	IUCD	Menorrhagia
	Anticoagulants	Bleeding from other sites Bruising
	Missed pills	Unplanned pregnancy

- cervicitis secondary to infection
- cervical ectropion
- atrophic vaginitis
- cervical cancer.

> **Cervical ectropion is a condition where the columnar epithelium of the endocervix extends into the upper vaginal wall, and undergoes metaplastic change to become stratified squamous epithelium.** It is a normal phenomenon in young women, but can make women prone to bleeding, especially on contact, e.g. with a tampon or after sex.

Postmenopausal bleeding (PMB)

This is vaginal bleeding in women who have completed the menopause and is commonly due to atrophic vaginitis. The postmenopausal lack of oestrogen leads to atrophy of the vaginal epithelium, which bleeds easily. Endometrial cancer is a rarer cause.

> **Patients presenting with PMB require an urgent transvaginal US of the uterus to check for endometrial cancer.** If the endometrium appears thickened, a small biopsy is taken using a transcervical Pipelle, which will confirm or exclude the cancer.

Variable cycle duration

A normal menstrual cycle is 21 to 35 days. Some women have irregular cycles for their entire reproductive lives, whilst others have very regular cycles. Psychosocial factors that affect cycle length are psychological stress, exercise, decreased food intake and acute illnesses and infections; all of these affect the hypothalamic–pituitary–ovarian axis. Some women simply have irregular cycle lengths as part of their normal physiology, which is usually a long-term cause of consternation.

If a woman's cycle suddenly becomes unpredictable it is usually due to the aforementioned psychosocial factors, and no tests or treatments are indicated. Physical conditions that cause a new disruption to a woman's menstrual cycle are:

- anovulatory cycles, which occur around the menarche and menopause
- polycystic ovarian syndrome (PCOS).

> **Many women find unpredictable menstrual cycles inconvenient and anxiety-inducing.** The oral contraceptive pill is a way of regulating the hormonal changes in the menstrual cycle, leading to a predictable menstruation pattern. Therefore not everyone taking the pill does so for contraception.

Polycystic ovarian syndrome. PCOS is a systemic disorder, where multiple ovarian cysts are seen on ultrasound in association with:

- elevated circulating androgen, leading to hirsutism and acne
- oligo- / amenorrhoea due to failure to ovulate
- subfertility
- insulin resistance, leading to type 2 diabetes and obesity.

Many of the symptoms are ameliorated by weight loss. Distressing androgenic features are treated with the combined oral contraceptive pill. Insulin resistance and subfertility occasionally require treatment with metformin.

Painful periods

Painful periods (dysmenorrhoea) are more commonly referred to as 'menstrual cramps' or 'period pain'. Primary (idiopathic) dysmenorrhoea is common and affects 40% of menstruating women. Secondary dysmenorrhoea is painful periods due to another illness. The commonest cause of secondary dysmenorrhoea is endometriosis.

Endometriosis

Endometriosis is the development of endometrial tissue outside the uterus, usually on the ovaries, uterine tubes and outer surface of the bladder and uterus. It causes inflammation, leading to chronic pelvic pain that exacerbates with menstruation. The inflamed tissue leads to adhesions – the reproductive organs become stuck to other abdominal organs, such as bowel loops. This leads to disruption of normal bowel movement and function. Laparoscopic surgery divides the adhesions, but there is no cure for the endometriosis.

Pelvic pain

Primary dysmenorrhoea is the commonest cause of pelvic pain. Other types of pain are divided into chronic or acute.

Chronic pelvic pain

Pain that is present for more than two menstrual cycles is chronic, and is due to:

- endometriosis
- pelvic venous congestion: dilation of pelvic veins, usually following pregnancy
- pelvic inflammatory disease (PID): chronic STI leads to generalised inflammation of the reproductive organs; it is associated with vaginal discharge and subfertility
- prolapse of pelvic organs.

Prolapse

This is the descent of pelvic organs through a weak pelvic floor (**Table 8.10**). The pelvic floor is a sheet of muscle that weakens with old age or following childbirth. Accompanying symptoms include:

- stress incontinence (involuntary urination on sneezing, coughing or laughing)
- a palpable lump in the vagina, or just outside (like sitting on a ball)
- a sensation of fullness or stretching within the vagina
- pain during sex.

Table 8.10 *Different types of prolapse*

Type of prolapse	Name	Associated features
The rectum prolapses through a weakened posterior vaginal wall	Rectocele	Constipation Tenesmus
The bladder prolapses through a weakened anterior vaginal wall	Cystocele	Stress urinary incontinence
The uterus descends downwards into the vagina	Uterine prolapse	Dyspareunia Pelvic pain
The urethra prolapses through a weakened anterior vaginal wall	Urethrocele	Stress incontinence Incomplete bladder emptying

Prolapse of the pelvic organs is very common in elderly patients and often requires surgical correction.

Acute pelvic pain

Acute severe pelvic pain requires urgent medical attention because many of the causes require surgery:

- Ovarian cyst torsion: a large cyst twists around and cuts off its own blood supply.
- Ectopic pregnancy: a fertilised ovum, rarely, implants into the wall of the uterine tube. When it reaches sufficient size, the tube ruptures.
- Appendicitis: causes RIF pain.

Pain on intercourse

This is called dyspareunia. The pain may be superficial (close to the vulva) or deep (within the pelvis). Superficial dyspareunia is usually due to vaginismus – an involuntary contraction of muscles surrounding the vagina on penetration. The cause is psychological or physical:

- psychological: fear or anxiety regarding intercourse
- physical: vulval or vaginal inflammation due to infection.

Superficial dyspareunia is also caused by atrophic vaginitis following the menopause. Deep dyspareunia is caused by:

- PID
- prolapse of pelvic organs
- cervicitis, e.g. due to infection
- endometriosis.

Vaginal discharge

This is fluid or semi-solid material expelled from the vagina. It appears white, cream-coloured or yellowish. It is commonly due to infection. Discharge is a sign of candidiasis or bacterial vaginosis, as well as of STIs.

Candidal vulvovaginitis

This is a yeast infection commonly called 'thrush'. It is not sexually transmitted. It causes vaginal itching and burning and a creamy discharge. It occurs in healthy women, but is more common during pregnancy, in those with diabetes, and those taking oral antibiotics for other infections.

Bacterial vaginosis

This is overgrowth of certain bacteria that naturally occur in the vagina. It is not an STI. It causes vaginal itching and burning, and thin grey or white discharge with an unpleasant fishy odour.

Abdominal distension

The reproductive organs lie deep within the pelvis. Benign and malignant growths of these organs do not cause a localised mass within the lower abdomen. Instead, the woman notices a generalised swelling, only when the growth is quite advanced.

Ovarian cancer

Classically, ovarian cancer affects middle-aged women, and causes non-specific symptoms of bloating, early satiety and abdominal distension.

> **Ovarian cancer is notoriously difficult to diagnose**, as the symptoms are vague and often attributed by patients and doctors to bowel disorders. This is due to the deep location of the ovaries within the pelvis.

Ovarian cysts

These are benign ovarian growths. They can reach massive sizes if left untreated.

Fibroids

These are benign growth of the endometrium. They are extremely prevalent, and are most common in middle-aged premenopausal women. In cases of multiple large fibroids, the woman notices an irregular swelling in the suprapubic area. They are associated with dysmenorrhoea and menorrhagia, which are usually the presenting complaints.

Ascites

Any malignancy of the reproductive system has the potential to cause a malignant ascites. This presents as generalised abdominal swelling.

Itching

Pruritus vulvae is itching of the vulva. In many cases, no cause is identified. Identifiable causes include:

- infection
- lichen sclerosus – itchy white patches on the vulval skin
- vulval carcinoma (rarely).

8.5.2 Taking a history

The gynaecology history explores symptoms related to the reproductive organs, and determines the woman's risk of developing cancer of the ovary, cervix and endometrium.

Past medical history

Ask about:

- endocrine disorders – thyroid disorders affect frequency and heaviness of periods (**Tables 8.7** and **8.8**)
- coagulopathy: patients with coagulopathy have menorrhagia
- previous obstetric history
- past surgical history – do they still have a uterus?
- the menopause, if the woman is of the appropriate age
- the age of menarche.

> **Just like breast cancer, the risk of endometrial cancer increases proportionate to the number of periods a woman has in a lifetime.** Women who had an early menarche, a late menopause and no pregnancies therefore carry the greatest risk.

Medications

Ascertain if they are using contraception (**Table 8.11**), anticoagulants or HRT.

Social history

Take a sexual health history, ascertaining whether the woman is sexually active. Ask if she has been previously screened for STIs. Smoking and excessive alcohol increase the risk of cervical cancer.

Family history

A family history of breast or ovarian cancer indicates an inherited gene mutation.

Systems review

A full systems review is shown in **Table 8.12**.

8.6 Gynaecology signs and examination

Despite changing public attitudes towards gynaecological health, there are many women who do not examine their external genitalia for abnormalities, so signs discovered in the examination may come as a surprise to the woman.

8.6.1 Signs

The main signs are general skin changes, vulval changes and abdominal distension.

Table 8.11 *Comparing contraception*

Type	What is it?	Mode of action	Benefits	Potential adverse effects
COC	Combined oral contraceptive (oestrogen and progesterone)	Inhibits ovulation	Predictable cycle length	VTE Unsuitable if: ■ >35 years ■ smoker ■ obese
POP	Progesterone-only pill	Thickens cervical mucus	Suitable for smokers, obese, >35 years	Irregular cycle lengths
IUS	Intrauterine system (contains levonorgestrel)	Prevents endometrial proliferation	Also excellent treatment for menorrhagia	Irregular bleeding for months after insertion Uterine perforation (rare)
IUCD	Intrauterine device (contains copper)	Toxic to spermatozoa	No hormonal effects Also effective emergency contraception	Menorrhagia for months after insertion Uterine perforation (rare)
Injectable contraceptive	Depot injection of progestogen	Inhibits ovulation	No pills needed Lasts 14 weeks	Weight gain May take 1 year to regain fertility after cessation
Contraceptive implant	Slow release of progesterone	Inhibits ovulation	No pills needed Lasts 3 years	Irregular cycle lengths
Condoms	Barrier method	Prevents spermatozoa from reaching ovum	Protects against STIs	Efficacy is related to 'perfect' use – suboptimal application leads to failure

Table 8.12 *Systems review as related to gynaecology*

System	Symptoms	Gynaecology-related causes
Cardiovascular	Chest pain	Pulmonary embolism due to gynaecological cancer
	Pedal oedema	Impaired lymphatic draining from legs due to pelvic mass
Respiratory	Breathlessness	Pleural effusion due to ovarian cancer (Meigs' syndrome) Lung metastases from gynaecological cancer Pulmonary embolism due to gynaecological cancer
Gastroenterological	Constipation Abdominal pain	Mass effect from gynaecological tumour
Genitourinary	Urinary incontinence	Mass effect from gynaecological tumour

Skin changes

Pallor
This is due to iron-deficiency anaemia, often seen with menorrhagia due to chronic blood loss.

Hirsutism
Excess body hair is noticeable on the forearms and in a beard distribution on the face.

Acanthosis nigricans
This is the presence of dark velvety patches in the axillae and is associated with insulin resistance, a common feature of PCOS.

Vulval changes
Common vulval abnormalities are listed in **Table 8.13**.

Abdominal distension
Large ovarian or uterine masses give rise to suprapubic or iliac fossa masses. The deep position of these organs means that such masses cause general abdominal distension rather than discrete 'lumps'.

8.6.2 Examination sequence

The examination sequence is detailed in **Table 8.14**.

'ID CHECK'
See *Section 3.2.1*.

This is an intimate examination. The woman must be assured that the examination will not be disturbed by your colleagues, and a female chaperone must be present. Let her undress behind a screen or curtain and lie on the bed, and ask her to call you when she has done so.

Do not watch her undress and lie down as this is very intimidating. Give her a blanket before she undresses so she can cover her lower half when she lies down. You can remove this blanket when you start the examination.

Endobedogram
Have a good look at the woman:
- Is she obese? Obesity increases the risk of breast and endometrial cancer. It is also a feature of PCOS.
- Is there any hirsutism?
- Does she have signs of a previous mastectomy? If she has had previous breast cancer she may have the gene mutation that predisposes to ovarian cancer.

Table 8.14 *The examination sequence for gynaecology*	
Element	**Details**
Inspection	Are there any vulval abnormalities?
	Is she clinically anaemic?
Palpation	Are there any masses in the abdomen?
	Are there any masses on bimanual examination?
	Is there any cervical motion tenderness?
	Is there any discharge?

Table 8.13 *Common vulval changes*		
	Disease	**Appearance**
Skin changes	Lichen sclerosus	White plaques
	Vulval carcinoma	Ulcerated lesion, usually on labia majora
	Candida infection	Thin white discharge, vulval skin erythematous
	Bartholin cyst	Inflamed swelling medial to labia majora
Urethral changes	Urethral caruncle	Fleshy growth over urethral meatus

Inspection

Check the abdomen for signs of distension. If it is distended, check for signs of ascites (**Table 6.17**). Ask her to bend her legs, keep her feet together, and 'flop' her knees apart to expose the vulva. Examine the vulva for abnormalities.

Bimanual pelvic examination

Apply lubricating gel to your right gloved hand (assuming that you are on the patient's right, as is usual). Advise her that you are about to perform the internal examination, and ask her to relax as much as she is able. Gently insert the second and third digits of the right hand into the vagina (**Figure 8.9**).

> **Make sure your hands are warm before any internal examination.** Cold hands are very uncomfortable for the woman and cause her to involuntarily contract her pelvic floor muscles, making the examination more difficult for you and more painful for her.

Gently palpate the cervix with your fingertips. Assess for cervical motion tenderness by carefully moving the cervix from side to side. This is a sign of PID.

Use your left hand to press on the abdominal wall, towards your right hand fingertips. Attempt to palpate the uterus between your two hands, noting if it feels bulky, correlating to fibroids or malignant masses. Palpate each ovary between your external left hand and internal right hand, noting the estimated size of each.

Withdraw your fingers and check for any blood or abnormal discharge.

Finishing off

Thank the patient and cover her lower half with a blanket. Leave the clinical area to allow her to get dressed.

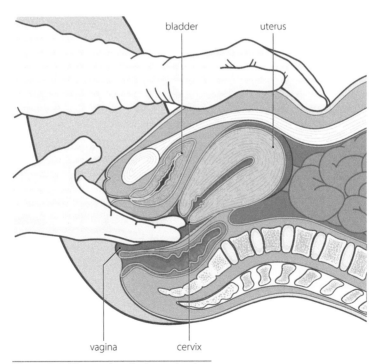

bladder   uterus

vagina   cervix

Figure 8.9 Bimanual vaginal examination.

8.7 Obstetric symptoms and history-taking

The obstetric history detects symptoms of pregnancy that fall outside of the norms, and indicate underlying pathology. Abnormal symptoms during pregnancy indicate problems with either mother or baby.

8.7.1 Symptoms

Many of the symptoms of pregnancy are related to normal physiological changes (**Table 8.1**).

Subfertility

This is failure to conceive despite regular sexual intercourse for 6 months (**Table 8.15**).

Antepartum haemorrhage

This is bleeding from the genital tract during pregnancy. The primary two causes are placenta praevia and placental abruption.

Table 8.15 *Female causes of subfertility*

Cause	Mechanism	Associated features
PCOS	Failure to ovulate	Hirsutism Obesity Insulin resistance Oligo- / amenorrhoea
Endometriosis	Structural changes to reproductive tract	Pelvic pain Menorrhagia Dysmenorrhoea
PID	Inflammation and damage to reproductive tract, especially in cases of chlamydia	May be asymptomatic Increased incidence of ectopic pregnancy Pelvic pain Vaginal discharge
Tobacco smoking	Impaired folliculogenesis and ovulation	Other smoking-related diseases
Underweight	Dysfunction of hypothalamic–pituitary–ovarian axis, resulting in failure to ovulate	Low BMI Oligo- / amenorrhoea
Obesity	Hormonal changes lead to failure to ovulate	High BMI Irregular periods
Iatrogenic	Chemotherapy causes ovarian failure	Other chemotherapy-related effects
Congenital / genetic abnormalities	Gonadal dysgenesis – failure of gonads to develop	Primary amenorrhoea
	Primary ciliary dyskinesia – failure of cilia to convey ovum down fallopian tube	Recurrent pneumonia due to inability to clear respiratory secretions
Hyperprolactinaemia	Suppression of FSH and LH, leading to anovulation	Galactorrhoea Headache if macroprolactinoma

Placenta praevia

This is when the placenta attaches to the lower uterine segment, near the internal os (the upper part of the cervix within the uterine cavity). It presents with painless bleeding.

Placental abruption

The placenta shears away from the uterine wall, causing haemorrhage. The mother develops cardiovascular shock, and the uterus feels hard and 'woody'.

Breathlessness

Many women report breathlessness during pregnancy. Progesterone stimulates the respiratory centres of the brainstem, causing respiratory alkalosis. A full-term foetus causes mild splinting of the diaphragm, limiting tidal volumes.

Sudden onset breathlessness with pleuritic chest pain signifies a pulmonary embolism.

Vomiting

Morning sickness is nausea and vomiting associated with pregnancy. It is normal, and usually occurs between weeks 7 and 12. Hyperemesis gravidarum is an extreme form of pregnancy sickness which requires IV rehydration and anti-emetics.

8.7.2 Taking a history

An obstetric history includes all previous pregnancy events, which include:
- pregnancies carried to term
- pregnancies that were terminated
- pregnancies resulting in miscarriage.

Ask whether any previous pregnancies were complicated by pregnancy-related diseases, including:
- gestational diabetes
- pregnancy-induced hypertension
- thyroid disease of pregnancy
- venous thromboembolism (VTE).

Past medical history

Ask about a history of VTE, as these patients require antenatal anticoagulation. Ask about autoimmune diseases, as these may either deteriorate or improve during pregnancy.

'**Gravida**' is the number of pregnancies a woman has had. '**Parity**' is the number of children a woman has delivered; this is often shorted to 'para'. This shorthand is used frequently in obstetric medicine. For example, a woman who has had one pregnancy that ended in miscarriage and a second pregnancy that resulted in a healthy baby would be described as gravida 2, para 1 (or even 'G2P1').

Medications

Some medications, such as anticonvulsants, are teratogenic and must be stopped during pregnancy. Therefore ask about current medications and those taken prior to pregnancy.

Social history

Explore whether there are social factors that may affect the pregnancy.

Socio-economic status

Women in lower socio-economic groups (with low income, low levels of education and no formal occupation) are at greater risk of:
- postnatal depression
- miscarriage
- perinatal death.

Smoking

Smoking causes intrauterine growth retardation and increases the risk of miscarriage and neonatal death.

Alcohol

It is recommended that women remain alcohol-free during pregnancy, although there is no evidence that infrequent intake is harmful to the foetus. Alcohol excess – drinking every day – leads to foetal alcohol syndrome.

Recreational drugs

Cocaine causes placental abruption. Amphetamines cause gestational hypertension and pre-eclampsia. Opiate abuse causes neonatal abstinence syndrome.

Social support

Social deprivation is a major risk factor for postnatal depression.

Don't make assumptions about whether the woman has a husband or a partner. The expectant mother may or may not be married, may have a male or female partner, or no partner at all; there are all sorts of families.

Family history
Ask about inherited diseases which could affect the foetus.

Systems review
A full systems review is in **Table 8.16**.

Table 8.16 *Systems review when taking an obstetric history*		
System	**Symptoms**	**Obstetric causes**
Cardiovascular	Chest pain	Pulmonary embolism
Respiratory	Breathlessness	Heart failure due to peripartum dilated cardiomyopathy (very rare)
Gastroenterological	Abdominal pain	Pre-eclampsia/HELLP syndrome
Endocrine	Excessive thirst Polyuria	Gestational diabetes
	Palpitations Sweating Insomnia	Thyrotoxicosis of pregnancy

8.8 Obstetric signs and examination

The obstetric examination looks for abnormal signs in the mother and the foetus.

8.8.1 Obstetric signs

The signs of pregnancy are either detectable in the mother (maternal signs), or by palpating the foetus itself (foetal-related signs). Maternal signs are skin changes and hypertension, and foetus-related signs are abnormal uterus size, abnormal position and abnormal lie.

Skin changes
Physiological and pathological skin changes in pregnancy are shown in **Table 8.17**.

Hypertension
This is blood pressure of >140/90mmHg, or 30/20mmHg greater than the blood pressure at the beginning of the pregnancy.

Pregnancy-induced hypertension (PIH)
This is hypertension after 20 weeks' gestation in a woman with no previous blood pressure problems. It results in intrauterine growth retardation, and must be treated with antihypertensives, such as labetalol (a beta blocker).

Pre-eclampsia
This is PIH with proteinuria and peripheral oedema. Proteinuria is detected on a urine dipstick. It occurs in the third trimester. It is associated with poor outcomes for both mother and foetus. A severe form of pre-eclampsia is HELLP syndrome, which stands for:

- **H**aemolytic anaemia
- **E**levated **L**iver enzymes
- **L**ow **P**latelets.

Patients with pre-eclampsia usually complain of headache, and exhibit signs of:

- papilloedema
- brisk tendon reflexes
- decreased conscious level.

Eclampsia
Eclampsia is a life-threatening condition causing maternal seizures resulting from untreated pre-eclampsia. Immediate delivery of the foetus, usually via an emergency caesarian, is mandated.

Table 8.17 *Skin changes in pregnancy*

	Condition	Cause
Physiological	Melasma	This is patches of discolouration that occur in sun-exposed areas in high-oestrogen conditions, including pregnancy. They usually fade several months postpartum, and are considered physiological.
	Linea nigra	This is a pigmented line that runs from the pubis to the umbilicus, and occasionally up to the xiphisternum. It reflects elevated levels of melanocyte-stimulating hormone, that is produced by the placenta. Like melasma, it fades after giving birth. It is a normal finding, affecting 75% of all pregnancies.
	Striae	The majority of women experience striae gravidarum, due to rapid stretching of the abdominal skin.
	Palmar erythema	Reddening of the palms is due to the high oestrogen state of pregnancy and is physiological.
	Excoriations	Obstetric cholestasis is the accumulation of bile salts, affecting 1% of pregnancies. It causes severe itching.
Pathological	Jaundice	Jaundice during pregnancy is always pathological, and signifies liver or gall bladder disease (*Section 6.5.1*)
	Pallor	Iron-deficiency anaemia is common in pregnancy, and is treated with supplemental iron until delivery.

Abnormal uterus size

The size of the uterus on examination is a surrogate for the size of the baby and the amniotic fluid. The uterus size increases throughout the pregnancy and its size is compared to the normal values for the relevant weeks of gestation.

An abnormally large or small uterus is due to abnormalities of the foetus, the amniotic fluid or the uterus itself.

The uterus size is quantified by measuring the symphyseal fundal height (SFH). This is the distance between the pubic symphysis and the uterine fundus. After 20 weeks of gestation the SFH in centimetres should be equivalent to the gestational age of the foetus in weeks, +/- 2cm.

Increased SFH

This is due to one of the following:
- polyhydramnios
- large for gestational age (LGA) foetus
- pre-existing fibroids
- multiple pregnancy.

Polyhydramnios. This is an increased volume of amniotic fluid; the causes are shown in **Table 8.18**.

LGA foetus. This is termed 'macrosomia'. A constitutionally large baby has a genetic predisposition towards a large birth weight (>4000g). The most common pathological cause of macrosomia is maternal hyperglycaemia, due to pre-existing or gestational diabetes. Macrosomic babies are at increased risk of delivery complications.

Pre-existing fibroids. Large fibroids distort the uterine anatomy and result in increased SFH.

Multiple pregnancy. Twins and triplets are identified on antenatal ultrasound.

Decreased SFH

This is due to either:
- oligohydramnios
- small for gestational age (SGA) foetus.

Oligohydramnios. This is a paucity of amniotic fluid; the causes are shown in **Table 8.19**.

Table 8.18 *The causes of polyhydramnios, usually due to impaired foetal swallowing*

Cause	Mechanism
Tracheo-oesophageal fistula	Foetus is unable to swallow amniotic fluid
Duodenal atresia	
Chromosomal abnormalities	Unknown
Brain defects	Impaired swallowing

Table 8.19 *The causes of oligohydramnios*

Cause	Mechanism
Foetal renal defects	Decreased foetal renal excretion of amniotic fluid
Drugs	Maternal ACE inhibitors or ARBs
Post-term babies	After 40 weeks' gestation, the amount of amniotic fluid decreases
Prelabour rupture of membranes	Draining of amniotic fluid from the ruptured amniotic sac through the cervix

SGA foetus. This is a foetus with a size below the 10th centile for its age, which may be due to physiological (i.e. a constitutionally small baby) or pathological factors, such as:
- chromosomal abnormalities
- maternal disease, such as CKD or hypertension
- maternal smoking or alcohol excess.

> **The terms intrauterine growth restriction (IUGR) and small for gestational age (SGA) are often used interchangeably, but actually mean different things.** IUGR indicates a slowing of growth over time, so multiple measurements of foetal size are required. A foetus that has IUGR may not be SGA.

Abnormal lie
The lie of the foetus is the relation of the long axis of the foetus in relation to the mother. It can be (**Figure 8.10**):
- longitudinal (this is the normal lie)
- oblique
- transverse.

Oblique and transverse lies are abnormal, but the foetus often moves to a longitudinal lie before or during labour.

Abnormal position
The position is the direction the foetus is facing, and is described in relation to the occiput. Most babies deliver in the occipitoanterior (OA) position. Occipitoposterior (OP) and occipitotransverse (OT) positions cause longer, complicated labours.

8.8.2 Obstetric examination

The following sequence follows the order of the examination itself (**Table 8.20**). Start with the 'ID CHECK' (*Section 3.2.1*).

Endobedogram
Have a good look at the woman:
- Does she look well or unwell?
- Is there any jaundice or pallor?

Inspection
Hands
Ask her to hold her hands out in front of her.
- Look for tar staining.
- Look for the peripheral stigmata of cardiovascular disease (see *Section 4.XX*)

LONGITUDINAL   OBLIQUE   TRANSVERSE

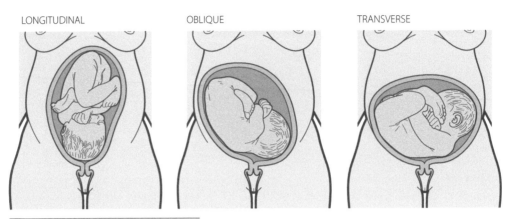

Figure 8.10 The three types of foetal lie.

Table 8.20 *The examination sequence of a pregnant woman*	
Element	**Details**
General inspection	Are there signs of smoking or chronic alcohol abuse?
	Is she breathless?
Wrist	What is the pulse rate and volume?
Arm	What is the BP?
Face	Is there any jaundice or pallor?
Abdomen	Is the SFH in keeping with gestational age?
	What is the lie and position?
	Is the head engaged or unengaged?
Feet	Is there any peripheral oedema?

Face
- Check the sclerae for jaundice and the conjunctivae for pallor.
- Note any patches of melasma (**Figure 8.11**).
- Check for any periorbital swelling, which indicates the generalised oedema of pre-eclampsia.

Blood pressure
Check the BP, to detect pregnancy-induced hypertension.

Abdomen
- Note whether the extent of abdominal distension is consistent with pregnancy.
- Check for the linea nigra and striae. Note if there is a transverse suprapubic scar, in keeping with a previous caesarian section.

Feet
Check for signs of peripheral oedema.

Palpation
Palpation of the abdomen allows you to estimate the size of the uterus.

SFH
With your left hand, palpate the uterine fundus. Start palpation at the xiphisternum and work your way down, until you encounter a firm mass. The uterine fundus becomes palpable in the abdomen at 12 weeks' gestation and at the level of the umbilicus at 20 weeks.

Place the tape measure over the fundus and measure the distance to the pubic symphysis, which is felt as a bony prominence under the mons pubis (**Figure 8.12**).

> **To avoid unconscious bias (i.e. 'making' the height match the gestational age), measure the SFH with the markers and numbers of the tape measure facing down toward the mother.** Once you are satisfied you have accurately measured the distance between the two landmarks, turn the tape measure over to reveal the SFH.

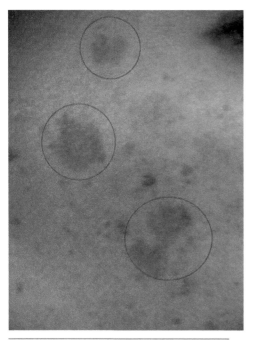

Figure 8.11 The dark skin patches of melasma seen in high oestrogen states (classically pregnancy).

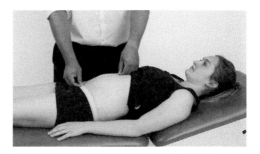

Figure 8.12 Measuring symphyseal-fundal height.

Determining the lie

Palpate the abdomen to establish the foetal lie.

Determining the position

Palpate the abdomen and note the bumps that represent the foetal limbs. Opposite to this, the abdomen feels smooth and 'full', correlating with the back of the foetus. If no limbs are palpated, then the foetus is likely to be in an OA position.

8.8.3 Finishing off

Thank the woman and offer to help her get dressed.

8.9 Common investigations

Gynaecological tests look for infection, malignancy and foetal health (**Table 8.21**).

8.9.1 Mammography

Mammography is X-ray imaging of the breast. It is the investigation used for breast cancer screening programmes internationally. In the UK, women are offered screening every 3 years after the age of 50.

8.9.2 Cervical smear

This is the sampling of cervical cells for analysis. It is the basis for cervical screening programmes. Patients with abnormalities detected on smear testing are referred for colposcopy. This is close macroscopic examination of the cervix (colposcopy) with biopsies. In the UK smear testing is offered every 3 years between the ages of 25 and 49 and every 5 years between ages 50 and 64.

Colposcopy is also performed to allow the practitioner to obtain cervical swabs to check for infection.

8.9.3 Transvaginal ultrasound

This is ultrasound scanning using a probe that is inserted into the vagina. It provides much better imaging resolution of the reproductive tract when compared to transabdominal ultrasound.

8.9.4 Hysteroscopy

A narrow flexible endoscope is passed through the cervix to visualise the interior of the uterus to investigate dysmenorrhoea, pelvic pain and postmenopausal bleeding.

Table 8.21 Common investigations in women's health			
	Investigation	**Benefits**	**Limitations**
Breast	Mammography	Non-invasive and well tolerated	Minimal ionising radiation Low sensitivity and specificity lead to false positive and negative results
Gynaecology	Transvaginal ultrasound	No ionising radiation	Invasive test – may be uncomfortable
	Cervical smear	Sensitive at detecting early malignancy	Invasive test – may be uncomfortable
Obstetrics	Cardiotocography	Non-invasive and well tolerated	Low specificity
	Foetal US	No ionising radiation	May not detect structural abnormalities of internal organs, such as cardiac defects

8.9.5 Foetal ultrasound

All pregnant women undergo transabdominal ultrasound scanning during pregnancy:

■ between 10 and 13 weeks' gestation to confirm normal development and gestational age
■ between 20 and 22 weeks to detect any foetal abnormalities.

8.9.6 Cardiotocography

This provides continuous monitoring the foetus during labour. The cardiogram records the foetal heart rate, and the tocogram monitors uterine contractions. This tracks the foetal heart rate continuously during contractions.

8.10 Answers to starter questions

1. Currently there are no adequate tests to screen for ovarian and uterine cancer. There are adequate tests for breast and ovarian cancer, however: women over the age of 50 are offered screening every 3 years for breast cancer and every 5 for cervical cancer, while women aged 25–48 are offered screening every 5 years for cervical cancer.

2. The effect that menstrual disorders, such as menorrhagia, have on the ability to perform daily activities should not be underestimated. Affected women are in agonising pain for several days or even bleed to such an extent that they cannot leave the house. Women with unpredictable cycles must be constantly vigilant in case they begin their period without having the appropriate sanitary protection available. These issues can cause feelings of embarrassment or shame if a woman is unable to predict the timing and severity of her period.

3. Expectant mothers with diabetes are at risk of several pregnancy complications, including macrosomia (oversized foetus), which causes difficult deliveries and an increased risk of postpartum haemorrhage. Maternal diabetes also increases the risk of congenital anomalies such as foot deformities, heart defects and spinal

malformations, and these women undergo regular screening to detect them.

4. While no adverse effects of minimal alcohol intake (1–2 units per week) during pregnancy have been proven, women should be advised that the safest course of action is to avoid alcohol altogether. Alcohol excess during pregnancy causes foetal alcohol syndrome.

5. Most complications of pregnancy are diagnosed on US or serum testing. However, abnormalities seen during an examination will point towards the diagnosis. For example, measuring SFH reveals whether a foetus is too small or large for its gestational age. Maternal diabetes is confirmed by examining the mother's fingertips for tiny pinpricks that indicate repeated capillary glucose testing (diabetic mothers must test their glucose levels several times a day).

6. Patients are routinely weighed in clinic because many gynaecological disorders are related to being over- or underweight. For examples, obesity is a risk factor for breast cancer, endometrial cancer and PCOS.

Chapter 9
Nervous system

Starter questions

1. Does everyone who has a seizure have epilepsy?
2. How do diseases of the somatic nervous system differ clinically from those of the autonomic nervous system?
3. What is a 'mini-stroke', and is it less serious than a stroke?
4. Why should we always shake our patient's hand?
5. Why don't neurologists use morphine to alleviate pain?

Answers to questions are to be found in *Section 9.8*.

9.1 Introduction

The neurological system detects all incoming information about the world, processes it, then determines a response. This incoming information is a constant stream of data related to pain, touch, vibration, temperature, hearing, sight and balance. These data may trigger a mood, a movement, a thought, or subtle variations in the body's many unconscious processes, such as breathing and pulse rate.

The human nervous system is the most developed of all animals. Due to the complexity of this system, neurological illnesses affect patients in very complex ways. Neurological disorders may be limited to one area, such as loss of hearing in one ear, to system-wide, such as a failure of sensory input from the entire body.

The word 'lesion' is used in neurological medicine to signify the site of disease or dysfunction. A lesion is an area of infarction, degeneration, inflammation, infection, haemorrhage or trauma. Although multiple different lesions in one patient are a possibility, clinical signs and symptoms can usually be linked together in a single unifying diagnosis.

The two critical questions to ask when making a neurological diagnosis are:
- Where is the lesion?
- What is the lesion?

Case 9.1   A patient with a headache

Presentation

Bella is a 24-year-old woman with a history of recurrent headaches. The most recent was two days ago. She is finding these headaches debilitating, and often has to take time off work due to the pain.

Initial interpretation

Headache has many causes. A continuous or slowly worsening headache would indicate a growing lesion within the brain, such as a tumour or idiopathic intracranial hypertension (IIH). IIH is a condition where abnormally large amounts of cerebrospinal fluid accumulate intracerebrally, causing increased pressure and pain. In this case, however, the headaches are intermittent, rather than continuous, so these diagnoses are unlikely. There are several intermittent headache disorders, and we need further history to differentiate between them.

History

The headaches started when Bella was 17 years old. They initially occurred once or twice a year, but now they happen every month. The pain is in the left side, but occasionally her entire head is affected. The pain is throbbing and severe. She feels nauseated, and occasionally vomits. During attacks, she can't bear any noise or bright lights, and has to lie down in a darkened, quiet room. Each attack lasts between 18 and 48 hours. The pain does not respond at all to paracetamol.

Interpretation of history

There are three main differentials at this point. Migraine is a chronic condition characterised by intermittent headaches. The 'classic migraine' is accompanied by neurological deficits, usually a transient visual impairment, called an 'aura'. 'Common migraines' are not accompanied by neurological impairments. Photophobia (intolerance of light) and phonophobia (intolerance of noise) are common features, as are nausea and vomiting. Migraine has a female preponderance.

A second possibility is cluster headache.

This disorder is characterised by 'clusters' of headaches occurring every few months or years. The headache is focused around the eye, is excruciating, and is unresponsive to normal analgesia. The affected eye becomes suffused and congested, with excessive lacrimation. However, a cluster headache usually lasts between 45 and 120 minutes, and has a male preponderance.

A third differential is tension headache. This is an episodic headache that causes a global sensation of pressure around the head. It is associated with psychological stress and sleep deprivation. It is not usually severe enough to cause the level of incapacitation experienced by Bella.

Further history

For the last two years each headache has been preceded by strange visual abnormalities. She sees vague flashing lights in the periphery of her vision, often accompanied by the impression of coloured lines in the far distance. When she experiences these visual changes, she knows that the headache is imminent.

She has not noticed that the pain is situated around the eye, nor had any excessive lacrimation or conjunctival injection. She cannot think of any triggers to the headache, although she realises on reflection that they occur around her period.

Examination

General examination of the patient reveals a slim young woman. Examination of the central and peripheral nervous system is completely normal, as is full examination of the cranial nerves. Fundoscopy is normal.

Interpretation of findings

Most headache disorders do not present any abnormal clinical findings in between attacks. The absence of papilloedema (swelling of the optic disc) on fundoscopy is reassuring that raised intracranial pressure is not the culprit here. Additionally, IIH is much more common in overweight patients.

Case 9.1 *continued*

Investigations

Blood testing is normal. A CT scan of the brain is performed, which is also normal.

Diagnosis

Bella has a diagnosis of migraine. She has the features of classical migraine, with a visual aura followed by a pain phase. Like many young female sufferers, her symptoms are linked to menstruation. The pathophysiology of migraine is poorly understood, and transient dysfunction of neurochemical pathways and changes to the cerebral vasculature are possible causes.

Treatment involves:
- prevention of attacks
- propranolol (a beta blocker) and topiramate (an anticonvulsant), which have proven to be the most effective medications for acute migraine prevention
- early termination of acute attacks

- early administration of triptans, which is effective in aborting an acute attack; triptans are tryptamine-based drugs that can be taken as a pill, or a nasal spray if the patient is vomiting
- analgesia during acute attacks
- a combination of paracetamol, aspirin and NSAIDs, which are most effective for pain relief
- anti-emetics are often required.

Other concerns

Young women with classical migraines with an aura are at higher risk of developing deep vein thrombosis (DVT). The risk is elevated even further if they take the combined oral contraceptive pill (OCP).

Topiramate, like most anticonvulsants, is teratogenic (causes foetal abnormalities). Women of childbearing age should take contraceptive precautions with topiramate. This is frustrating to patients, as the OCP is contraindicated.

Hemiplegic migraines are a rare and severe form of migraine. They are associated with transient weakness affecting one side of the body, mimicking an acute stroke.

9.2 System overview

The nervous system is divided anatomically into the central nervous system (CNS), composed of the brain and the spinal cord, and the peripheral nervous system (PNS), composed of nerve roots and peripheral nerves (**Figure 9.1**).

The PNS is also divided functionally into the somatic and autonomic system.
- The somatic nervous system is responsible for sensation and voluntary movements.
- The autonomic nervous system controls homeostasis and unconscious processes.

The cranial nerves and ophthalmology are discussed in detail in *Chapter 10*.

9.2.1 Central nervous system

The brain

The brain is the control centre of the body. It receives all sensory information and instigates voluntary and involuntary movement. It is the seat of 'higher order' functions, such as decision-making, mood, cognition and complex planning. It interacts with all hormonal axes of the body, thus controlling digestion, metabolism and respiration. The main structures are the cerebrum, cerebellum, basal ganglia, thalamus and brainstem.

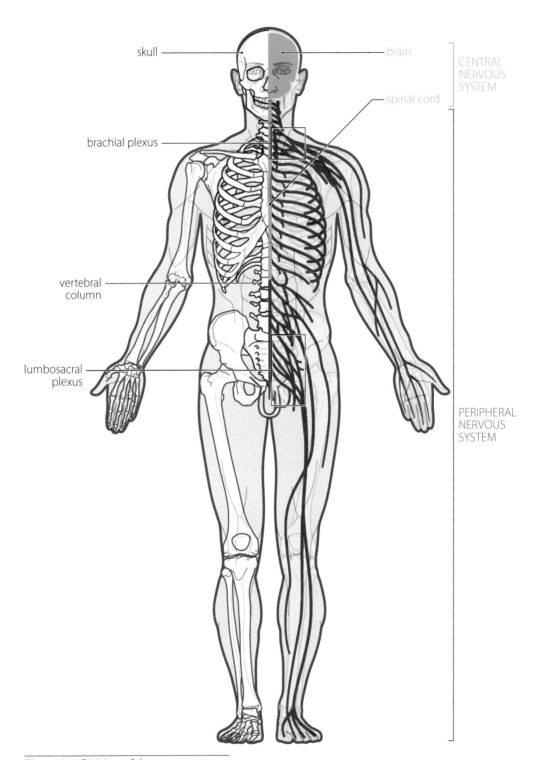

Figure 9.1 Divisions of the nervous system.

Cerebrum

This is divided into separate lobes (**Figure 9.2**):

Frontal lobe. This is responsible for:

- executive function, decision-making and making judgements
- controlling voluntary body movements
- speech formation (in Broca's area).

Disease of the frontal lobe causes:

- motor weakness
- personality change, disinhibition, socially incongruous behaviour
- expressive dysphasia.

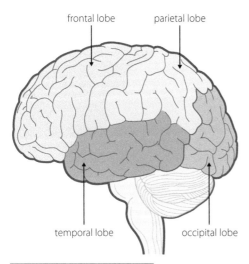

Figure 9.2 Lobes of the brain.

Temporal lobe. This is responsible for:

- processing auditory information
- memory creation
- language comprehension (in Wernicke's area).

Disease of the temporal lobe results in:

- complex hallucinations
- receptive dysphasia.

Normal speech involves Broca's area and Wernicke's area. Patients with lesions of Wernicke's area are unable to interpret speech, so hear spoken language as incomprehensible gibberish (receptive dysphasia). Patients with lesions of Broca's area are unable to formulate speech and speak either unintelligibly (expressive dysphasia) or cannot speak at all (aphasia).

Parietal lobe. This is responsible for processing sensory information. Disease of the parietal lobe results in sensory loss and dyspraxia (inability to sequence complex motor tasks).

Occipital lobe. This is responsible for processing visual information from the retinas. Disease of the occipital lobe results in visual loss.

Brainstem

The brainstem sits at the base of the brain. It controls basic, unconscious bodily functions, including:

- respiratory rate and tidal volumes
- heart rate
- sleeping and wakefulness.

It also contains the nucleus of several of the cranial nerves (see *Section 10.2.1*).

Motor and sensory fibres cross over from left to right (and vice versa) at different points in the brainstem (with the exception of pain fibres, which cross over within the cord). The right cerebral hemisphere controls and responds to the left side of the body and vice versa. The exception to this is the cerebellum. Each cerebellar hemisphere controls the ipsilateral side of the body.

Spinal cord

The cord is a large bundle that carries fibres between the brain and peripheral nervous system. There are 31 segments, each named after their corresponding vertebra. Each segment has a left and right spinal nerve root, which carries motor impulses from the cord to the body, and sensory inputs from the body to the cord (**Figure 9.3**).

Vertical tracts within the cord carry sensory nerve fibres up towards the brain, and motor fibres down to the body (**Figure 9.4**):

- The spinothalamic tract carries pain and temperature sensation.
- The dorsal column carries fine touch and vibration sensation.
- The corticospinal tract carries motor impulses.

Lesions of different anatomical sites within a cord segment therefore result in different clinical signs (**Figure 9.5**).

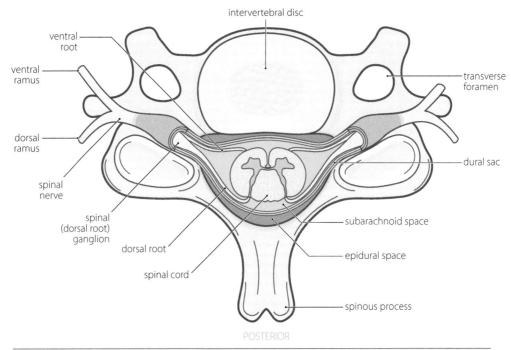

Figure 9.3 Cross-section of the cervical spine. The spinal cord sits within the bony vertebra. The dorsal root carries sensory information from the PNS, and the ventral root carries motor impulses from the brain. These two roots combine to form the spinal nerve.

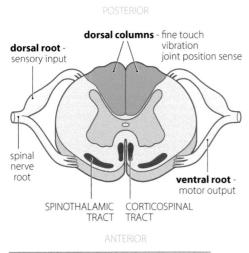

Figure 9.4 Cross-section of the spinal cord showing the motor and sensory tracts.

Lesions of the spinal cord can be:

- traumatic: such as following a severe car accident
- infarction: occlusion of a spinal artery (also known as a spinal stroke)
- inflammatory: multiple sclerosis (MS) is a condition that causes patches of inflammation in different sites in the CNS
- infective: some diseases cause a transverse myelitis (inflammation across the entire cord segment), such as Lyme disease and HIV
- neoplastic: primary tumours of the spine are rare, but it is a common site of metastasis. Metastases cause compression of the spinal cord.

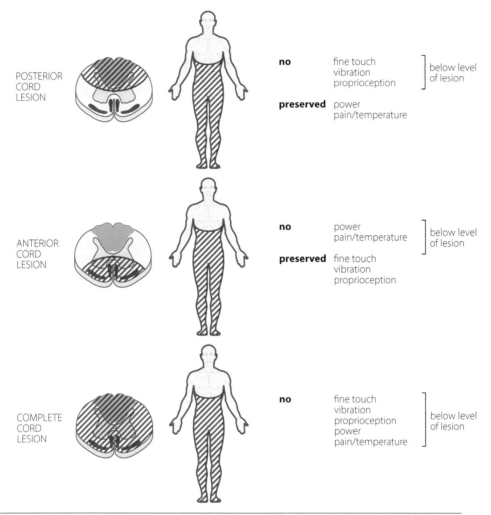

Figure 9.5 Lesions of different anatomical sites within a cord segment (in this example, T6) result in different clinical signs.

9.2.2 Peripheral nervous system

The spinal nerve roots are named after their originating segment:
- 8 cervical nerves (C1–C8)
- 12 thoracic nerves (T1–T12)
- 5 lumbar nerves (L1–L5)
- 5 sacral nerves (S1–S5).

The cord terminates at vertebrae L2–3, and the remaining spinal nerve roots form the cauda equina ('horse's tail') (**Figure 9.6**).

The spinal nerve roots are composed of:

- afferent pathways, which transmit sensory information from the dorsal peripheral nerves to the dorsal horn of the spinal cord
- efferent pathways, which transmit motor signals from the ventral horn to the peripheral nerves.

Use the acronym **SAD-MEV** to remember the anatomy and function of the spinal nerve roots:
- **S**ensory, **A**fferent, **D**orsal
- **M**otor, **E**fferent, **V**entral

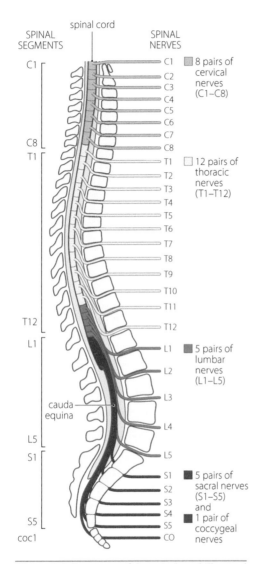

spinal cord

SPINAL SEGMENTS	SPINAL NERVES	
C1	C1	■ 8 pairs of cervical nerves (C1–C8)
	C2	
	C3	
	C4	
	C5	
	C6	
	C7	
C8	C8	
T1	T1	□ 12 pairs of thoracic nerves (T1–T12)
	T2	
	T3	
	T4	
	T5	
	T6	
	T7	
	T8	
	T9	
	T10	
	T11	
T12	T12	
L1	L1	■ 5 pairs of lumbar nerves (L1–L5)
	L2	
cauda equina	L3	
	L4	
L5	L5	
S1	S1	■ 5 pairs of sacral nerves (S1–S5) and
	S2	
	S3	
	S4	■ 1 pair of coccygeal nerves
S5	S5	
coc1	CO	

Figure 9.6 Segments of the spinal cord. The cord terminates between L2 and L3.

Sensory pathways

The sensory pathways begin in the sensory receptors in the skin and joints.

■ Skin receptors detect pain, temperature, fine touch and vibration.

■ Joint receptors detect the joint position and movement (proprioception).

Sensory impulses are transmitted via the peripheral nerves and nerve roots to the spine, where they are conveyed via spinal pathways to the parietal lobe.

Each spinal nerve receives sensory input from a different area of the skin. These areas are called dermatomes. Spinal nerves combine to make up peripheral nerves. When assessing sensory loss, mapping out the affected areas of skin reveals whether there is a nerve root problem (causing sensory loss in a dermatomal pattern) or a peripheral nerve problem (sensory loss in the distribution of a peripheral nerve) (**Figure 9.7**).

Motor pathways

Motor pathways begin in the motor cortex in the frontal lobe. They pass down the corticospinal tract in the anterior cord to the ventral horn of the relevant cord segment. The motor neurons in the brain and the cord are upper motor neurons. Motor impulses pass down the spinal nerve root to the peripheral nerve, terminating at the neuromuscular junction (NMJ). Motor neurons between the ventral horn and the NMJ are lower motor neurons.

Myotomes are groups of muscles that perform one movement, such as elbow flexion. Each myotome is innervated by a spinal nerve, whereas a peripheral nerve innervates one particular muscle. When assessing motor loss, mapping out the pattern of muscle weakness reveals whether there is a lesion of the spinal nerve or the peripheral nerve (**Tables 9.1** and **9.2**). Lesions of the spinal nerve will usually have a corresponding dermatome sensation loss.

9.2.3 Cognitive function

Cognitive neurology incorporates recognition, thought and reasoning processes, speech and comprehension, and memory. The major components are explored in **Table 9.3**.

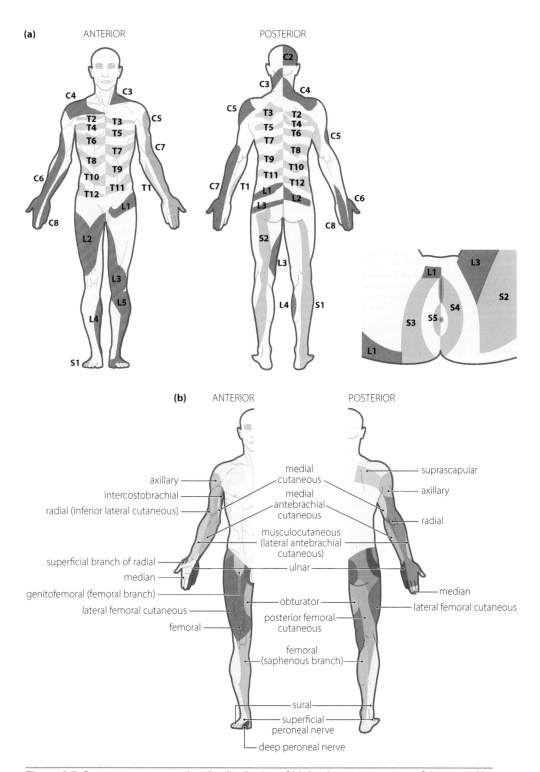

Figure 9.7 Sensory maps comparing the distribution of (a) the dermatomes, areas of skin sensed by each spinal nerve, and (b) the peripheral nerves.

Table 9.1 *Spinal nerves and their associated dermatomes*

Peripheral nerve	Nerve roots	Motor innervation	Sensory innervation
Median nerve	C5–T1	Forearm flexors Muscles of the thenar eminence	Lateral 2½ fingers on palmar aspect
Ulnar nerve	C8, T1	Small muscles of the hand, except those supplied by median nerve	4th/5th fingers and medial border of the hand
Radial nerve	C5–T1	Triceps Brachoradialis Forearm extensors	Lateral aspect of dorsum of hand
Musculocutaneous nerve	C5–C7	Biceps brachii Brachialis	Lateral surface of forearm (as the lateral cutaneous nerve of the forearm)
Sciatic nerve	L4–S3	Anterior and lateral muscles of thigh	Foot Lower leg (except medial border)
Branches of the sciatic nerve:			
Common peroneal nerve	L4–S2	Anterior and lateral lower leg muscles	Lateral lower leg
Tibial nerve	L4–S3	Calf muscles	Lateral sole Lateral 1½ toes
Femoral nerve	L2–L4	Anterior thigh / knee extensors	Anterior and medial thigh Medial lower leg
Obturator nerve	L2–L4	Thigh adductors	Medial thigh

Table 9.2 *Spinal nerves and their associated myotomes*

Spinal nerve	Movement	Spinal nerve	Movement
C5	Shoulder abduction	L3	Knee extension
C6	Elbow flexion	L4	Ankle dorsiflexion
C7	Elbow extension	L5	Big toe extension and ankle dorsiflexion
C8	Wrist flexion		
T1	Finger abduction	S1	Ankle plantarflexion
L2	Hip flexion	S2	Knee flexion

Table 9.3 *Disorders of cognitive function and their features*

Cognitive function	Areas of CNS affected	Clinical features
Language	Wernicke's area	Incomprehension of language
	Broca's area	Inability to form language
Decision-making and problem-solving	Frontal lobe	Impaired executive function
Memory	Complex synergistic processes mainly in the frontal and temporal lobe	Impaired creation and retrieval of memories
Praxis 'the doing of things'	Prefrontal area of frontal lobe	Dyspraxia – inability to sequence and complete complex motor tasks
Gnosis 'the knowing of things'	Parietal lobe	Stereoagnosia – the inability to recognise familiar objects by touch
	Fusiform gyrus in occipitotemporal lobes	Prosopagnosia – the inability to recognise familiar faces
	Parieto-occipital area	Agnosia – the inability to recognise familiar objects

9.3 Symptoms of neurological disease

The commonest features are weakness, impaired coordination, impaired sensation, cognitive disorders, headaches, seizures and gait disorders.

9.3.1 Weakness

Muscular weakness is due to a lesion of the upper or lower motor neurons. Upper motor and lower motor weakness have different characteristics.

Noting the pattern of the weakness will point you towards the location of the lesion or lesions (**Table 9.4**).

Patterns of weakness

Determine whether the weakness pattern is compatible with a single neurological lesion (**Table 9.5**) (**Figure 9.8**).

Table 9.4 *Comparing UMN and LMN lesions*

	UMN lesion	LMN lesion
Tone	Increased – spastic or rigid	Decreased – flaccid
Power (strength)	Reduced	Reduced
Reflexes	Exaggerated	Diminished / absent
Fasciculations	Absent	Present
Plantar reflex	Extensor	Flexor
Clonus	Present	Absent

Table 9.5 *Patterns of weakness*

Pattern	Affected areas	Causes	Common diseases
Hemiparesis	Only the left or the right side of the body affected	Unilateral cerebral infarction	Stroke
		Unilateral cerebral mass	Brain tumour
			Intracranial bleed
		Unilateral cerebral inflammation	Multiple sclerosis
Proximal weakness	Weakness of the proximal muscles, with normal power in the distal groups	Proximal myopathy	Endocrinopathy
			Hyperthyroidism
			Hypercortisolism
			Myositis
			Long-term steroid treatment
			Genetic muscular dystrophy
Peripheral weakness	Peripheral neuropathy	Peripheral axonal damage	Diabetes mellitus
			Chronic alcohol abuse
		Peripheral demyelination	Guillain–Barré syndrome
Fatiguable weakness	Power that gets worse with repeated movement	NMJ damage	Myasthenia gravis
Lower limb weakness (paraparesis)	Weakness of legs, with sparing of arms, due to lesion within vertebral column	Flaccid paraparesis due to cauda equina disease	Cauda equina syndrome
		Spastic paraparesis due to spinal cord disease	Spinal trauma
			Multiple sclerosis
			Spinal metastases
Localised weakness	One muscle affected	Mononeuropathy	Neural trauma
			Neural inflammation
	One muscle group affected	Spinal nerve root disease (radiculopathy)	Nerve root compression due to degenerative spinal disease

Hemiparesis

This is paralysis of either left or right side of the body. It is due to a lesion in the brain. Lesions in the right cerebral hemisphere cause left hemiparesis, and vice versa.

The commonest cause of hemiparesis is a stroke. Less common causes are brain tumour, brain trauma, or cerebral inflammation due to multiple sclerosis.

Stroke. A stroke causes a sudden neurological deficit. The deficits are dependent on the area of brain affected, but the commonest signs include:

- acute slurred speech (dysarthria)
- acute hemiparesis
- acute receptive dysphasia.

Unless the brainstem is involved, the patient retains consciousness throughout. Most strokes are ischaemic, caused by sudden lack of cerebral

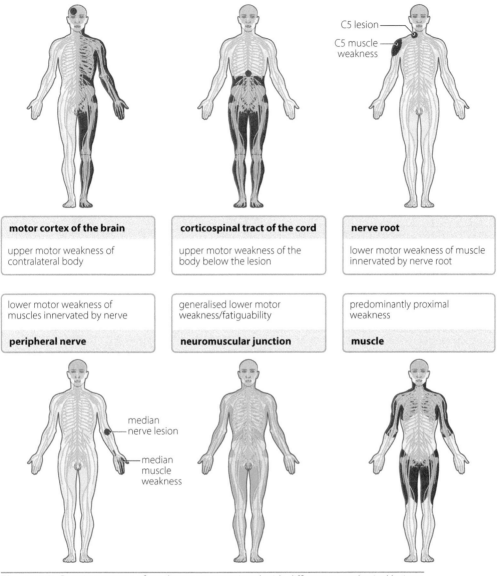

motor cortex of the brain	corticospinal tract of the cord	nerve root
upper motor weakness of contralateral body	upper motor weakness of the body below the lesion	lower motor weakness of muscle innervated by nerve root

lower motor weakness of muscles innervated by nerve	generalised lower motor weakness/fatiguability	predominantly proximal weakness
peripheral nerve	**neuromuscular junction**	**muscle**

Figure 9.8 Certain patterns of weakness are associated with different neurological lesions.

blood flow. Less common are haemorrhagic strokes, due to a spontaneous intracerebral bleed.

Paraparesis

This is leg weakness with sparing of the arms. It is either flaccid or spastic paraparesis. It is due to a lesion of the spinal cord or the cauda equina.

Flaccid paraparesis. This is due to a lower motor lesion. Cauda equina syndrome is caused by compression of the cauda equina. It comprises:

- flaccid tone
- weakness
- reduced or absent reflexes
- flexor plantar response
- bladder or bowel sphincter dysfunction
- sensory loss in the L2–S5 dermatomes – 'saddle anaesthesia'.

Spastic paraparesis. An upper motor lesion affecting the legs indicates bilateral cord disease. The patient will have:

- spastic tone
- weakness
- hyperreflexia
- extensor plantar response
- clonus.

If the entire cord is affected, the patient will also have sensory loss below the level of the lesion.

Localised weakness

This is suggestive of either spinal nerve pathology or a peripheral mononeuropathy – only one nerve is affected (**Table 9.5**). Mononeuropathies are usually due to mild trauma (neuropraxia) (**Table 9.6**).

Non-traumatic mononeuropathies are usually caused by systemic inflammatory diseases, probably due to microcirculatory defects to the nerve. A useful mnemonic to remember the causes of mononeuropathy is **WARDS PLC**:

- **W**egener's disease (granulomatosis with polyangiitis)
- **A**myloidosis
- **R**heumatoid arthritis
- **D**iabetes
- **S**arcoidosis
- **P**olyarteritis nodosa
- **L**eprosy
- **C**hurg–Strauss disease (eosinophilic granulomatosis with polyangiitis) / carcinomatosis.

Fatiguable weakness

Patients have normal muscle strength, but become profoundly weak if they repeat the movement. It is the hallmark of myasthena gravis, an autoimmune disease of the NMJ. Patients struggle to chew food, as their muscles of mastication weaken with repeated contraction. Patients also report double vision (diplopia) and a quiet voice towards the end of the day, as their extra-ocular muscles and laryngeal muscle fatigue.

9.3.2 Poor coordination

Coordination is controlled by the cerebellum, which constantly receives motor input from the cerebrum and ensures motor functions are carried out smoothly.

Disease of the cerebellum causes dyscoordination, tremor, gait abnormalities (ataxia), unwanted movements of the limbs (dyskinesia), abnormal tone (dystonia) and loss of balance.

Causes of cerebellar disease are:

- chronic alcohol excess
- phenytoin (an anti-epileptic)
- rare inherited diseases, including Friedreich's ataxia and spinocerebellar ataxia
- cerebellar strokes
- cerebellar tumours.

Table 9.6 *Common traumatic mononeuropathies and their clinical features*

Nerve affected	Common causes	Motor dysfunction	Sensory loss
Ulnar	Trauma to nerve at the posterior elbow (to the 'funny bone')	Weakness of finger abduction	Medial 2 fingers
Radial	Trauma to the nerve at the posterior mid-humerus	Weakness of wrist extension	Dorsum hand – lateral aspect
Median	Compression in the carpal tunnel in the wrist (carpal tunnel syndrome)	Weakness of thumb abduction	Lateral 3 fingers
Peroneal	Trauma to nerve in the lateral knee	Weakness of ankle plantarflexion ('foot drop')	Lateral lower leg
Femoral	Pelvic fracture	Weakness of knee extension	Anterior thigh

Other causes of poor coordination are:

- acute intoxication
- sensory ataxia: impaired proprioception means patients cannot ascertain their body position in space
- vestibular disorders (see *Section 10.6.8*).

9.3.3 Impaired sensation

This signifies a lesion in the pathway between the sensory receptors in the skin and the brain (**Table 9.7**).

A peripheral sensory neuropathy is known as a 'glove and stocking' neuropathy due to its anatomical distribution. They are a consequence of multisystem disease, as peripheral nerves are more vulnerable to microcirculatory damage (**Table 9.8**).

9.3.4 Cognitive disorders

Disorders of cognition are either due to a discrete lesion in the brain (**Table 9.3**) or a more global dysfunction, such as dementia or delirium.

> **Lesion of a spinal nerve root is called a radiculopathy.** The primary symptom of a radiculopathy is pain along the corresponding dermatome. Other symptoms are dermatomal numbness and myotomal weakness. Nerve roots are vulnerable to compression as they exit the spinal cord, due to degenerative spine disease or an intervertebral spinal disc herniation (a 'slipped disc').

9.3.5 Headache

Migraines develop over hours, whereas headaches due to growing intracranial lesions have an insidious onset over days and weeks (**Figure 9.9**).

Raised intracranial headaches are much worse in the mornings. They are associated with nausea. The pain worsens when patients increase their intracranial pressure by coughing, sneezing, laughing or straining on the toilet (**Table 9.9**). The pain is worse when lying flat, as this increases intracranial pressure. Causes of raised intracranial pressure include tumours, slow venous bleeds or IIP.

Table 9.7 *Patterns of sensory impairment and their causes*

Pattern of sensory impairment	Site of lesion	Other features
Dermatomal pattern	Radiculopathy: damage or compression of a nerve root as it leaves the spinal column	Pain along the affected dermatome Weakness in associated myotome
Region of a peripheral nerve	Mononeuropathy	Motor dysfunction of affected nerve
Hemisensory loss	Cerebral hemisphere	Associated hemiparesis
'Glove and stocking' distribution	Peripheries of arms and legs	Legs are more affected May be associated with peripheral motor neuropathy
Pain / temperature below a specific dermatome	Anterior spinal cord	May have sphincter dysfunction Associated upper motor paresis below affected cord segment
Fine touch / vibration / proprioception below a specific dermatome	Posterior spinal cord	May have sphincter dysfunction

Table 9.8 *Causes of peripheral neuropathy*	Axonal	Demyelinating
Acute onset	Rare axonal forms of Guillain–Barré syndrome	Guillain–Barré syndrome: rare disease leading to acute immune-mediated destruction of nerves
Chronic onset	Chronic alcohol abuse Diabetes mellitus Vitamin B12 deficiency Chronic renal failure Drugs Hereditary sensorimotor neuropathy	Chronic inflammatory demyelinating polyneuropathy: autoimmune inflammation and demyelinating disease affecting peripheral nerves Hereditary sensorimotor neuropathy

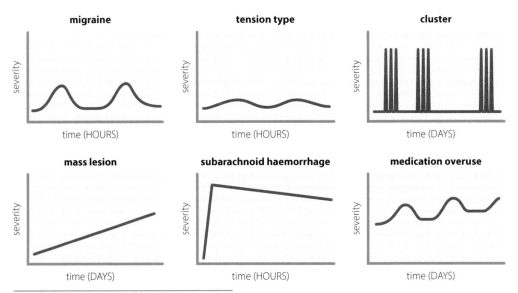

Figure 9.9 The timings of different headaches.

The 'thunderclap' headache goes from non-existent to maximum pain in seconds, and is due to a subarachnoid haemorrhage – a sudden arterial bleed in the subarachnoid space around the brain. The pain is usually combined with features of meningism: photophobia, neck stiffness and vomiting. Thunderclap headaches are spontaneous, without head trauma, and are a neurosurgical emergency.

9.3.6 Seizures

If the patient presents with seizures, ask them how they know they had a seizure; it is impossible to know without a witness history (**Table 9.10**). Non-epileptic attack disorder (NEAD - sometimes referred to as 'pseudoseizures') is a functional disorder characterised by attacks that look very similar to epileptic seizures.

Table 9.9 Causes and features of headache			
Headache type	**Cause**	**Character of pain**	**Associated features**
Migraine	Likely neurochemical changes in the cerebrum	Throbbing, pulsing	Phonophobia Photophobia Vomiting
Raised intracranial pressure	Tumour Bleed IIH	Global Worse on Valsalva manoeuvres	Abducens nerve palsy Visual changes due to papilloedema Vomiting
Cluster headache	Unknown	Sharp, piercing, 'boring through the eye'	Ipsilateral lacrimation and nasal congestion
Tension headache	Psychological stress Sleep deprivation	Pressure Bilateral	Fatigue Irritability
Temporal arteritis	Vasculitis of cranial vessels	Unilateral, temporal area	Jaw claudication Visual loss if severe Polymyalgia rheumatica
Facial pain			
Sinus disease	Infection Allergy Polyp formation	Pressure and pain over affected sinus	Cough Sore throat Nasal congestion
Trigeminal neuralgia	Vascular compression of trigeminal nerve	Stabbing 'electric shocks'	Exacerbated by touching face

There are different types of epileptic seizures which have different clinical phenotypes (**Table 9.11**).

Seizures are usually idiopathic. However, they also result from a state of severe metabolic dysfunction, such as:

- hypoglycaemia
- hypoxia
- electrolyte derangement
- fever
- severe acidosis
- drug overdose
- hepatic encephalopathy.

They are also associated with an acute brain injury, such as intracranial bleed, or head trauma or chronic brain structural damage. For this reason, they are more common in patients who have experienced:

- stroke
- brain surgery
- brain tumours.

A patient suffering a single unprovoked seizure must inform the DVLA immediately and desist from driving for 6 months.

Table 9.10 *Obtaining a witness history of a seizure to differentiate between true seizures and non-epileptic attack disorder (NEAD)*

Questions	Epileptic seizure	NEAD
How was the patient before the seizure?	Triggered by periods of physiological stress, e.g. infection, sleep deprivation	Triggered by emotional or psychological distress
Did the patient slump to the floor, or collapse outright?	Sudden, unpreventable collapse Patient often sustains injuries	Usually non-injurious to the patient
What did the patient look like during the event?	Jerking movements of limbs Partial seizures may retain some level of consciousness Unresponsive and mute Often cyanosed	Jerking movements of limbs Unresponsive, may cry out Eyes closed, resists eye opening
Did the patient bite their tongue or become incontinent of urine?	Common	Uncommon
What was the patient like after the attack?	Post-ictal state: withdrawn, irritable, disoriented, confused Severe headache Sleepy	Oriented, able to engage in conversation
Can the patient remember the attack?	No memory of the attack Retrograde amnesia (no memory of events leading up to the seizure)	Able to recall the attack

Table 9.11 *Comparing different types of epilepsy*

Seizure type	Features	Consciousness
Partial seizures		
Simple	Focal motor or sensory symptoms	Maintained
Complex	Automatisms, such as lip smacking, plucking at clothes, chewing	Impaired
Generalised seizures		
Tonic	Generalised hypertonia	Impaired
Clonic	Generalised limb jerking	Impaired
Tonic-clonic	Mixture of hypertonia and limb jerking	Impaired
Absence	Vacant stare, unresponsive	Impaired

9.3.7 Gait disorders

This is a change in the way the patient walks. Normal gait results from complex interactions between the sensory, motor, coordination and vestibular sections of the nervous system.

Common gait disorders are listed in **Table 9.12**.

Table 9.12 *Gait disorders*

Gait	Description	Cause
Ataxic	Broad-based, unsteady Staggering	Cerebellar disease
Festinant	Stooped posture Small shuffling steps Reduced / absent arm swing	Parkinson's disease Parkinsonian syndromes
Myopathic	Tilting pelvis side to side to lift each leg off the floor 'Waddling'	Proximal myopathy / weakness of hip girdle muscles
Antalgic	'Dot-dash' walking: short time on one leg, longer time on the other	Pain in affected leg
Foot drop	High stepping gait on the affected side so dropped foot can clear the floor	L4 lesion Common peroneal nerve palsy Peripheral neuropathy Cauda equina syndrome
Sensory gait	'Stamping' gait	Proprioception loss in peripheral neuropathy

9.4 The neurological history

Remember that neurological terms have different meanings in lay terms. For example, the phrase 'loss of power' is quite confusing for patients, and 'headache' often denotes pain anywhere between the neck and the face.

9.4.1 Past medical history

Ask about hypertension, diabetes and high cholesterol, as these are risk factors for stroke disease.

Ask whether they ever had a seizure before – even as a child. Febrile convulsions in infancy are linked to epilepsy in later life.

Ask about immunodeficiency syndromes. Immunocompromised patients are at higher risk of developing CNS infections.

9.4.2 Medications

Make note of anti-epileptics, and ask about compliance (**Table 9.13**). Some patients do not take their medication due to intolerable side-effects. Poor medication compliance is the commonest cause of seizures in known epileptics.

If the patient reports headaches, ask if they are taking regular analgesia, how much and how frequently. Medication overuse headache is a paradoxical syndrome that occurs as a side-effect of regular analgesia, including paracetamol, NSAIDs and opiate-based medications. The only treatment is to stop all analgesics for a period of weeks – a prospect that horrifies patients with the condition. The cause is unknown.

Drug	Side-effect
Table 9.13 *Common anti-epileptics and their side-effects*	
Drug	**Side-effect**
Carbamazepine	Teratogenic
	Aplastic anaemia
	Agranulocytosis
Sodium valproate	Teratogenic
	Deranged liver function
Topiramate	Teratogenic
	Weight loss
	Fatigue
Levetiracetam	Fatigue
	Neuropsychiatric symptoms, e.g. agitation, depression
Phenytoin	Teratogenic
	Gum hyperplasia
	Excess body hair

Antipsychotic medications often cause parkinsonian symptoms, due to impaired dopamine transmission. Signs include rigidity, tremor and tardive dyskinesia (repetitive movements such as lip smacking).

> **Many anti-epileptic medications are also used as mood stabilising drugs** in psychiatric disorders, particularly bipolar affective disorder. If a patient takes anti-epileptic drugs (AEDs), do not assume that they have epilepsy.

9.4.3 Social history

This explores the ways in which the patient and their lifestyle and environment interact with their medical conditions.

Smoking

Tobacco smoking is the biggest independent risk factor for cerebrovascular disease.

Alcohol

Excessive alcohol has multiple deleterious effects on the nervous system:

- axonal injury to peripheral nerves, causing peripheral neuropathy
- neurotoxic effects to the brain and cord
- Wernicke's encephalopathy
- cerebellar degeneration, causing ataxia, speech problems and dyscoordination
- alcohol withdrawal: agitation, tremor, sweating, vomiting and tachycardia – if left untreated, it progresses to delirium tremens: visual hallucinations, seizures and even death.

> **Wernicke's encephalopathy** is a reversible disease due to thiamine (vitamin B1) deficiency and alcohol abuse. It is a triad of:
> - ophthalmoplegia (disorder of eye movements)
> - ataxia
> - confusion.
>
> If untreated, it progresses to Korsakoff's syndrome, an irreversible neuropsychiatric disorder characterised by the inability to create new memories. This disability leads the sufferer to invent explanations and events to cover their inability to remember (confabulation).

Illicit drugs

There is increasing evidence that chronic use of psychoactive drugs such as cannabis and lysergic acid diethylamide (LSD) leads to impairments of higher cognitive function.

Functional capacity

Chronic neurological diseases are associated with severe disabilities. Neurodegenerative diseases lead to an irreversible decline in function which requires regular reassessments of the patient's care requirements.

Enquire how the patient is currently living their day-to-day life, paying particular attention to:

- how they cope with their activities of daily living
- whether they require carers, and if so, how many and how often
- how they transfer from bed to chair – do they need a hoist?

In patients with an intractable neurological decline, addressing their functional capacity and ability to enjoy life is the most useful thing a doctor can do.

9.4.4 Family history

Hereditary neurological diseases include:

- Huntington's disease: early dementia and severe chorea (jerky involuntary movements)
- hereditary sensorimotor neuropathy: inherited peripheral neuropathy
- myotonic dystrophy: a chronic disease causing progressive muscle wasting and myotonia (inability to relax muscles).

9.4.5 Systems review

Ask about other symptoms the patient has noticed, which are related to a neurological problem (**Table 9.14**).

Table 9.14 *Full systems review*		
System	**Symptoms**	**Neurological causes**
Respiratory	Breathlessness	Respiratory muscle weakness
GI	Dysphagia	Weakness of pharyngeal and oesophageal muscles
	Faecal incontinence	Sphincter dysfunction due to sacral nerve / spinal cord disease
Genitourinary	Overactive bladder	Autonomic detrusor dysfunction
	Urinary incontinence	Sphincter dysfunction due to sacral nerve / spinal cord disease

9.5 Signs of neurological disease

9.5.1 Skin changes

There are two major neurocutaneous disorders: neurofibromatosis and tuberous sclerosis.

Neurofibromatosis

This is an inherited condition (**Figure 9.10**), consisting of:

- multiple 'café-au-lait spots' on body (dark pigmentation)
- numerous neurofibromas
- axillary freckling
- learning difficulties
- epilepsy.

Tuberous sclerosis

This is a rare multisystem disease, consisting of:

- abnormal cerebral growths
- facial adenofibromas (red bumps)
- 'ash leaf spots' – areas of hypopigmentation on the body
- learning difficulties
- epilepsy.

9.5.2 Abnormal tone

Tone is the muscle's resting state. Normal muscle tone aids body position and posture, and offers a slight resistance to passive stretching. Hypertonic muscles are contracted, and hypotonic muscles are soft and 'floppy'.

Causes

Hypertonia

Disease of upper motor neurons causes increased tone. There are two types of hypertonia: spastic and rigid (**Table 9.15**).

Spastic hypertonia. This is caused by diseases of the brain or corticospinal tract.

Spastic muscles exhibit a 'clasp-knife' response to stretch: the muscle will be hypertonic up until a certain point of extension, and then will give way.

> In the upper limbs, spastic hypertonia affects the flexor muscles more than the extensors, so the patient holds their arm in a fixed flexed position.
>
> In the lower limbs, spastic hypertonia affects the extensor muscles more than the flexors, so the patient holds their leg in a fixed extended position.

Rigid hypertonia. This is caused by disease of the extrapyramidal system in the brain. The

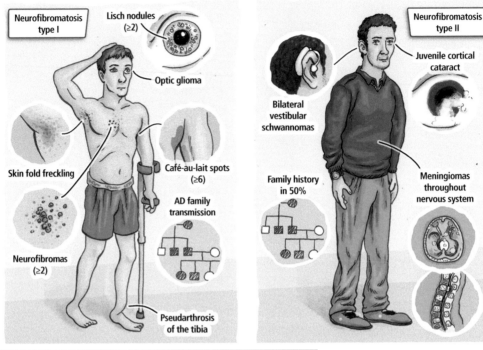

Figure 9.10 The clinical features of neurofibromatosis type 1 and 2.

extrapyramidal system controls coordination and fluidity of movements.

In extrapyramidal hypertonia, the muscle will be rigid in all positions and degrees of flexion / extension ('lead pipe rigidity'). Lead pipe rigidity, together with the resting tremor of Parkinson's syndrome, causes 'cog-wheeling': the impression that the joint is composed of cog-wheels locking together, causing a juddering movement.

Hypotonia

This is due to disease of lower motor neurons. It is also called flaccid tone. It is accompanied by fasciculations – tiny spontaneous twitches in the muscle bulk.

Rarer causes of hypotonia are severe hypothyroidism and severe cerebellar disease.

9.5.3 Tremor

As discussed above, tremor is either resting or action.

Resting tremor

A unilateral resting tremor is classical for Parkinson's disease, whereas bilateral resting tremor is associated with a parkinsonian syndrome.

Other causes of a resting tremor include:
- alcohol withdrawal
- hyperthyroidism
- anxiety
- phaeochromocytoma

Action tremor

The commonest cause is essential tremor, which has a genetic cause. It is usually bilateral and most noticeable when the patient holds their hands out in front of them. Parkinson's disease is sometimes indistinguishable from essential tremor, or a parkinsonian syndrome.

Cerebellar disease causes an intention tremor, which is noticeable when the patient reaches out towards a target.

Table 9.15 *Causes of hypertonia and clinical features*

Cause	Aetiology	Hypertonia type	Associated features
Parkinson's disease	Degeneration of substantia nigra in the basal ganglia	Rigid	Shuffling gait Hypomimia Pill-rolling tremor Bradykinesia
Multiple sclerosis	Inflammation of upper motor neurons in brain and cord	Spastic	Optic neuritis Sphincter dysfunction Depression
Stroke	Infarction of upper motor neurons	Spastic	Cerebral stroke: ■ hemiparesis ■ higher cognitive impairments Spinal stroke: ■ paresis and sensory loss below level of stroke
Tumour	Malignant or benign growth	Spastic	Raised intracranial pressure symptoms
Motor neurone disease	Degeneration of ventral horn of cord, affecting upper and lower motor neurons	Spastic when upper motor neurons affected Flaccid tone when lower motor neurons affected	Chronic decline Preserved cognitive function Preserved sensation

9.5.4 Decreased power

The pattern of the power loss is crucial in reaching a diagnosis (**Table 9.5**). Deficiencies in power must be reconciled with the patient's muscle tone, in order to decide whether it is due to an upper or lower motor lesion.

> **Motor neurone disease is a neuro-degenerative disorder which affects the ventral horn of the spinal cord.** It causes a mix of upper and lower motor signs. Dysphagia (due to lower motor disease of the cranial nerves) is a common feature.

9.5.5 Impaired reflexes

A reflex is a neurological impulse loop, starting as a sudden stretch of a muscle, and resulting in a brief contraction of the same muscle. This 'reflex arc' is mediated by the spinal cord, without motor impulses from the brain. It combines both the CNS and the PNS (**Figure 9.11**).

Hyporeflexia
Absent or weak reflexes indicate either:
■ a peripheral sensory disorder (stretch impulses are not reaching the cord)
■ a lower motor neuron (LMN) problem.

Hyperreflexia
Exaggerated, or 'brisk' reflexes indicate an upper motor neuron (UMN) problem. Severe hyperthyroidism causes slow-relaxing reflexes.

9.5.6 Visual disturbances

These are explored in *Chapter 10*.

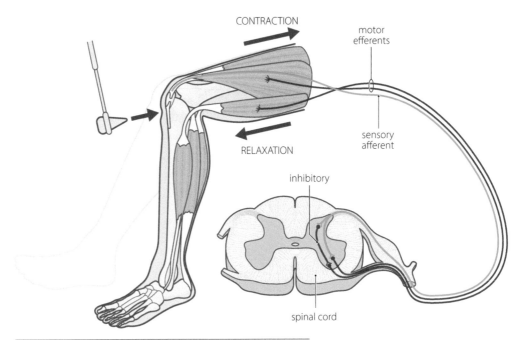

Figure 9.11 The spinal reflex arc, as it pertains to the knee jerk.

9.5.7 Movement disorders

These are unwanted movements or problems in initiating and carrying out voluntary movements. Movement disorders are due to disease of the basal ganglia, which form the extrapyramidal system.

Parkinson's disease

This is an idiopathic neurodegenerative disease of the substantia nigra in the basal ganglia. The classical signs are:
- bradykinesia
- resting 'pill-rolling' tremor
- rigid hypertonia.

There are many other features, which may not all be present:
- hypomimia: lack of facial movements
- festinant gait (tiny shuffling steps with no arm swinging and difficulty turning)
- micrographia: small handwriting
- anosmia
- rapid eye movement (REM) sleep behavioural disorder

- visual hallucinations.

Treatment is focused on dopamine therapy.

Parkinson-plus syndromes

These are diseases that have many features of Parkinson's ('parkinsonism'), but with extra signs.

Multi-system atrophy

This is parkinsonism with signs of autonomic nervous system dysfunction, such as blood pressure dysregulation.

Progressive supranuclear palsy

This is parkinsonism with frequent falls and vertical gaze defects.

Drug-induced parkinsonism

Drugs which affect dopamine neurotransmission within the extrapyramidal system produce the bradykinesia, tremor and rigidity seen in Parkinson's disease. Patients with drug-induced parkinsonism often have a bilateral tremor, whereas idiopathic Parkinson's disease presents with a unilateral tremor in the early stages.

Dystonia

Dystonia is an involuntary contraction of a muscle or muscle group. It is either a genetic disorder, or acquired. Acquired causes include drug side-effects or brain trauma. One common form of focal dystonia is spasmodic torticollis: a painful intermittent contraction of the neck muscles.

Chorea

This is a sudden series of uncoordinated and jerky movements affecting one, several or all four limbs. They occur in the upper or lower limbs. It is a presenting feature of Huntington's disease, a rare autosomal dominant disorder that leads to dementia and personality changes. Severe, thrashing forms of chorea are termed 'ballismus'.

Tourette's syndrome

This is a disease of uncertain aetiology which causes multiple motor and vocal tics in affected patients.

9.6 Examination of the neurological system

The neurological examination assesses five domains: tone, power, reflexes, sensation and coordination (**Table 9.16**).

9.6.1 'ID CHECK'

This is detailed in *Section 3.2*.

9.6.2 Endobedogram

Have a good look at the patient.
- Are they fully conscious? If not, then assess their conscious level, as described in *Section 15.2.6*.
- Are they comfortable?
- Is their muscle bulk symmetrical? Or is there any wasting?
- Is there an obvious tremor, or any other abnormal movements?
- Around the bedside, are there any walking aids or a wheelchair? Are there any other aids, such as an ankle foot orthosis?

The sequence for examining the neurological system is remembered by the mnemonic **I**s **T**he **P**hysician **R**eally **S**o **C**ool?:
- **I**nspection
- **T**one

Table 9.16 *The sequence of the neurological examination*

Element	Details
Inspection	Appearance: is there any muscle wasting or abnormal movements?
	Environment: does the patient require walking aids due to a gait disturbance?
Tone	Is there increased or decreased tone in the arms and legs?
	If there is increased tone in the legs: is there clonus?
Power	Does the patient have normal power in their arms and legs?
Reflexes	Are the reflexes normal, increased or decreased?
	Is the plantar response extensor or flexor?
Sensation	Is the sensation intact?
	If it is impaired, is it in a dermatomal, peripheral nerve, cord lesion or central pattern?
Coordination	Is the coordination intact?
	Is the gait normal?

- **P**ower
- **R**eflexes
- **S**ensation
- **C**oordination.

This order is important, as a patient with decreased power will not be able to perform the tasks needed to assess coordination.

9.6.3 Inspection

Look at the patient in a relaxed pose on the bed. A flaccid paralysis is noted by the wasting of the affected limbs. Patients with spastic tone hold the upper limb in flexion, and the lower limb in extension. Look for the classic pill-rolling tremor of Parkinson's syndrome.

Inspect the large muscle groups – quadriceps, biceps and triceps – for any fasciculations.

Examine the skin for signs of a neurocutaneous disorder.

9.6.4 Tone

Ask the patient to hold both arms out in front of them, with their palms turned up to the ceiling, and close their eyes. Spastic tone causes pronator drift: slow pronation of the outstretched hand over several seconds on the affected side.

Upper limbs

Hold the patient's relaxed arm. Flex and extend the elbow whilst supinating and pronating the forearm, feeling for abnormal tone or cog-wheeling.

Lower limbs

Grasp the thigh and roll the leg side to side. In normal tone the feet will flop gently side to side. Next, slide your forearm under the patient's knees, and ask the patient to relax and let you take the weight off their legs. Briskly raise the knees up from the bed. In normal tone, the feet will slide up the bed towards the buttocks; in increased tone the feet will rise up into the air.

Finally, quickly dorsiflex the foot and feel for clonus: reflexive downward beats of the foot against the hand that indicate spastic hypertonia.

9.6.5 Power

Test each individual muscle group individually, comparing left with right. Test the upper limbs (**Table 9.17**, **Figures 9.12–9.17**), then the lower limbs (**Table 9.18**, **Figures 9.18–9.23**).

> **Patients will need a lot of encouragement when you are testing their power.** They find pushing and pulling against a doctor quite strange and inhibiting, and rarely use their full strength to start with. In order to properly assess their power, constantly encourage them through the different movements ('Push, push, push! Harder!')

For each muscle group you test, award a score from 0 to 5, based on the Medical Research Council (MRC) scale:

- 0 No movement at all
- 1 Flicker of movement
- 2 Able to move whilst resting on surface, not against gravity
- 3 Able to overcome gravity, but gives way on resistance
- 4 Able to move against some resistance
- 5 Normal power.

9.6.6 Reflexes

Deep tendon reflexes are used to test certain nerve roots, and to differentiate between upper motor and lower motor diseases.

Check the biceps, triceps, supinator, knee and ankle jerk (**Figures 9.24–9.28**). When eliciting a reflex, use only a small amount of force, not much more than the reflex hammer's own weight, or you will hurt the patient (**Table 9.19**).

> **Remembering the nerve roots responsible for deep tendon reflexes is as easy as 1, 2, 3.**
> - S1, 2 Ankle jerk
> - L3, 4 Knee jerk
> - C5, 6 Biceps jerk / supinator jerk
> - C7, 8 Triceps jerk

Table 9.17 *Upper limbs motor examination sequence*

Movement	Muscle group	Nerve root	Peripheral nerve	Instruction for patient
Shoulder abduction	Deltoid	C5	Axillary nerve	'Hold your elbows up like a chicken. Now don't let me push them down.'
Elbow flexion	Biceps	C6	Musculocutaneous nerve	'Hold your arms in tight like a boxer, and don't let me pull you towards me...'
Elbow extension	Triceps	C7	Radial nerve	'... now try and push me away.'
Wrist extension	Wrist extensors	C6, C7	Radial nerve	'Cock your wrists back, and don't let me push them down.'
Finger abduction	Interossei	C8, T1	Ulnar nerve	'Spread your fingers out wide, and don't let me push them back together.'
Thumb abduction	Abductor pollicis brevis	C5–T1	Median nerve	'Put your hand out, palms upward. Now point your thumb straight up to the ceiling, and don't let me push it back down.'

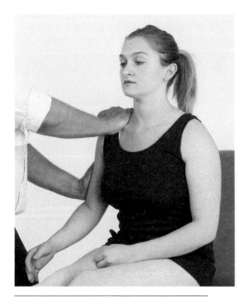

Figure 9.12 Testing shoulder abduction.

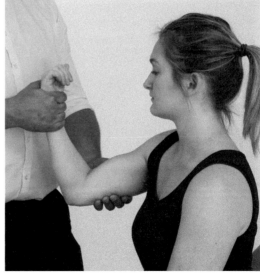

Figure 9.13 Testing elbow flexion.

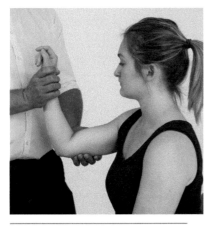

Figure 9.14 Testing elbow extension.

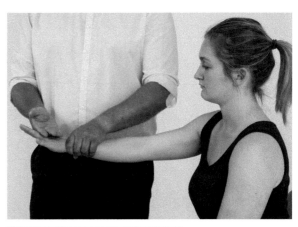

Figure 9.15 Testing wrist extension.

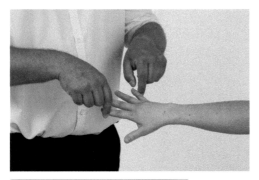

Figure 9.16 Testing finger abduction.

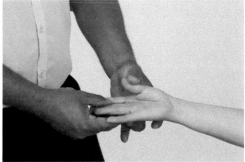

Figure 9.17 Testing thumb abduction.

Table 9.18 *Lower limbs motor examination sequence*

Movement	Muscle group	Nerve root	Peripheral nerve	Instruction for patient
Hip flexion	Ileopsoas muscle	L2, 3, 4	Femoral nerve	'Lift your leg up off the bed, and don't let me push it back down.'
Hip extension	Gluteus maximus	L5, S1	Inferior gluteal nerve	'Push your leg down into the bed and don't let me lift it up.'
Knee flexion	Hamstring	L5, S1	Sciatic nerve	'Bend your knee to 90°, and keep your foot on the bed. Now try to pull me in towards you with your heel…'
Knee extension	Quadriceps	L2, 3, 4	Femoral nerve	'… and now try to kick me away.'
Ankle dorsiflexion	Anterior tibialis	L5	Peroneal nerve	'Pull your feet up towards your head, and don't let me pull them down.'
Ankle plantarflexion	Gastrocnemius	S1	Sciatic nerve	'Now point your toes like a ballerina, and don't let me push them up.'

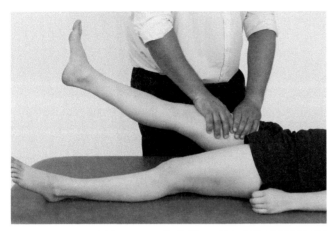

Figure 9.18 Testing hip flexion.

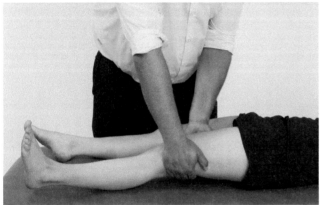

Figure 9.19 Testing hip extension.

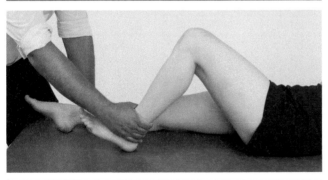

Figure 9.20 Testing knee flexion: ask the patient to pull their heel in towards their buttock.

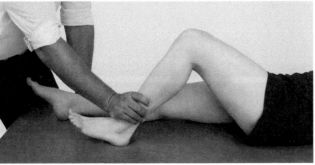

Figure 9.21 Testing knee extension: ask the patient to try to kick your hand away.

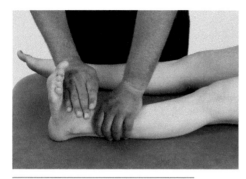

Figure 9.22 Testing ankle dorsiflexion.

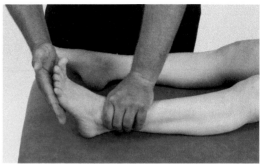

Figure 9.23 Testing ankle plantar flexion.

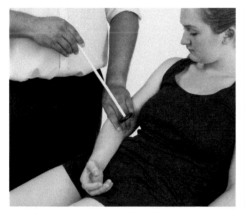

Figure 9.24 Testing the biceps jerk.

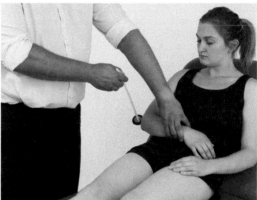

Figure 9.25 Testing the triceps jerk.

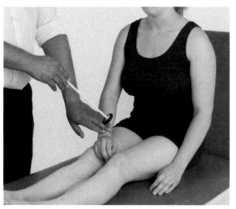

Figure 9.26 Testing the supinator jerk.

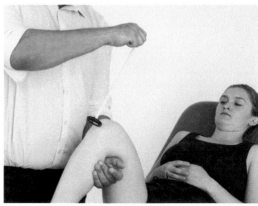

Figure 9.27 Testing the knee jerk.

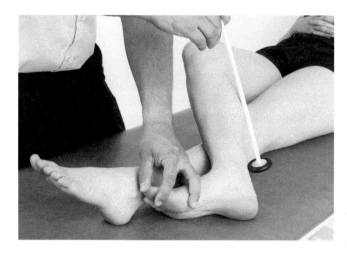

Figure 9.28 Eliciting the ankle jerk.

Reflex	Tendon	Location	Technique
Table 9.19 *Eliciting the deep tendon reflexes*			
Ankle jerk	Calcaneal (Achilles tendon)	Superior to patient's heel	Strike the tendon with the foot slightly plantarflexed, and watch for contraction of the gastrocnemius
Knee jerk	Patellar	Below patella	Strike the tendon with knee flexed to 45°
Biceps jerk	Biceps tendon	Antecubital fossa	Strike the tendon with patient relaxing their forearm across their abdomen
Triceps jerk	Triceps tendon	Superior to olecranon	
Supinator jerk	Supinator tendon	Lateral border of radius	

Plantar response

Gently stroke the sole of the patient's foot with a blunt instrument, from the heel to the sole (**Figure 9.29**). Carefully watch the big toe:

- A normal response is downward flexion of the toe.
- Upward movement of the toe (usually associated with spreading of the remaining toes) is called an 'upgoing plantar', 'extensor plantar' or Babinski's sign, and indicates a UMN lesion.

If you are not able to elicit a reflex, try to 'reinforce' it by asking the patient to perform a different simultaneous motor task. If you can't elicit an upper limb tendon reflex, ask the patient to grit their teeth at the exact moment you strike the tendon. In the lower limb reflexes, try reinforcing them by asking the patient to interlock their fingers and pull them apart the moment you strike the tendon.

9.6.7 Sensation

When testing sensation, remember that you are testing two separate spinal tracts: the dorsal columns, which detect fine touch and vibration, and the anterolateral columns (aka the spinothalamic tracts), which detect pain and temperature.

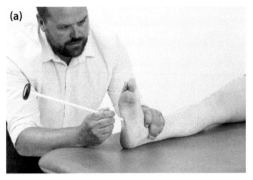
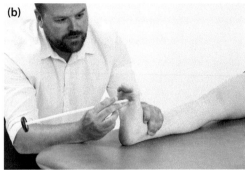

Figure 9.29 (a) Elicit the plantar response by stroking the sole of the foot firmly with a blunt instrument from heel to toe; (b) flexion of the big toe is a normal response.

Testing the dorsal columns

Testing vibration sense using a 256Hz tuning fork on bony prominences:

■ Start by striking the tuning fork, then hold it over the patient's sternum, and ask: 'can you feel it buzzing?'

■ Place the vibrating tuning fork over the lateral malleolus and ask: 'can you feel it buzzing here? Does it feel the same as it did on your chest?'

■ Repeat at the patella and anterior superior iliac spines, asking the same questions.

Testing fine touch using cotton wool or a microfilament:

■ Start by touching the cotton wool to the sternum and asking the patient 'does this feel soft?'

■ Starting distally, touch the cotton wool to the skin in each dermatome, always comparing left with right. Each time, ask the patient whether it feels the same on both sides, and whether both sides feel the same as the sternum.

Testing proprioception (joint position sense) (**Figures 9.30** and **9.31**):

■ In the upper limbs, hold the patient's index finger with the metacarpophalangeal joint extended, and the proximal interphalangeal joint flexed.

■ With your other hand, gently move their distal phalanx a few millimetres up, saying 'this is up'; then move it a few millimetres down, saying 'this is down'.

■ Now tell the patient to close their eyes, and ask them 'am I moving it up or down?' Gently

move the joint up and down in a random sequence, asking the patient to tell you the direction each time.

■ For the lower limbs, repeat the sequence using the big toe.

Testing the spinothalamic columns

Testing pain:

■ Start by touching the neurotip to the sternum and asking the patient 'does this feel sharp?'

■ Starting distally, touch the neurotip to the skin in each dermatome, always comparing left with right. Each time, ask the patient whether it feels the same on both sides, and whether both sides feel the same as the sternum.

> **Only use neurotips to assess pain**. These have been designed to produce a mild pinprick sensation without breaking the skin. Never use hypodermic needles, which are designed to break the skin, or any other sharp object.

9.6.8 Coordination

The coordination part of the examination tests cerebellar function. The sequence of the cerebellar examination is remembered by the acronym DANISH (**Table 9.20**).

9.6.9 Gait

Ask the patient to walk for a few metres, turn around, and walk back towards you, observing for any gait disturbance (**Table 9.12**).

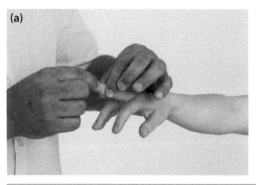
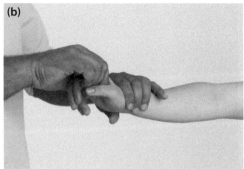

Figure 9.30 Testing proprioception in the upper limbs at (a) the distal interphalangeal joint, and, if impaired, (b) at the wrist.

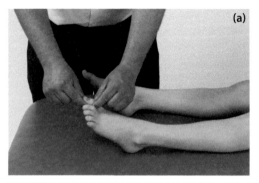
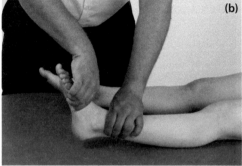

Figure 9.31 Testing proprioception in the lower limbs at (a) the interphalangeal joint, and, if affected, (b) at the ankle.

Table 9.20 *The features of cerebellar dysfunction are remembered using the DANISH mnemonic*		
Feature	**Clinical appearance**	**How to examine**
Dysdiadochokinesis	Impaired coordination when trying to rapidly supinate / pronate forearm	'Twist your hand back and forth like you're turning a key in a door.'
Ataxia	Unsteady, broad-based gait	'Can you walk a few steps for me?' 'Lie on your back, touch your left heel to your right knee, then run the heel up and down your shin.'
Nystagmus	Jerky eye movements in lateral gaze	'Follow my finger all the way to the left, then the right.'
Intention tremor	Hand tremor worsening as it approaches a target	'Touch your nose, then my finger, and continue alternating between the two.'
Speech problems	Broken, staccato speech	'Repeat these words: British constitution, baby hippopotamus.'
Hypotonia	Generally flaccid tone	Elicited during the limb examination

This is also an opportunity to further assess coordination by asking the patient to walk heel-to-toe. Problems of plantar- and dorsiflexion of the ankle are better observed by asking the patient to walk on their tiptoes and their heels, respectively.

9.6.10 Higher mental function

Cognition is not routinely assessed during the standard neurological examination, unless there is a suspicion of cognitive dysfunction.

A quick and informal assessment of cognition can be carried out by checking the following:

- Orientation to time, person and place.
- Attention and concentration, e.g. spelling a five-letter word backwards, or the serial sevens test. Record how long it takes and how many errors are made.
- Memory:
    - short-term: ask the patient to name and remember three objects, such as clock, pen, phone, then carry out the serial sevens test, then ask them to recall the objects
    - recent: ask them what they last ate
    - remote memory: ask them where they grew up or similar

- Grasp: ask the patient to name the current prime minister or monarch.

If cognitive impairment is suspected, you can carry out the Mini-Mental State Examination (MMSE), a 30-point questionnaire that tests aspects of cognition. A score of less than 24 out of 30 indicates a cognitive impairment.

Whilst specific anatomical lesions of the brain result in specific deficits in the MMSE (for example, a lesion of Wernicke's area causing a receptive dysphasia will result in the inability to follow the 3-stage command), globally poor scores in all areas point to dementia.

A shortened version of the MMSE is the abbreviated mental test score. This is used as a rapid screening tool for cognitive impairment. There are ten questions, each worth one point (**Table 9.21**). A score of <8 indicates cognitive impairment.

9.6.11 Finishing off

A complete neurological examination also includes a cranial nerve examination (see *Chapter 10*).

Table 9.21 *The abbreviated mental test score. A score of <8 indicates cognitive impairment*

Question	Point
What is your age?	1
What is the time?	1
Remember this address: 42 West Street	–
What is the year?	1
Where are we right now?	1
What is your date of birth?	1
What job do I do? What about this person? (a nurse / carer / other healthcare worker)	1
When did the Second World War start / finish? (other countries / cultures may ask other important dates the patient is more likely to know)	1
Who is the current monarch?	1
Can you count backwards from 20 to 1?	1
What was the address that I asked you to remember?	1

9.7 Common investigations

Neurological investigations examine the structure and function of the nervous system (**Table 9.22**).

9.7.1 Computed tomography

CT of the brain:
- assesses the structure of the brain
- identifies space-occupying lesions
- identifies intracranial haemorrhages, such as extradural, subdural and subarachnoid bleeding.

9.7.2 Magnetic resonance imaging

MRI of the CNS:
- examines the brain and cord parenchyma
- displays the nature and appearance of CNS masses
- identifies areas of inflammation (whether infective or non-infective in aetiology).

9.7.3 Lumbar puncture

Lumbar puncture (LP) involves passing a needle between the L2–L3 vertebrae under local anaesthetic to obtain cerebrospinal fluid (CSF). CSF circulates continuously between the brain and spinal column.

LP measures the pressure within the subarachnoid space, which is equivalent to the intracranial pressure, thus diagnosing idiopathic intracranial hypertension, and other disease processes that raise the intracranial pressure.

CSF analysis measures protein and glucose levels, and identifies infective pathogens.

9.7.4 Electroencephalogram

An electroencephalogram (EEG) measures the electrical activity within the brain, and is the diagnostic test for epilepsy.

9.7.5 Nerve conduction studies and electromyography

Nerve conduction studies (NCS) and electromyography (EMG) identify diseases of the peripheral nerves and muscles, respectively.
- NCS measure nerve conduction velocity and amplitude and diagnose peripheral neuropathic disorders.
- EMG measures the electrical activity within a muscle, and diagnoses neuromuscular disorders, including diseases of the neuromuscular junction and myopathies.

Table 9.22 *Choosing investigations in neurological disease*

	Indication	Benefits	Limitations
CT	Assess intracranial structure Identify intracranial bleeding	Non-invasive	Ionising radiation No fine detail on CNS parenchyma
MRI	Examine CNS parenchyma	Non-invasive	Contraindicated in patients with surgical metalwork
LP	Analysis of CSF Measurement of intracranial pressure	Identifies pathogens in severe CNS infection	Invasive Small risk of infection, bleeding, post-LP headache
EEG	Diagnosis of epilepsy	Non-invasive	Not useful test between seizure events
NCS/EMG	Investigation of peripheral nerve or myopathic diseases	Non-invasive	Provides descriptions of abnormalities – may not provide ultimate diagnosis

9.8 Answers to starter questions

1.   One seizure does not make a diagnosis of epilepsy, as 5–10% of the population will experience an epileptic seizure in their lifetime, which does not require long-term treatment. Therefore, AEDs are not routinely instigated following a single seizure; a second seizure is required to establish the diagnosis.

2.   Dysfunction of the somatic nervous system leads to impairment of voluntary motor tasks, and of sensation. Dysfunction of the autonomic nervous system causes impairments of involuntary bodily functions. Common autonomic disturbances include gut dysmotility, abnormal heart rate and fluctuating BP, bladder instability and sexual dysfunction and impotence.

3.   A stroke is the clinical manifestation of a brain infarct. It results in a permanent neurological dysfunction, although the severity of the dysfunction can improve over time with medical therapy and physiotherapy. Transient ischaemic attacks (TIAs) are often called 'mini-strokes'. A TIA causes identical symptoms to a stroke, but the symptoms are reversible, and completely resolve within 24 hours of onset (they usually resolve within the hour).

4.   As well as extending basic courtesy, a handshake reveals information about a patient's neurological status. The action of reaching out their hand may reveal an action tremor. The patient may be unable to extend their hand due to hemiparesis. You may see the classic bradykinesia and difficulty in movement initiation associated with Parkinson's disease. Shaking the hand is the first glimpse into the patient's nervous system.

5.   Many neurological diseases cause neuropathic pain. This type of pain is due to disease of the sensory nerve fibres. Neuropathic pain is described as sharp, stabbing, 'electric shock' or burning. It is mostly insensitive to opiates. Alternative drugs, including anti-epileptics and antidepressants, are more successful in managing neuropathic pain.

Chapter 10
Cranial nerves and ophthalmology

Starter questions

1. Can a doctor see a patient's brain without using a scalpel?
2. Is poor eye abduction always caused by an abducens nerve palsy?
3. Why might a head injury cause loss of smell?
4. Why would someone with Bell's palsy not go to a rock concert?
5. Why do some people walk with a white walking stick?

Answers to questions are to be found in *Section 10.10*.

10.1 Introduction

The cranial nerves are the neurological control for the head and neck. They allow the special senses of taste, hearing and, along with the visual system, sight. They are essential in the processes of speech and swallowing. Dysfunction of the cranial nerves and visual system can be a primary disorder, as part of a syndrome or as a consequence of systemic disease.

Cranial nerve disease and examination are often thought of as complicated and difficult. An understanding of the basic anatomy and organisation of the nerves, along with a stepwise logical examination technique, helps to overcome this.

Case 10.1 Monocular visual loss

Presentation

Mrs Tan is 75 years old. She is referred to the Ophthalmology clinic with blurred vision.

Initial interpretation

Visual blurring has many causes including:

- cataracts
- myopia / hyperopia (short- and long-sightedness, respectively)
- glaucoma
- retinal disease
- ophthalmoplegia
- giant cell arteritis

- stroke
- optic nerve inflammation or damage
- ischaemia to the ophthalmic nerve or artery.

Given Mrs Tan's age, any of these could be possible. More information is required to ascertain the diagnosis.

History

Mrs Tan's vision has been deteriorating over the last year. She finds words are blurred when reading, which improves if she closes or covers her left eye. She often gets headaches if she reads for too long.

Interpretation of history

Visual blurring that improves when an eye is closed implies abnormal vision in that eye. Systemic diseases affecting the retina, such as poorly controlled diabetes mellitus and hypertension, usually affect both eyes equally, so are less likely in this case.

Ischaemia tends to cause sudden or rapid deterioration of vision. Visual impairment due to stroke is also sudden and is often associated with other neurological deficits such as facial palsy and limb weakness. Giant cell arteritis is painful and progresses rapidly. Similarly, optic nerve disease tends to present acutely or subacutely. None of these pathologies fits with the clinical presentation.

The remaining differentials have slower progression. Headache from glaucoma can occur as intraocular pressure increases, whereas headache from the other causes can be due to straining for prolonged periods of time.

Further history

Mrs Tan suffers from diet-controlled type 2 diabetes mellitus and hypertension, for which she takes amlodipine. As a child growing up in Malaysia she suffered recurrent ear infections requiring many courses of antibiotics. She does not smoke or drink alcohol. She is usually active and takes regular exercise.

Examination

Mrs Tan looks well and is not in discomfort. Her facial appearance is normal and her gaze is aligned. On examination of the eyes she has no global tenderness or obvious deformity of the orbit or eyelids. Visual fields, pupillary reflexes and colour vision are all normal. There is no visual neglect. Visual acuity is 6/6 in the right eye but 1/3 in the left eye. On fundoscopy, the red reflex is absent in the left eye and the left retina is not clearly visualised. On the right, cotton wool spots and microaneurysms are seen. Observed eye movements are normal.

Interpretation of findings

Mrs Tan has reduced visual acuity, a reduced red reflex and difficulty viewing the retina in the left eye. These fit with her having a cataract. Cataracts are clouding of the lens and are associated with:

- age (most common)
- trauma
- diabetes mellitus
- alcohol
- tobacco
- sunlight exposure.

Being 75 years of age, having diabetes and having grown up in Malaysia are all risk factors here. Of note, she also took multiple courses of antibiotics as a child. Tetracyclines, which were widely used previously, are also associated with the development of cataracts.

Of concern, the visualised right retina shows cotton wool spots and microaneurysms. These are most commonly found with hypertensive retinopathy and background diabetic retinopathy, respectively, thus indicating poor control of her hypertension and diabetes.

Investigations

Mrs Tan undergoes phacoemulsification (cataract removal) of the left eye, her blurred vision resolves and her visual acuity improves to 6/6. Retinal photography performed two weeks after her procedure confirms hypertensive and background diabetic retinopathies. Her HbA1c is raised at 52mmol/mol and 24-hour ambulatory BP monitoring reveals a persistently raised BP of around 155/90mmHg.

Diagnosis

Mrs Tan had a cataract which was treated with a simple procedure, restoring her vision. She is likely to develop a cataract in the other eye and should be reviewed regularly for this.

Both her diabetes and hypertension are poorly controlled. This is not only detrimental to her vision but also to her cardiovascular, renal and neurological health. She should be started on medication for diabetes (such as metformin) and her antihypertensives should be increased – ideally with the addition of an ACE inhibitor. She should be followed up by her GP with regular BP and HbA1c monitoring to ensure good pharmacological control.

She should be seen regularly in a diabetic retinopathy clinic to monitor her retinal disease with sequential retinal photography. In advanced disease, laser photocoagulation therapy can prevent progression to blindness.

10.2 System overview

10.2.1 Cranial nerves

Unlike spinal nerves, which arise from the spinal cord, cranial nerves arise from the brain and brainstem. There are two of each cranial nerve (CN), one on the left and one on the right.

The majority of cranial nerve bodies are situated in nuclei and are numbered according to their position of origin along the forebrain and brainstem (**Figure 10.1**). The cranial nerves exit the skull at different points and supply motor and sensory function (or both) to the head and neck, with the vagus nerve (CN X) also providing parasympathetic innervation to the organs of the thorax and abdomen (**Table 10.1**). The function of the individual nerves is described below.

Olfactory nerve (CN I)

The olfactory nerve is sensory and detects smells from the nose and carries recognition of these to the brain.

Optic nerve (CN II)

The optic nerve is sensory. It receives visual stimuli from the retina and conveys them to the visual centres within the occipital lobes.

Oculomotor, trochlear and abducens nerves (CN III, IV and VI)

These three nerves have motor function and control the muscles of the eyelids and eyes. They work together to control the movement of the eyes to allow a person's gaze to move. Each nerve innervates particular muscles to allow this:

■ CN III: muscles of the eyelid and all intrinsic muscles of the eye except superior oblique and lateral rectus
■ CN IV: superior oblique
■ CN VI: lateral rectus.

The oculomotor nerve also has parasympathetic function and supplies the ciliary muscles within the pupil which promote pupillary constriction.

Trigeminal nerve (CN V)

The trigeminal nerve has both motor and sensory function. It innervates the muscles of mastication (the masseters, temporalis and pterygoids) as well as conveying sensation over the face via three sensory branches:

■ Ophthalmic nerve (V1)
■ Maxillary nerve (V2)
■ Mandibular nerve (V3); this branch also carries touch and temperature sensation from the mouth, but not taste.

These branches correspond to distinct areas over the skin of the face (**Figure 10.2**):

Facial nerve (CN VII)

The facial nerve's motor function controls the muscles of the face that allow facial expression. The sensory fibres detect taste from the anterior two-thirds of the tongue and oral cavity. Salivary,

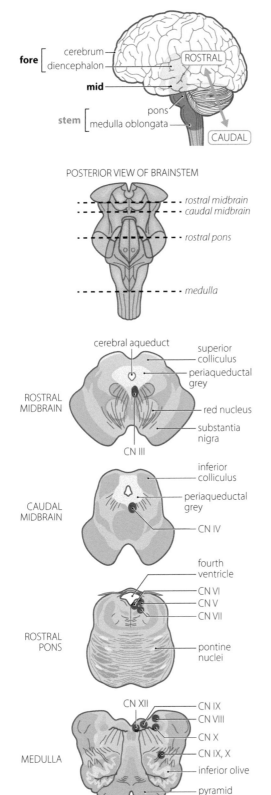

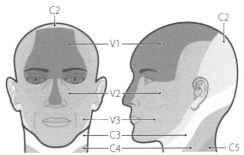

Figure 10.2 Sensory innervation of the face and head by cervical nerves C2 and 3 and three branches of CN V (trigeminal nerve).

lacrimal and nasal cavity glands are stimulated by the facial nerve's parasympathetic fibres.

Vestibulocochlear nerve (CN VIII)

The vestibulocochlear nerve is purely sensory. It detects sound and balance sensations from the inner ear.

Glossopharyngeal nerve (CN IX)

The glossopharyngeal nerve has mixed function. The motor fibres innervate the stylopharyngeus muscle (responsible for elevation of the larynx and pharynx during speech and swallowing) and sensory fibres transmit touch sensation from the tonsils, pharynx, middle ear and posterior third of the tongue, as well as taste sensation from the posterior third of the tongue. Parasympathetic fibres stimulate parotid gland secretion.

Vagus nerve (CN X)

The vagus nerve carries sensation from the pharynx and back of the throat. Parasympathetic fibres innervate all the organs (except for the adrenal glands) from the neck to the transverse colon. Consequences of vagus nerve signalling include slowing of the heart rate and gastrointestinal peristalsis.

Accessory nerve (CN XI)

The accessory nerve provides motor innervation to the sternocleidomastoid and trapezius muscles.

Figure 10.1 The brainstem and origin of cranial nerves.

Table 10.1 *Summary of cranial nerves*

	Nuclei position	Exit point	Sensory or motor function?	Function
Olfactory nerve (CN I)	Forebrain	Cribriform plate	Sensory	Sensation of smell
Optic nerve (CN II)	Forebrain	Optic foramen	Sensory	Sensation of vision
Oculomotor nerve (CN III)	Midbrain	Superior orbital fissure	Motor	Eye movement Eyelid elevation Pupil constriction
Trochlear nerve (CN IV)	Midbrain	Superior orbital fissure	Motor	Eye movement
Trigeminal nerve (CN V)	Pons	V1 – superior orbital fissure V2 – foramen rotundum V3 – foramen ovale	Both	Sensation of facial skin Movement of mastication muscles
Abducens nerve (CN VI)	Pons	Superior orbital fissure	Motor	Eye movement
Facial nerve (CN VII)	Pons	Internal auditory canal	Both	Facial expression Taste
Vestibulocochlear nerve (CN VIII)	Pons	Internal auditory canal	Sensory	Sound and balance perception
Glossopharyngeal nerve (CN IX)	Medulla	Jugular foramen	Both	Speech and swallowing Taste
Vagus nerve (CN X)	Medulla	Jugular foramen	Both	Throat and pharynx sensation
Accessory nerve (CN XI)	Medulla	Jugular foramen	Motor	Neck and shoulder movement
Hypoglossal nerve (CN XII)	Medulla	Hypoglossal canal	Motor	Tongue movement

Hypoglossal nerve (CN XII)

The hypoglossal nerve innervates all the muscles of the tongue, except for the palatoglossus.

10.2.2 Visual system

The visual system is responsible for sight and encompasses the eyes, visual cortices and their communicating pathways (**Figure 10.3**).

The eyes

Light reception

Light waves enter the eye and are refracted by the cornea (**Figure 10.4**). They pass through the pupil and are further refracted through the lens to produce an inverted image upon the retina. The size and shape of the pupil and lens are controlled by the iris and ciliary bodies respectively, and accommodate for distance and light levels.

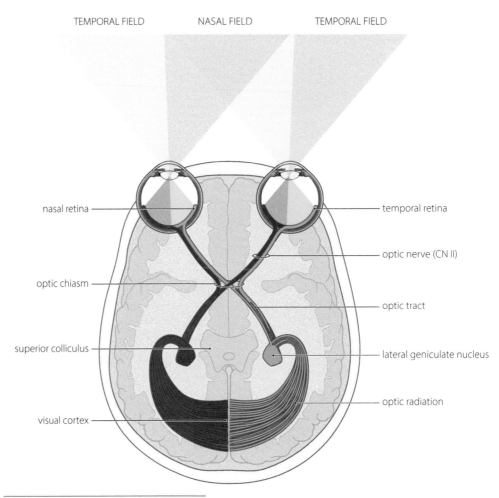

TEMPORAL FIELD   NASAL FIELD   TEMPORAL FIELD

nasal retina

temporal retina

optic nerve (CN II)

optic chiasm

optic tract

superior colliculus

lateral geniculate nucleus

optic radiation

visual cortex

Figure 10.3 Pathways of the visual system.

Light detection

Photoreceptor cells on the retina (rod and cone opsins) absorb photons and produce electrical impulses. Different types of rod opsin detect different wavelength photons, allowing for colour vision. These impulses generate action potentials which are carried to the optic nerves.

Communicating pathways

The optic nerves receive and convey detected light signals from the eyes to the visual cortices. At the optic chiasm, information is split according to visual field so that signals from corresponding fields in each eye are carried to the same area of the cortex. After the optic chiasm, unilateral field information (i.e. left and right vision) from both eyes traverses the optic tracts, lateral geniculate nuclei and optic radiations to the visual cortices within the occipital lobes.

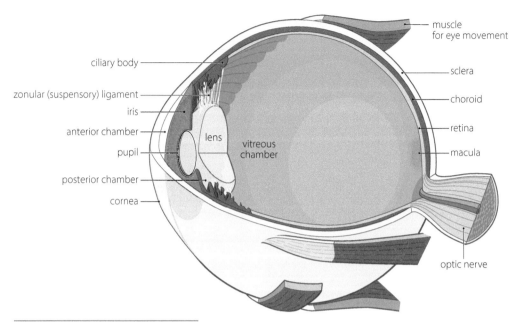

Figure 10.4 Gross anatomy of the eye.

10.3 Symptoms of cranial nerve and ophthalmological disease

The commonest features of cranial nerve and visual system disease are visual impairment, impaired taste and smell, hearing loss, altered facial appearance, speech and swallowing difficulty and impaired balance.

The symptoms of cranial nerve disease are relatively self-explanatory. They each have specific functions and if affected, the particular function is reduced or lost. For all cranial nerves, there is a core group of pathologies that affect all of them. To avoid repetition, they are discussed here first. Otherwise, specific causes that do not fit this pattern are discussed later in this section.

Nerve compression

Like any other nerve, cranial nerves can be externally compressed. This can occur either at the nucleus or anywhere along the course of the nerve, impairing signal transmission. Space-occupying lesions (SOLs) such as tumours or vascular aneurysms are the commonest causes. Specific SOLs affect particular cranial nerves:

- Optic glioma – CN II compression
- Pituitary tumours – CN II compression; those extending into the cavernous sinus can compress CN III, VI and VI
- Acoustic neuroma – CN VII and VII compression
- Posterior communicating artery aneurysm – CN III compression.

High intracranial pressures compress the cranial nerves against the skull. This is commonly associated with headache. Causes include intracranial haemorrhage, severe benign intracranial hypertension, severe hydrocephalus and cerebral oedema. A cranial nerve lesion caused by raised intracranial pressure is referred to as a 'false localising sign'. This describes a clinical finding that appears like a problem related to the area of the brain that is affected (e.g. a tumour compressing a particular nerve nucleus) but is actually due to a problem somewhere else (the cause of the raised pressure).

Ischaemia

Impaired blood supply to the cranial nerve nucleus, such as with a brainstem stroke, starves the cells of oxygen. This leads to cell necrosis and causes nerve damage.

Demyelination

Loss of the myelin sheath around cranial nerve fibres slows impulse conduction and impairs nerve function. Causes include:
- multiple sclerosis
- optic neuritis
- Devic's disease (neuromyelitis optica).

Trauma

Trauma can occur either at the nucleus or along the course of the nerve, impairing signal transmission. Whilst this is unusual overall, it is more likely that trauma affects a nerve's course rather than its nucleus.

Non-traumatic mononeuropathies

This is the term used for damage to or dysfunction of a single nerve that does not correspond with anything above. The common causes for a mononeuropathy are outlined in **Table 10.2**.

10.3.1 Visual impairment

Vision relies on the ability to receive, detect, transmit and interpret light entering the eye, and the causes of visual impairment should be thought of in the same way.

Cranial nerve

Lesions of cranial nerves III, IV or VI can disrupt eye alignment and cause double vision (diplopia).

Intraocular disease

Anterior chamber

Corneal damage or bleeding and infection within the anterior chamber disrupt light passage to the lens, reducing visual acuity.

Lens and pupil

Iritic damage or inflammation and pupillary muscle dysfunction prevent appropriate pupillary response in accommodation and visual focusing. Opacification of the lens (due to a cataract) reduces and blurs light images refracted to the retina.

Table 10.2 *Causes of non-traumatic mono- and polyneuropathies*

Category	Examples
Endocrine / metabolic	Diabetes mellitus
	Chronic kidney disease
	Porphyria
	Amyloidosis
	Hypothyroidism
Inflammatory	SLE
	MS
	Lyme disease
	Vasculitis
	Sarcoidosis
Toxins	Vincristine
	Phenytoin
	Metronidazole
	Isoniazid
	Heavy metals
	Alcohol
	Chemotherapeutics
Deficiencies	Vitamin A
	Vitamin B1
	Vitamin B12
Other	HIV
	Paraneoplastic syndromes
	Herpes simplex virus
	Radiation

Posterior chamber

Raised intraocular pressure (glaucoma) compresses blood flow to the retina and optic nerve. Over time this damages the retina and optic nerve. When this happens suddenly, a condition called acute angle-closure glaucoma, it must be treated as an emergency as visual loss is rapid.

Infection and bleeding within the posterior chamber disrupt the passage of light to the retina.

Retina

Retinal diseases reduce the volume of rod opsins available to receive light. These include retinitis pigmentosa, macular degeneration and retinoblastoma. Microvascular disease prevents adequate blood flow to the retina. The two biggest causes are poorly controlled hypertension and diabetes mellitus. Retinal detachment can occur spontaneously or after injury and is an ophthalmological emergency requiring urgent reattachment.

Optic tract disease

Lesions occurring between the optic nerves and visual cortices have characteristic patterns of visual loss (**Figure 10.5**). The causes for these are similar to those of primary cranial nerve disease.

Cerebral disease

The occipital lobes 'process' impulses carried by the optic nerves to give the perception of vision. Infarction (stroke), tumours or neuronal degeneration within these lobes cause regional visual loss.

Vascular

Vasculitis

Giant cell arteritis (or temporal arteritis) is a vasculitis causing inflammation of the temporal artery. It is painful and usually unilateral. It causes occlusion of the ophthalmic artery, resulting in visual impairment to the affected eye. If untreated, this leads to permanent blindness.

Central retinal artery occlusion

Occlusion of the retinal artery blocks blood delivery to the retina, causing sudden, painless visual loss in the affected eye. It is most commonly due to atherosclerotic disease.

Central retinal vein occlusion

The retinal vein provides sole drainage of blood from the retina. Its occlusion causes retinal oedema and damage, leading to blindness and glaucoma.

Pharmacological

Many drugs affect sight. The commonest examples are:

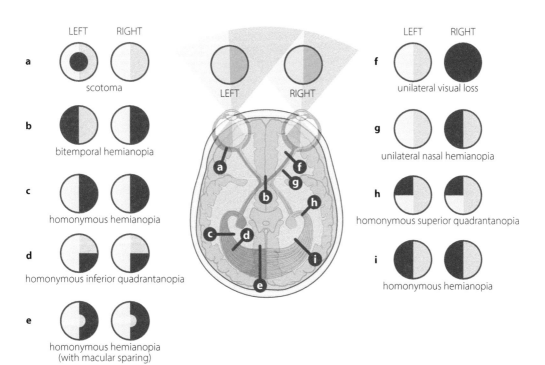

Figure 10.5 Patterns of visual loss according to lesion within the visual system pathways.

- ethambutol – optic neuritis
- topiramite – acute angle-closure glaucoma
- sildenafil – blue vision discolouration
- digoxin – yellow vision discolouration
- diuretics – progression to glaucoma.

10.3.2 Impaired taste and smell

Cranial nerve
As discussed above, any lesion syndrome affecting CNs I, VII and IX alters the sensations of taste and smell.

Cerebral disease
Any cerebral disease affecting the gustatory cortex and olfactory bulb (within the frontal lobe and forebrain, respectively) can disrupt taste and smell sensation.

Trauma
Trauma to the nose and oral cavity damages chemoreceptors and reduces the ability to perceive sensation.

Infections
Severe oral candidiasis coats the tongue and prevents the sensation of taste. Upper respiratory tract infections stimulate increased mucus production, resulting in nasal blockage and a reduced sensation of smell.

Pharmacological
Many drug side-effects include impaired or abnormal taste and smell; these are described in **Table 10.3**.

10.3.3 Hearing loss

Age
Hearing loss is a common and normal part of ageing. Presbyacusis is the name given to this progressive loss of high frequencies with age.

Noise exposure
Noise-induced hearing loss accounts for nearly half of all cases of hearing loss. It can be temporary or permanent and there is no treatment to regain it once lost.

Cranial nerve
CN VIII lesions cause hearing impairment.

Table 10.3 *Common drugs associated with abnormal taste and smell*	
	Examples
Antibiotics	Ampicillin
	Macrolides
	Quinolones
	Trimethoprim
	Tetracyclines
Cardiology	Diltiazem
	Enalapril
	Nifedipine
	Spironolactone
	Aspirin
	Propranolol
	Pravastatin
Endocrinology	Propylthiouracil
	Carbimazole
	Metformin
Neurology	Carbamazepine
	Phenytoin
	Baclofen
	Dantrolene
Rheumatology	Colchicine
	Dexamethasone
	Gold
	Methotrexate
Psychiatry	Amitriptyline
	Lithium
	Clozapine
Other	Chlorpheniramine
	Chemotherapeutics

Infection
Viral illnesses causing labyrinthitis result in both temporary and permanent hearing loss. Maternal infections, such as measles, mumps and herpes simplex, are associated with hearing impairment in the newborn. Chronic or recurrent middle ear infections damage the tympanic membrane and small bones.

Pharmacology

Common medications implicated in deafness include:

- NSAIDs
- quinine
- antibiotics – macrolides, aminoglycosides
- platinum-based chemotherapeutic agents.

Genetic disorders

Some inherited disorders are associated with congenital deafness. These include:

- Stickler syndrome
- Alport's syndrome
- neurofibromatosis type 2.

10.3.4 Abnormal facial appearance

Cranial nerve

Facial nerve lesions can be of the upper or lower motor neurons. An upper motor neuron (UMN) lesion spares the muscles of the forehead (giving a preserved frown), whereas a lower motor neuron (LMN) lesion involves these muscles also.

Bell's palsy

Bell's palsy is the commonest cause of an idiopathic LMN CN VII lesion. The cause is unknown but diabetes mellitus is an important risk factor.

Cerebral disease

Stroke

An ischaemic event within the motor cortex of the frontal lobe causes an ipsilateral UMN CN VII lesion. If the stroke involves areas of the motor cortex that do not control the muscles of the face, it is associated with a limb weakness on the contralateral side.

Infection

Ramsay Hunt syndrome

Reactivation of herpes zoster virus within the geniculate ganglion causes Ramsay Hunt syndrome. The classical presentation is with a triad of:

- LMN CN VII lesion
- facial vesicles
- ear pain.

Lyme disease

Lyme disease is a *Borrelia* infection acquired through tick bites. These ticks are typically found on deer and most patients with Lyme disease have been in a forested area some time before their symptoms arise. The classical symptoms of Lyme disease are:

- LMN CN VII lesion
- erythema migrans – a spreading red-ringed rash
- fevers
- headache
- lethargy
- arthralgia.

10.3.5 Speech and swallowing difficulty

Cerebral disease

Intracerebral diseases affecting Broca's area (the centre for language production) cause aphasia (inability to communicate). Neurodegenerative diseases are associated with a decline in language and the ability to coordinate swallowing.

Cerebellar disease

Cerebellar lesions cause slurred speech due to impaired muscular coordination (see **Table 9.20**).

Vocal cord disorders

Vocal cord dysfunction can prevent or disrupt speech. Causes include neoplastic invasion, infections and strain from overuse. The vocal cords are innervated by the recurrent laryngeal nerves. These pass close to both main bronchi and are susceptible to damage from invading bronchial tumours.

> **Impaired swallowing is a clinically important symptom**. If muscular contraction is not coordinated with closure of the epiglottis, oral contents (such as food and secretions) can enter the lungs and cause infection. This is called aspiration pneumonia.

10.3.6 Impaired balance

Cranial nerve
CN XIII lesions affect the sensation of balance.

Cerebellar disease
Cerebellar lesions disrupt balance through impaired proprioception (see *Section 9.2.2*).

Inner ear pathology
The labyrinth within the inner ear senses balance via the movement of perilymph. Vertigo is a sensation caused by a mismatch between visual perception and sensation from the labyrinth. Causes include:

- labyrinthitis – infection of the inner ear
- Ménière's disease – associated with tinnitus and deafness
- motion sickness.

10.4 The cranial nerve and ophthalmology history

10.4.1 Past medical history

Ask about previous neurological illness such as stroke, as this can result in facial weakness or visual disturbance.

Conditions such as MS, diabetes and inflammatory conditions (such as sarcoidosis) can cause neuropathies which may present as cranial nerve palsies. If the patient has cancer, particularly those of lung, breast and renal origins, metastases to the brain cause neurological symptoms.

Diabetes and hypertension are the commonest causes of acquired blindness in the UK through cataracts and retinal disease.

Ask about any markers of their control (i.e. renal disease, neuropathy, HbA1c levels) and how often the patient has these checked.

Ask about previous surgery or trauma to the eyes, head or neck.

10.4.2 Medications

Chronic conditions leading to cranial nerve and ophthalmic disease require good compliance and regular review. Ask about the drug regimens and whether the patient takes them as prescribed.

Drugs causing neurological side-effects are explored in **Table 10.4** and those with ophthalmic side-effects in **Table 10.5**.

Table 10.4 *Common drugs affecting cranial neuropathy*

Category	Examples
Anti-epileptics	Phenytoin
Chemotherapeutics	Cisplatin
	Vincristine
Anti-arrhythmics	Amiodarone
Antimicrobials	Nitrofurantoin
	Metronidazole
	Ciprofloxacin
	Isoniazid

Table 10.5 *Common drugs affecting the visual system*

Ophthalmic complaint	Examples
Uveitis and scleritis	Bisphosphonates
	Moxifloxacin
Retinal toxicity	Hydroxychloroquine
Optic neuritis	Ethambutol
Acute angle-closure glaucoma	Topiramate
Discoloured vision	Sildenafil (blue vision)
	Digoxin (yellow vision)
Progressive glaucoma	Diuretics

10.4.3 Social history

Smoking
Tobacco smoking promotes atherosclerosis, implicated in worsening neurovascular disease and retinal disease.

Alcohol
High and sustained alcohol exposure is neurotoxic and can lead to the development of peripheral neuropathies.

Employment
People working with machinery or metal are at risk of having foreign bodies entering and damaging the eye. Ask about the use of eye protection.

Physical activity
Physical activity helps prevent the onset or progression of cardiovascular disease and diabetes. Blindness and hearing impairment can impede independence and confidence in people when outside in busy areas. They may avoid leaving their home because of it.

Functional capacity
Enquire about how the patient is currently living:
- How do they cope with their activities of daily living?
- Are they able to see enough to safely move around indoors and outside?
- Do they have difficulty communicating or swallowing?
- Are they able to hear and interact with other people?

10.4.4 Family history

Ask about maternal infections during pregnancy such as mumps, measles and rubella, as these are associated with foetal deafness. There are many rare syndromes and diseases that cause the symptoms discussed above, including:
- hereditary sensorimotor neuropathy: inherited peripheral neuropathy
- retinitis pigmentosa: progressive retinal degeneration (affecting rod photoreceptors)
- Alport's syndrome: glomerulonephritis, end-stage kidney disease and sensorineural hearing loss.

10.4.5 Systems review

Ask about other symptoms which may be related to cranial nerve or ophthalmic disease. These are discussed in **Table 10.6**.

Table 10.6 *Full systems review: symptoms that may indicate an underlying cause for cranial nerve or visual system dysfunction*

System	Symptoms	Possible associations
Neurological	Headache	Giant cell arteritis
		Glaucoma
		Raised intracranial pressure
	Weakness	Stroke
		MS
Musculoskeletal	Rash and lumps	Granulomas associated with sarcoidosis
	Arthralgia	Lyme disease
Cardiovascular	Exertional chest pain	Atherosclerotic disease
Gastrointestinal	Nausea and vomiting	Vitamin deficiencies
	Weight loss	Underlying malignancy (giving metastases or paraneoplastic syndrome)
Genitourinary	Reduced urine production	CKD

10.5 Signs of cranial nerve disease

The signs of cranial nerve disease are relatively straightforward and best thought of according to the individual nerve's function.

10.5.1 Olfactory nerve (CN I)

Olfactory nerve lesions disrupt smell. A partial loss of smell is called parosmia, whereas a total loss is called anosmia.

10.5.2 Optic nerve (CN II)

Visual loss occurs from optic nerve damage. This can be total or partial, depending on the location of the lesion along the course of the optic nerve (**Figure 10.5**).

10.5.3 Oculomotor, trochlear and abducens nerves (CN III, IV and VI)

Lesions of these three nerves impair the function of the ocular muscles. The malalignment of the eyes from this is termed 'ophthalmoplegia'. This is described in **Table 10.7**.

10.5.4 Trigeminal nerve (CN V)

Due to its multiple functions, lesions of the trigeminal nerve cause a cluster of symptoms. If particular fibres (i.e. sensory or motor only) are affected, then just those functions are lost. The classical signs of trigeminal nerve impairment are weakness and decreased bulk of the muscles of mastication, sensory loss over the ipsilateral half of the face (for lesion at the nerve nucleus) or over the corresponding branch area (for a branch lesion) and loss of touch and temperature sensation from the mouth (for a lesion involving V3). Trigeminal nerve problems commonly present with facial pain (called trigeminal neuralgia) and can often mimic severe headaches.

10.5.5 Facial nerve (CN VII)

Facial nerve palsies present with weakness of facial muscles, giving loss of expression, with or without forehead involvement. There is also associated loss of taste from the anterior two-thirds of the tongue and oral cavity, and impaired salivary and lacrimal secretions, giving a dry mouth and dry eyes.

10.5.6 Vestibulocochlear nerve (CN VIII)

Vestibulocochlear nerve palsies present with reduced hearing, impaired balance and dizziness.

Table 10.7 *Characteristic symptoms of ophthalmoplegia*

	Eye position of affected eye (when looking straight ahead)	Impaired movement of the affected eye	Extraocular motor impairment	Parasympathetic impairment
Oculomotor (CN III)	Turned "down and out"	Unable to look inwards	Ptosis	Dilated pupil that does not constrict
		Unable to look up or down		Loss of pupillary accommodation reflex
Trochlear (CN IV)	Normal	Unable to turn inwards or down	Nil	Nil
Abducens (CN VI)	Normal / turned inwards	Unable to turn outwards	Nil	Nil

10.5.7 Glossopharyngeal nerve (CN IX)

Glossopharyngeal nerve diseases usually present with an alteration in the person's voice (dysphonia). They can also cause impaired swallowing, altered taste over the posterior third of the tongue and reduced parotid gland secretion.

10.5.8 Vagus nerve (CN X)

Vagus nerve palsies present much differently than the other cranial nerve problems. Patients report palpitations, either fast or slow:

- Tachyarrhythmia and fast GI transit in nerve lesions

- Bradyarrhythmia and slow GI transit in nerve hyperstimulation.

On examination, the gag reflex is lost.

10.5.9 Accessory nerve (CN XI)

Accessory nerve palsies result in impaired neck rotation and shoulder elevation. Wasting of trapezius and sternocleidomastoid muscles is noted.

10.5.10 Hypoglossal nerve (CN XII)

Hypoglossal nerve palsies reduce the ability to protrude the tongue and move it from side to side. Tongue wasting and fasciculations are often seen.

10.6 The cranial nerve examination

Like all examinations, a consistent and thorough approach is required (**Table 10.8**).

10.6.1 'ID CHECK'

- This is detailed in *Section 3.2*.
- The patient should be sitting in a chair and have their head, neck and shoulders exposed.

10.6.2 Endobedogram

Have a good look at the patient:

- Are there any obvious facial abnormalities?
- Are the eyes aligned?
- Is there any speech abnormality?
- Are there mobility aids to suggest neurological disease elsewhere?
- On the patient and around the bedside, are there any medications, spectacles, false eyes or hearing aids?
- Are there any scars on the head or neck?
- The cranial nerve examination follows a different structure to other examinations by examining each nerve function in turn, according to the level of their origination.

10.6.3 Olfactory nerve (CN I)

Ask the patient if they have noticed any change in their sense of smell.

10.6.4 Optic nerve (CN II)

The acronym **'FRANCO'** (**F**ields, **R**eflexes, **A**cuity, **N**eglect, **C**olour, **O**phthalmoscopy) is a good memory aid to examining the optic nerve.

Visual fields

Examining visual fields is easy to perform but difficult to explain to the patient. Be clear and consistent in your instructions.

- Sit directly opposite the patient at a distance of 1m.
- Ask the patient to cover their right eye with their right hand.
- Cover your left eye with your left hand.
- Tell the patient to look directly into your right eye throughout the examination.
- Hold your right forefinger at the upper and outer part of your visual field. Ensure your hand is positioned equally between you and the patient.
- Slowly draw your finger towards the centre of vision and ask the patient to tell you when they see it in their peripheral vision. The patient must continue to look directly into

Table 10.8 Summary of cranial nerve exam	
Cranial nerve	**Test**
Olfactory (CN I)	Ask about smell
Optic (CN II)	Assess visual fields
	Check pupillary reflexes
	Assess for visual neglect
	Test colour vision
	Perform fundoscopy
Oculomotor, trochlear and abducens (CN III, IV and VI)	Check for ptosis
	Check eye alignment
	Assess eye movements
	Assess for nystagmus
Trigeminal (CN V)	Assess facial sensation
	Test muscles of mastication and jaw movement
	Test jaw jerk
	Consider testing corneal reflex
Facial (CN VII)	Assess facial expressions
Vestibulocochlear (VIII)	Test general hearing
	Rinne's test
	Weber's test
	Vestibular testing
Glossopharyngeal and vagus (CN IX and X)	Check for uvular deviation
	Consider gag reflex
	Assess cough
Accessory (XI)	Assess neck rotation and shoulder elevation
Hypoglossal (XII)	Check for tongue fasciculations
	Assess tongue movement

your eye during this test and you may need to remind them to do so (**Figure 10.6**).
- Repeat this process in the lower and outer, upper and inner and the lower and inner quadrants of vision.
- Repeat this assessment on the other eye.

Pupillary reflexes

Turn the lights down, warning the patient that you are doing so.

Direct pupillary reflex

Shine a light directly into the eye and check for pupillary constriction (**Figure 10.7**). This should occur within a second. Delayed, 'sluggish' constriction indicates nerve or brainstem pathology.

Repeat this for the other eye.

Consensual pupillary reflex

Shine a light directly into one eye and check for constriction of the contralateral pupil. Delayed or absent constriction indicates optic nerve or Edinger–Westphal nucleus pathology.

Swinging light test

Swing the light between both eyes. In this test, both pupils should constrict and stay constricted. If one pupil dilates, this indicates a relative afferent pupillary defect which is caused by damage to the tract between the optic nerve and optic chiasm.

Accommodation reflex

- Ask the patient to focus on a distant object.
- Place your finger 20cm in front of the patient.
- Ask them to switch their vision to your finger.
- The pupils should constrict and converge on your finger.

Visual acuity

Visual acuity is measured by standing the patient 6m in front of a Snellen chart (**Figure 10.8**). If they use glasses, these should be worn for the assessment.

- Ask the patient to cover one eye and read down the chart as far as they can. The result is recorded as the distance away from the chart over the lowest full line read. If letters are incorrect, these are recorded as 'minus' the bottom number. For example, for a patient who stands 6m away and reads the 6/6 line with one letter wrong, this would be recorded as 6/6 (–1).
- If the patient cannot read to the 6/6 line, repeat the test using a pinhole. If acuity is

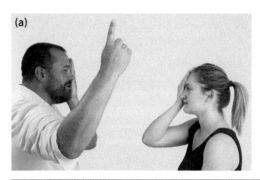
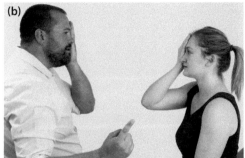

Figure 10.6 Testing the visual fields: use your forefinger to map out the limits of the patient's visual field by comparing it with your own.

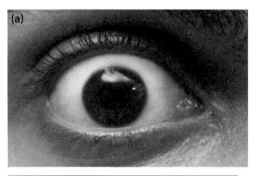
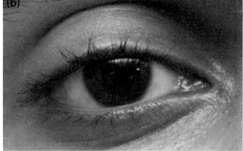

Figure 10.7 (a) Dilated and (b) constricted pupil.

E	1	20/200
F P	2	20/100
T O Z	3	20/70
L P E D	4	20/50
P E C F D	5	20/40
E D F C Z P	6	20/30
F E L O P Z D	7	20/25
D E F P O T E C	8	20/20
L E F O D P C T	9	
F D P L T C E O	10	
P E Z O L C F T D	11	

Figure 10.8 A Snellen chart.

improved, this reflects a refractive error in acuity.

- If the patient still cannot read the chart, move them to 3m away, then 1m.
- If they still cannot read the chart, try finger counting, then hand movements, then ability to see light. An inability to see light indicates blindness in that eye.
- Repeat this for the opposite eye.

Visual neglect

Visual neglect is also known as 'visual inattention'.

- Sit directly opposite the patient at a distance of 1m.
- Ask them to look directly at your face throughout.
- Hold both your arms equally between you and the patient in their peripheral vision.
- Move the fingers on one hand and ask the patient which side is moving in their

peripheral vision. Remember, they must be looking directly at you and not at your hands.

■ Then move the fingers on the other hand and ask them which side is moving.

■ Then move the fingers on both hands and ask them which side is moving.

■ Inability to perceive both sides moving at once indicates a visual neglect on the absent side.

Colour vision

Ishihara charts, if available, can be used to assess red–green colour vision.

Fundoscopy (ophthalmoscopy)

Fundoscopy is performed in a dimly lit environment. Consider using short-acting mydriatic eye drops to dilate the pupil. (These drops should never be used in confirmed or suspected glaucoma as they may cause acute angle-closure glaucoma.) The patient should remove their spectacles or contact lenses.

■ Standing away from the patient, shine the light at their eye and look through the fundoscope. The 'red reflex' is positive if the pupil appears red. If absent, this indicates the presence of a cataract.

■ Place a hand on the patient's forehead and slowly move towards their eye whilst looking through the fundoscope until the retina is visualised (**Figure 10.9**).

■ Locate the optic disc and note the colour, contour and the presence of any disc margin cupping.

■ Next follow the four main retinal vessels and note the presence of any cotton wool spots, arteriovenous nipping or neovascularisation (**Figure 10.9b**).

■ Finish by asking the patient to look directly at the light to assess the macula for drusen (indicating macular degeneration) (**Figure 10.9b**).

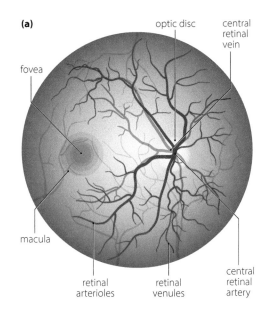

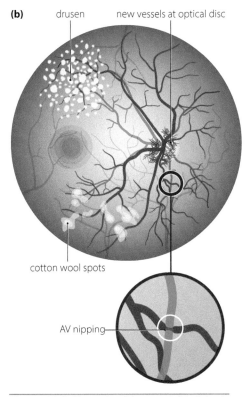

Figure 10.9 The retina: (a) normal; (b) diabetic retinopathy.

10.6.5 Oculomotor, trochlear and abducens nerves (CN III, IV and VI)

Ptosis

Note the presence of a drooping eyelid (ptosis) from oculomotor nerve pathology.

Eye movements

- Ask the patient to keep their head still throughout the test.
- Hold out a finger and move it to make an 'H' shape.
- Ask the patient to follow your finger and report any double vision.
- Watch both eyes for restricted movement or nystagmus.
- The pattern of abnormality reflects the affected cranial nerve (**Table 10.7**).
- Note any pain on eye movement which could reflect orbital or global pathology.

Nystagmus

Accentuate nystagmus by quickly moving your finger from one side of vision to the other. This can be performed horizontally and vertically.

10.6.6 Trigeminal nerve (CN V)

Sensory function

Comparing each side, assess sensation to light touch and pinprick in the three branches of the trigeminal nerve.

Motor function

- Ask the patient to clench their jaw and feel for the muscle bulk of both masseters and temporalis muscles.
- Ask the patient to open their mouth whilst you resist them, noting any deviation (the jaw will deviate towards the side of the nerve lesion).

Reflexes

Jaw jerk

Ask the patient to open their mouth and relax their jaw. Place your finger on their chin and tap it with a tendon hammer. The jaw should close slightly. Complete closure of the jaw indicates a UMN lesion.

Corneal reflex

This is an uncomfortable test and should only be performed by a trained professional. It involves touching the cornea with cotton wool. A normal reflex causes both eyes to blink immediately.

10.6.7 Facial nerve (CN VII)

Facial movements

Ask the patient to perform specific facial movements (**Figure 10.10**) noting any asymmetry:

- "Raise your eyebrows."
- "Screw your eyes shut and don't let me open them." Try to open the patient's eyes against resistance.
- "Blow out your cheeks and don't let me 'pop' them." Try to press in the patient's inflated cheeks against resistance.
- "Smile to show me your teeth."
- "Purse your lips."

10.6.8 Vestibulocochlear nerve (CN VIII)

Gross hearing

Explain this test to the patient before continuing.

- Stand behind the patient and hold your hand next to their left ear, rubbing your fingers and thumbs together.
- Whisper a number or word 60cm away from their right ear.
- Ask them to repeat what you have said.
- Repeat in the opposite ear.

Rinne's test

- Tap a 512Hz tuning fork and hold it over the external auditory meatus (testing air conduction), asking the patient if they can hear it.
- Now place the base of the fork on the ipsilateral mastoid process (testing bone conduction).
- Normally, air conduction should be louder than bone conduction (**Figure 10.11**).
- If bone conduction is louder, this indicates a conductive deafness.
- If neither are heard, this indicates a neural deafness.

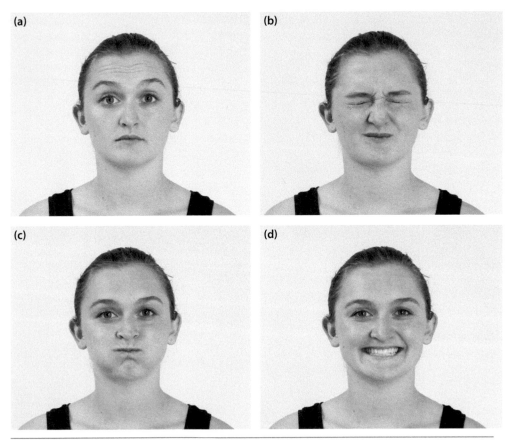

Figure 10.10 Facial expressions: (a) frontalis muscle raises the eyebrows; (b) orbicularis oculi screws the eyes closed; (c) buccinator keeps the lips closed with the cheeks puffed out; (d) risorius bares the teeth and allows smiling.

Weber's test

- Tap a 512Hz tuning fork and place it in the middle of the forehead (**Figure 10.12**).
- Normally, this should be heard equally in both ears.
- With neural deafness, the sound is louder in the normal ear.
- With conductive deafness, the sound is louder in the affected ear.

Vestibular testing

Ask the patient to close their eyes, hold their hands out in front of them and march on the spot.

- Normally, the patient should maintain their position.
- A vestibular lesion will cause them to turn towards the affected side.

10.6.9 Glossopharyngeal and vagus nerves (CN IX and X)

Inspection

- Ask the patient to open their mouth and say "ahhh". Note any uvular deviation (away from the side of the lesion) and normal elevation.

Gag reflex

- As with the corneal reflex, testing the gag reflex is uncomfortable and not routinely performed. It involves touching a stick to the back of the oral cavity to induce gagging.

Function

- Ask the patient to cough. A 'bovine' cough is heard with nerve lesions.

(a) 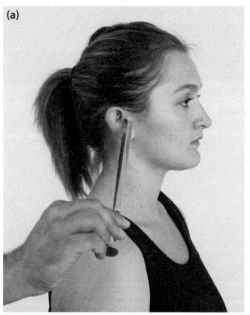(b)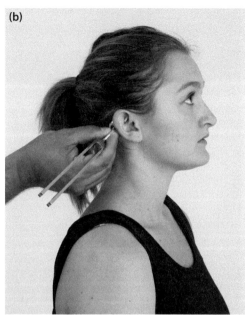

Figure 10.11 Performing Rinne's test: ask the patient whether the tuning fork is louder via (a) air conduction, or (b) bone conduction.

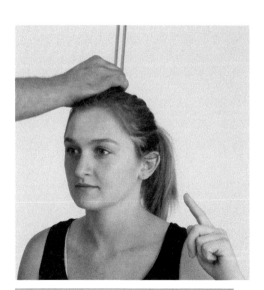

Figure 10.12 Performing Weber's test: ask the patient on which side the tuning fork is louder.

- Ask the patient to swallow and note any delay or coughing.

10.6.10 Accessory nerve (CN XI)

Test the trapezius muscle by asking the patient to shrug their shoulders against your resistance. Then test their sternocleidomastoid muscles by asking them to turn their head both ways against resistance.

10.6.11 Hypoglossal nerve (CN XII)

- Ask the patient to open their mouth and look for tongue fasciculations.
- Ask them to protrude their tongue; it will deviate towards the side of the lesion.

10.6.12 Finishing off

"To complete my examination, I would like to perform a full neurological examination of the upper and lower limbs and consider further investigations."

10.7 The visual system examination

The ophthalmic examination has a large crossover with the cranial nerve examination.

10.7.1 'ID CHECK'

This is detailed in *Section 3.2*.

The patient should be seated in a chair with their eyes exposed.

10.7.2 Endobedogram

- Are the eyes aligned?
- Is there any speech abnormality?
- Are there mobility aids to suggest neurological disease elsewhere?
- On the patient and around the bedside, are there any medications, spectacles, contact lenses or false eyes?
- Are there any scars on eyelids indicating previous surgery?

10.7.3 Inspection

Begin by looking at and around both eyes for any abnormalities.

Orbit
- Assess for any deformity or redness and swelling, indicating infection. Periorbital cellulitis is a serious condition and may rapidly spread to the eye. It requires urgent intravenous antibiotics.

Globe
- Look at the eyes anteriorly, laterally and superiorly for orbital protrusion. Posterior orbital cavity pathologies or severely raised intracranial pressure cause the eyes to be pushed abnormally far forward. Hyperthyroidism is a common cause of posterior orbital muscle and adipose tissue inflammation that makes the eye appear 'bulging'.

Eyelids
- Look for ptosis, eyelid masses or any infection within the eyelash follicles. The eyelash follicles can become blocked, inflamed and painful – this is called a stye.

Conjunctiva
- Inflammation and discharge from the conjunctiva is known as conjunctivitis. Gently pull the lower eyelid down to assess properly. Conjunctivitis is highly contagious so be careful to wash your hands again afterwards if the patient has it. Look also for any masses. Foreign objects (e.g. splinters, hairs, leaves and insects) are often blown into the eye and lodge within the conjunctival recesses.

Sclera
- Look at the whites of the eye (the sclera) for injection (prominent blood vessels making the eye red), masses and foreign bodies. Scratches or abrasions of the sclera are difficult to see but become much more visible with the instillation of fluorescein dye drops and shining a blue light.

Iris
- Look at the shape of the iris. An irregular shape can be due to an oculomotor nerve lesion. Inflammation of the iris gives a nodular appearance; this is called iritis. Pus or blood over the lower iris are sometimes seen and signify acute anterior uveitis and trauma, respectively. A syndrome called rubeosis iridis causes blood vessels to grow over the iris.

Pupil
- Look at the pupils and note their size. A normal pupil is around 2–4mm in a brightly lit room. Small pupils are seen with Horner's syndrome (usually unilateral), intracranial haemorrhage (particularly those occurring at the pons) and opioid toxicity. Asymmetry of both pupils is called anisocoria. This is usually benign but can indicate a unilateral Horner's syndrome or intracranial bleed.

10.7.4 Functional testing

- Functional testing of the eye involves examining CN II, III, IV and VI as described above. Characteristic fundoscopic findings are described in **Table 10.9**.

Table 10.9 Common fundoscopy findings

	Disc	Retina	Vessels	Macula / fovea	Other findings
Normal	Clear outline Pale cup	Red / orange Dark macula Macula ~2 disc diameters from disc	A/V ratio 2:3	Normal	
Background diabetic retinopathy	Normal	Flame haemorrhages Hard exudate	Microaneurysms	With or without maculopathy	
Preproliferative diabetic retinopathy	Normal	Flame haemorrhages Hard exudate Cotton wool spots	Microaneurysms Venous loops	With or without maculopathy	
Proliferative diabetic retinopathy	Neovascularisation	Flame haemorrhages Hard exudate Cotton wool spots	Microaneurysms Venous loops	With or without maculopathy	Preretinal fibrosis Retinal detachment
Laser photocoagulation	Neovascularisation	Flame haemorrhages Hard exudate Cotton wool spots	Microaneurysms Venous loops	With or without maculopathy	Regular, widespread pale areas associated with laser therapy
Hypertensive retinopathy	Normal	Hard exudates Retinal oedema	AV nipping Silver wiring	Normal	
Central retinal artery occlusion	Normal	Pale	Less visible	Normal	Cherry red spot Cholesterol emboli
Central retinal vein occlusion	Normal	'Stormy sunset'	Engorged	Normal	Widespread haemorrhage
Optic atrophy	Pale and featureless	Normal	Normal	Normal	
Papilloedema	Blurred disc margin	Normal	Obscured vessels (severe)	Normal	
Macular degeneration	Normal	Normal	Normal	Drusen	

10.8 Common investigations

Investigations used in cranial nerve diseases are aimed at identifying or confirming the cause of the nerve problem. Much of the investigations for cranial nerves are the same as those in *Chapter 9* that investigate peripheral nerve pathologies. They are not discussed again here.

10.8.1 Computed tomography

CT gives non-invasive views within the brain which identifies mass lesions. The addition of IV contrast can assess for vascular lesions, less obvious solid mass lesions, intracranial bleeds and vascular abnormalities such as arterial aneurysms. However, CT does not give great detail of the brainstem.

10.8.2 Magnetic resonance imaging

MRI gives far more detailed images of the brainstem and cranial nerve nuclei. As with CT, IV contrast can be given to enhance lesions and blood vessels.

10.8.3 Slit lamp examination

Slit lamp examination allows for an experienced ophthalmologist to make a more detailed examination of the retina.

10.8.4 Retinal photography

Special cameras are used to photograph the patient's retina. This gives detailed images to aid both diagnosis and monitoring of any progression of retinal disease.

10.8.5 Tonometry

Tonometry is the measuring of intraocular pressure using a warm puff of air blown at the patient's eye. Glaucoma is defined as a pressure exceeding 20mmHg.

10.8.6 Retinal artery and vein angiography

Angiography using IV fluorescein images the blood supply to the retina when diagnosing retinal vein occlusion.

10.9 System summary

Dysfunction of the cranial nerves and visual system impacts greatly on individuals' lives. Such disorders affect safe eating and drinking, reduce the ability to communicate, see or hear and alter physical facial appearance. Most causes are reversible if diagnosed and treated early. Understanding the underlying processes and how to identify them is the first step in helping patients with such problems.

10.10 Answers to starter questions

1. Seeing the brain of a living person outside of the neurosurgical theatre is usually abnormal and they should be offered a speedy method of getting to hospital. However, in many circles, the retina is considered a part of the CNS, given its direct connection to visual centres within the brain. Therefore, it is argued that a physician need only pick up an ophthalmoscope and look in someone's eye to be able to see the brain.

2. An abducens nerve (CN VI) palsy does cause inability to abduct the eye on the affected side. However, the abducens nerve course is long and tortuous and it is subject to compression caused by raised intracranial pressure. This focal sign without direct nerve injury is termed a 'false localising sign'. Raised intracranial pressure can be missed if investigation focuses purely on the direct causes of abducens nerve palsy.

3. The olfactory nerve (CN I) passes through the cribriform plate on its course to the brain. Head injuries causing bony fractures sometimes damage the small nerve fibres, leading to loss of smell (anosmia). Additionally, the olfactory centres lie within the frontal lobes and are particularly susceptible to injury from traumatic brain injuries, especially those where the injury is sustained from behind. Up to 8% of traumatic brain injuries are associated with anosmia which is usually permanent. Non-neurological causes of anosmia include blockage of the nasal passages (such as from upper respiratory tract infections and nasal polyps), Paget's disease of the bone and Kallmann's syndrome (a genetic hypogonadotrophic hypogonadism and incomplete puberty with anosmia).

4. Bell's palsy is an idiopathic disease of the facial nerve (CN VII). One of the functions of the facial nerve is to dampen the stapedial muscles of the inner ear. Loss of innervation to these muscles may lead to hyperacusis – intolerably loud hearing.

5. A white walking stick holds no benefit to mobility and should not be considered a mobility aid. People with visual impairment use white canes to tap on objects in their path to guide them as they walk. It is also a universally recognised sign to people with normal vision to identify those with visual impairment so that they may help them or remove themselves and objects from their path.

Chapter 11
Musculoskeletal system

Starter questions

1. Should patients with rheumatoid arthritis see a physician, surgeon or occupational therapist?
2. Why should you always look a patient in the eye?
3. Why do patients with ankylosing spondylitis have difficulty on November 5th?
4. Why are some rheumatological conditions treated in the Respiratory clinic?

Answers to questions are to be found in *Section 11.9*.

11.1 Introduction

The musculoskeletal (MSK) system comprises the skeleton, a collection of 206 bones, and the muscles that move them. Muscles attach to bones via tendons, whereas bones attach to other bones via ligaments.

Together, the MSK system performs several major functions, as it:

- provides structural support to allow upright posture
- provides movement and locomotion
- provides physical protection to major organs
- produces cells of the blood
- provides a homeostatic store for calcium, phosphate and glucose.

Diseases of the MSK system present at any time of life, as a consequence of primary disease or associated with multisystemic diseases. Indeed, MSK manifestations are often the first presentation of some diseases.

MSK diseases can be severely debilitating and painful, causing psychological distress and social isolation.

Clinical assessment of the MSK system includes quantifying the severity of disease and the impact on the patient's day-to-day life.

Case 11.1 A swollen knee

Presentation

Mr Lock is 21 years old. He presents to his GP with a painful and swollen right knee.

Initial interpretation

The causes of joint swelling are loosely categorised as:

- infection (e.g. septic arthritis) – a medical emergency
- inflammation, including rheumatological disease, seronegative arthropathies and crystal arthropathies
- injuries including fractures, dislocations and tendon or ligamental damage
- non-injurous including spontaneous haemarthrosis in patients with coagulation disorders.

Infections happen at any time and must be confidently ruled out. Rheumatological disease is uncommon in younger people and if present, tends to affect females more than males. Injuries are the commonest cause of joint complaints in younger people.

History

Mr Lock has just returned from a skiing season in the French Alps. He is normally very active and was working as a ski instructor for the last four months. Since returning he has noted that his right knee was aching for a few days and then that it was swollen when he woke up three days ago. It is painful to walk and tender to touch. He cannot recall injuring himself at any point. He feels generally well in himself and denies any systemic symptoms of fevers or sweats. He denies any other symptoms on systems review. He has had no joint problems in the past.

Interpretation of history

Mr Lock's knee swelling is acute and appears to have occurred without injury. He is very active and has been taking part in a sport that puts a lot of strain on the knees over a prolonged period. This would put him at risk of stress or overuse injury although his symptoms would tend to be worse when performing the particular movement (i.e. bending his knees).

Reassuringly, he does not describe any symptoms of severe infection, and his knee symptoms have been present for a week, making septic arthritis unlikely. He is young and describes pain and swelling in a single joint, making rheumatological disease unlikely.

Reactive arthritis remains a possibility and should be excluded in a patient with unexplained joint inflammation.

Further history

Mr Lock has no past medical history and takes no regular medications. He does not smoke but admits to occasional binge drinking with friends. He is sexually active and admits to unprotected intercourse with a regular partner over the last four months but denies any urethral symptoms. He is not aware of any family history of joint disease.

Examination

He looks well and is comfortable sitting in the chair but was noted to 'hobble' into the consultation room. His right knee is swollen, erythematous and warm to touch. Knee flexion and extension are painful but the range of movement is not reduced. The opposite knee appears normal and there is no other inflammation elsewhere. He has no rashes on his body and his eyes appear normal.

Interpretation of findings

Mr Lock has clear evidence of inflammation in his right knee and no evidence of any other joint being affected. This makes primary rheumatological disease much less likely. He has no evidence of skin or eye involvement, which supports this.

Reactive arthritis and injury remain the most likely causes for his knee swelling. There is little to differentiate them from the history and examination. He requires imaging of the joint, primarily with plain X-rays to rule out bony injury. He should have the fluid aspirated to both provide samples for laboratory analysis and relieve his pain. This should be performed by an experienced practitioner in a sterile environment to prevent introducing infection into the joint space.

Irrespective of his joint disease, Mr Lock should seek sexual health screening after having unprotected intercourse with a new partner, even if he does not have active symptoms.

Investigations

Mr Lock's knee X-ray is normal and shows no fractures or dislocation. Routine blood tests show a slightly raised white blood cell count and normal C-reactive protein. His erythrocyte sedimentation rate (ESR) is normal. The fluid aspirated from his joint is a creamy / straw colour and slightly turbulent. Urgent Gram staining shows no bacteria and microscopy shows a large

amount of pus cells. His urine antigen tests are negative for *Neisseria gonorrhoeae* and positive for *Chlamydia trachomatis.*

Diagnosis

Mr Lock has reactive arthritis, a condition caused by immune cross-reactivity to an infection elsewhere in the body. Whilst treating the underlying infection, the joint is treated symptomatically with a course of NSAIDs – these should be used with caution in those with severe asthma or GI disease. Of those with reactive arthritis, around a third recover with no further symptoms, a third suffer a recurrent arthritis and a third develop a chronic or progressive arthritis. He should be educated on safe sexual practices and be screened for other sexually transmitted diseases such as HIV and hepatitis.

11.2 System overview

11.2.1 Bones

The human skeleton has around 270 bones at birth. As we grow some bones fuse together, leaving 206 in the adult skeleton. Between the sexes there are some marked differences in the shape of the skeleton, such as a wider pelvis in the female skeleton to allow for childbirth. The skeleton supports movement and posture as well as providing protection to the organs and structures underneath. The bone marrow produces the blood cells and is a vital part of the immune system.

Composition
Bones are formed of cells held within an extracellular matrix composed of:
- osteoid – a collagen-rich, organic scaffold giving structure and elasticity
- ground substance – a mineral-rich material giving rigidity.

Bones contain three parts:
- Cortical bone – a hard outer layer with extracellular matrix arranged in columns (osteons): 80% of skeletal mass
- Cancellous bone – a spongy network of bone: 20% of skeletal mass
- Bone marrow – there are two types:
  - □ red marrow – responsible for the production of red and white blood cells and platelets (haematopoiesis); found within flat bones and areas of cancellous bone in long bones
  - □ yellow marrow – mainly fat cells; replaces red marrow with age but can be converted back if increased production of blood cells is required; found in the medullary cavity of long bones.

The distribution of these parts varies depending on the type of bone (**Table 11.1**).

Growth
Bones grow in two ways:
- Intramembranous ossification – a non-cartilaginous, connective tissue model is replaced with bone (ossification)

Table 11.1	*Types of bone*			
Type	**Description**	**Function**	**Examples**	**Growth type**
Long bones	Rounded heads (epiphyses) of cancellous bone at either end of a shaft (diaphysis) of compact bone. Shaft contains a hollow medullary cavity containing yellow marrow.	Movement / locomotion	All limb bones excluding carpal / tarsal bones and patellae	Endochondrial ossification
Short bones	Generally cubic bones with a thin layer of compact bone around cancellous bone	Joint stability	Carpal (wrist) bones Tarsal (ankle) bones	Endochondrial ossification
Flat bones	Thin and curved bones with a thin layer of compact bone around cancellous bone	Mechanical cages / protection	Skull Sternum Ribs	Intramembranous ossification
Sesamoid bones	Bones embedded within tendons	Hold tendons away from joint to allow increased muscle leverage	Patella Pisiform	Endochondrial ossification
Irregular bones	Bones that do not fit into above categories Consist of a thin layer of compact bone around cancellous bone		Vertebrae Pelvis Mandible	Endochondrial ossification

- Endochondrial ossification – a cartilage model of bone in two stages:
  - □ primary ossification – cartilage model is replaced by bone during foetal development, leaving epiphyseal plates at either end
  - □ secondary ossification– new bone growth at epiphyseal plates allowing bone lengthening.

Remodelling

Bone is a dynamic tissue under the influence of different cells:

- Osteoblasts – bone-forming cells responsible for primary and secondary ossification
- Osteocytes – osteoblasts that have become surrounded by bone and are no longer functional
- Osteoclasts – bone-destroying cells responsible for resorption.

In healthy bone, osteoclasts migrate towards and resorb damaged or strained areas. Osteoblasts are then activated to reform healthy "remodelled" bone.

Osteoclastic activity is also under hormonal control to allow the increased release of calcium and phosphate from bone to allow homeostasis.

11.2.2 Joints

Joints between bones are classified by the movement permitted (**Table 11.2**).

The articular surfaces of bones within synovial joints are covered in a shock-absorbing layer of cartilage that allows smooth movement against another bone. Loss of cartilage within a joint reduces shock absorbance and allows bones to rub against each other, leading to formation of osteophytes (abnormal bony growths), subchondral bone inflammation and joint destruction. This is extremely painful.

Joint classification	Mobility	Description	Examples
Synarthrosis	Minimal / nil	Direct fibrous linkage between bones	Skull sutures
Amphiarthrosis	Slight	Direct cartilaginous linkage between bones	Intervertebral discs
Synovial	Free	Indirect linkage of bones contained within a fluid-filled cavity and ligaments	Elbow joints Hip joints Shoulder joints

Table 11.2 *Classification of joints*

Ligaments are fibrous bands of connective tissue that act to stabilise the joint and limit excessive movement causing over-articulation and dislocation.

> Movements across a joint have different terms (**Figure 11.1**):
> ■ Flexion is the reduction of the angle between bones of a joint; extension is when this angle increases.
> ■ Abduction is the movement of a bone away from the centre of the body; adduction pulls the bone towards the body.
> ■ Elevation occurs when a body part is raised superiorly (such as shrugging the shoulders); depression refers to inferior movement.
> ■ Rotation is either internal (medial, towards the body) or external (lateral, away from the body).

11.2.3 Muscles

There are three types of muscle, which perform different functions within the body:
■ Skeletal muscle. These muscles are attached to bones via tendons and are under voluntary control to coordinate movement. The muscles referred to in this chapter are skeletal muscles.
■ Smooth muscle. These are the muscles that are found within organs and other body structures outside of the skeletal system. They are not under voluntary control (i.e. a person cannot consciously activate smooth muscles).
■ Cardiac muscle. These are the muscles of the heart. They are more similar in structure to

skeletal than smooth muscle but are not under conscious control. These are discussed in more detail in *Chapter 4*.

Individual skeletal muscle cells (myocytes) contain mitochondria to produce energy in the form of adenosine triphosphate (ATP) from stored glycogen, myoglobin to bind and store oxygen and filaments of actin and myosin arranged in sarcomeres.

Myocytes are grouped into fascicles which are surrounded and grouped by the epimysium to give muscles. At each end, the epimysium becomes tendon and attaches the muscle to bone. Muscular contraction pulls the attached bones at either side of the joint towards each other.

There are two types of skeletal myocytes:
■ Slow twitch – fibres containing plenty of myoglobin and mitochondria to allow prolonged but relatively weak contraction during aerobic respiration.
■ Fast twitch – fibres containing minimal myoglobin and mitochondria for short periods of strong contraction during anaerobic respiration.

Skeletal muscle contraction is under the control of motor pathways. Lesions of these pathways give stereotypical weakness (see **Table 9.5** in *Chapter 9: Neurology*). In muscle contraction, an action potential travels along a neuron, releasing acetylcholine at the neuromuscular junction, causing calcium to flood the myocyte. This allows actin and myosin to bind and, with ATP acting as an energy source, form sequential cross bridges that lead to muscle fibre shortening.

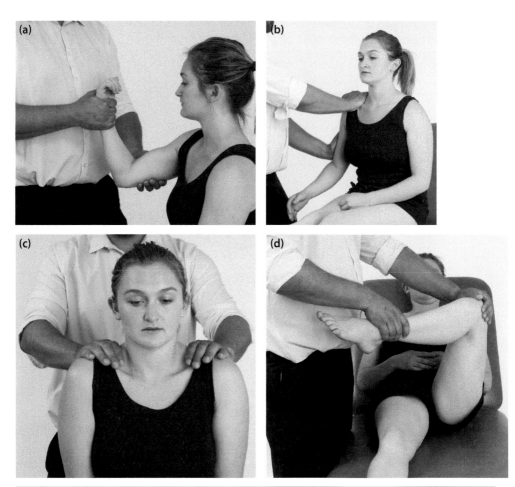

Figure 11.1 Joint movements: (a) elbow flexion and extension; (b) shoulder abduction and adduction; (c) shoulder elevation and depression; (d) hip internal and external rotation.

11.2.4 Musculoskeletal disease

The musculoskeletal system is particularly susceptible to damage from either trauma or overuse. The ability to remodel bone reduces with age and articular cartilage cannot be replaced if worn down.

Rheumatic disease (**Table 11.3**) encompasses most disease of the musculoskeletal system, and includes other disorders such as vasculitis. Some rheumatic diseases are immunological, where a patient possesses an antibody or antibodies that recognise a normal antigen within the body as foreign. This triggers an immune response that causes inflammation and damage to the body's own tissue. These diseases are chronic and disabling and have no cure. The mainstay of treatment is alleviating the symptoms and disrupting or suppressing the immune response.

Table 11.3 *Overview of immunology in rheumatological diseases of the MSK system*

Disease	Associated antibodies	Antigen	Note
Rheumatoid arthritis	Rheumatoid factor Anti-CCP	HLA DR4	Symmetrical, polyarticular disease
SLE	Anti-dsDNA Anti-Ro Anti-La Anti-Sm Anti-RNP		Multisystem disease
Diffuse scleroderma	Anti-Scl70 Anti-centromere		Multisystem disease
Limited scleroderma	Anti-centromere		CREST syndrome = Calcinosis, Raynaud's syndrome, oEsophageal dysmotility, Sclerodactyly, Telangiectasia
Reactive arthritis		HLA B27	Inflammatory arthritis in response to infection elsewhere in the body
Osteoarthritis	None	None	'Wear and tear' of articular cartilage
Gout	None	None	Negatively birefringent crystal arthropathy
Pseudogout	None	None	Positively birefringent crystal arthropathy
Septic arthritis	None	None	Bacterial infection within synovial cavity
Polymyalgia rheumatica		HLA DR4	Muscle inflammation causing pain and stiffness
Polymyositis	Anti-Jo		Inflammation of proximal skeletal muscles
Dermatomyositis	Anti-Jo		Inflammation of proximal skeletal muscles with skin rash
Ankylosing spondylitis		HLA B27	Inflammatory arthritis of spine
Psoriatic arthritis		HLA B27	Arthritis may occur before onset of visible psoriasis
Sjögren's syndrome	Anti-Ro Anti-La		Dry eyes, mouth and skin

11.3 Symptoms of musculoskeletal disease

The key symptoms of musculoskeletal disease are pain, swelling, deformity, weakness and fatigue. Symptom terminology is described in **Table 11.4**.

11.3.1 Pain

Muscular

Myalgia is typically an aching sensation that is worse on movement or palpation of the affected muscle. It occurs with:

- injury / trauma
- overuse (repetitive strain injury)
- rhabdomyolysis
- fibromyalgia
- autoimmune disorders
- metabolic disorders (such as Conn's syndrome, adrenal insufficiency, diabetes mellitus and thyroid disease).

> **Fibromyalgia** is a syndrome of chronic widespread pain, increased pain response to pressure, sleep disturbance, profound tiredness and memory problems. The cause is unknown but it has been linked to stress, trauma and some infections.

Joint

Any damage within a joint causes arthralgia (**Table 11.5**) through a combination of:

- loss of cartilage on articular surfaces allowing bones to rub against each other
- inflammation of soft tissues around joints
- increased fluid (including blood and pus) within the joint space stretching synovial membranes.

Arthralgia can also be triggered by the immune response to certain infections (particularly viral ones) and vaccinations.

Bone

The periosteum is highly sensitive and is stimulated by:

- damage – bone fractures, tumour invasion
- irritation – infection, ischaemia, rheumatological conditions.

In other diseases, such as osteomalacia, rickets and osteonecrosis, the cause for ostalgia is not fully understood but is thought to involve non-periosteal neural pathways.

Tendon / ligamental pain

Enthes- and tendinopathies are usually caused by overuse and irritation (such as plantar fasciitis, Achilles tendinitis or patellar tendinitis). Enthesitis is associated with HLA B27 arthropathies (ankylosing spondylitis, psoriatic arthritis, reactive arthritis).

Nerve entrapment

Inflammation and thickening of the ligaments

Table 11.4 *Prefixes and suffixes in MSK disease. These are combined to describe a particular sign or symptom. For example, myo- and -algia combine to form 'myalgia' meaning muscle pain, 'arthro-' and '-itis' form arthritis, meaning joint inflammation*			
Prefix		**Suffix**	
Myo-	Muscle	-algia	Pain
Arthro-	Joint	-itis	Inflammation
Osteo-	Bone	-opathy	Disease or disorder
Tendin-	Tendons		
Entheso-	Connective tissue joining tendon or ligament to bone		
Dermato-	Skin		

Table 11.5 *Disease processes causing joint pain*

Process	Example	Mechanism
Destruction of articular surfaces	Osteoarthritis	Wear and tear of cartilage
	Gout, pseudogout	Crystal deposition causing inflammatory response
	Rheumatological diseases	Autoimmune destruction of articular cartilage
Inflammation and thickening of joint capsule	Rheumatological diseases	Autoimmune attack on joint capsule
Soft tissue inflammation	Sports injury, trauma	Abnormal strain on particular tendon / ligament
Increased fluid	Haemarthrosis, septic arthritis	Increased fluid volume within synovial cavity

enclosing the small passages through which nerves pass compress the nerve, causing pain and distal weakness and numbness (**Table 11.6**).

Causes include:
- trauma or repetitive use
- rheumatoid arthritis
- endocrinopathies (diabetes mellitus, hypothyroidism and acromegaly)
- pregnancy
- obesity.

11.3.2 Swelling

Joint swelling

Excess fluid (effusion) within the joint space causes swelling. This is usually painful due to stretching of the synovial membranes. Effusions associated with active inflammation appear red, hot and tender.

Septic arthritis
Infection within the joint space is an orthopaedic emergency and must be excluded in any acute knee effusion. The patient is usually systemically unwell with fevers and lethargy, or even has sepsis.

Crystal arthropathies
Deposition of crystals (such as uric acid in gout) causes a recurrent acute inflammatory process.

Other arthropathies
Any condition which causes an immune reaction within a joint can cause effusions.

Haemarthroses
Bleeding into a joint space will cause swelling. This can be traumatic or due to disorders of coagulation (e.g. haemophilia).

Table 11.6 *Common nerve entrapment syndromes*

Syndrome	Affected nerve	Site of compression
Carpal tunnel syndrome	Median nerve	Wrist
Cubital tunnel syndrome	Ulnar nerve	Elbow
Guyon's canal syndrome	Ulnar nerve	Wrist
Radial tunnel syndrome	Radial nerve	Forearm

11.3.3 Weakness

Weakness from musculoskeletal disease is due to:
- primary muscular disease
- functional limitation from pain
- functional limitation from muscle wasting
- functional limitation from lethargy.

11.3.4 Deformity

Changes in physical appearance occur from:
- chronic or repetitive joint inflammation and erosion
- weakness or wasting of muscles around a joint causing malalignment.

11.3.5 Fatigue

Fatigue is the sensation of tiredness during or after completing tasks that are usually a normal part of life (such as washing and dressing) and that inhibits normal social and physical functioning. It is separate from weakness in that it improves with rest. It is particular to the individual and is sometimes severely depressing. The exact cause of fatigue in MSK disease is a multifactorial combination of:
- inflammatory and metabolic burden from chronic disease
- a direct consequence of disease
- a side-effect of treatments / medications
- low mood from chronic disease.

> **Chronic fatigue syndrome** is defined as fatigue for more than six months. It can be relapsing or persistent, and is associated with many chronic medical conditions.

11.4 The musculoskeletal history

The commonest cause of MSK system symptoms is through injury or trauma. These usually affect joints, as there are tendons and ligaments that are susceptible to stretch injuries but do not have the elasticity to tolerate this and become irritated or torn. If a patient has injured themselves, ask about the mechanism of the injury – how it happened and how the joint was affected. Ask:
- What position was the joint / limb in before the injury?
- What happened to the joint / limb during the injury?
- Were there any sounds (crunching, clicking or popping)? This could indicate a bony injury.
- Was there pain immediately after the injury or did this take time? Bone fractures and tears to tendons or ligaments tend to be painful immediately, whereas irritations hurt after a time.
- Are they able to walk on or use the affected joint / limb? This guides the clinician in how to best support the patient with coping with the injury whilst it heals.

11.4.1 Past medical history

MSK disease presents in a multitude of ways. Acute injuries have an obvious onset and cause, whilst some rheumatological conditions have a more insidious onset. Symptoms of ache, lethargy and feeling generally unwell often occur over years before a patient presents for investigation. Understanding a long-term timeline of symptoms is key in understanding the disease process.

The distribution of symptoms around the body differs according to disease. Establish if joint disease affects large joints, small joints or both. Is the distribution of joints affected symmetrical? Does muscle weakness affect a particular limb or just the arms or legs, and are the muscles proximal or distal?

Some diseases of the MSK system are preceded by an acute infection. Sometimes, as with rheumatic disease and rheumatic fever, the infection is in childhood.

11.4.2 Medications

Medications used in treating rheumatological conditions have severe side-effects, with immunosuppression and allergic reactions. Many patients trial and escalate through different treatment courses, so establish why these treatments were changed. Drugs used in rheumatological diseases have many side-effects (**Table 11.7**). Analgesia is a key component of managing MSK disease and varies widely between patients. Be especially aware of GI side-effects from NSAIDs.

There are many medications with MSK side-effects (**Table 11.8**); always enquire about previous treatment courses predating the onset of symptoms.

Table 11.7 *Side-effects of common drugs used in rheumatology*

Drug	Use in MSK disease	Side-effect
Steroids	Immunosuppression in active disease	Increased susceptibility to infection Osteoporosis Cushing's syndrome Bruising Thin skin GI irritation
NSAIDs	Anti-inflammatory painkillers	GI irritation Worsening asthma Kidney injury Contraindicated in heart disease
Methotrexate	DMARD	GI irritation Immunosuppression Mouth ulcers Liver injury Lung fibrosis
Sulfasalazine	DMARD	GI irritation Bone marrow suppression Liver injury Kidney injury
Ciclosporin	DMARD	Hypertension Kidney injury Excessive hair growth
Hydroxychloroquine	DMARD	GI irritation Headache Muscle weakness
Biological therapies	Interference of antigen–antibody response in disease	Allergic reactions (including anaphylaxis) Lymphoma Reactivation of latent infections (e.g. TB)

Table 11.8 *Medications with MSK side-effects*

Drug	Use	MSK side-effect
Statins	Cholesterol-lowering	Muscle aches Rhabdomyolysis
Vaccinations (especially influenza)	Immune defence against disease	Muscle aches
Granulocyte colony-stimulating factor	Accelerated neutrophil release in neutropenic sepsis	Bone ache
Fluoroquinolones (ciprofloxacin)	Antibiotic	Tendinitis, especially Achilles tendinitis

11.4.3 Social history

This focuses on establishing the presence of modifiable risk factors and how the patient's health is impacting on their life.

Smoking
Tobacco smoking is detrimental to preservation of bone density, especially in post-menopausal women.

Alcohol
High alcohol intake also detracts from bone and muscle health. The poor nutritional state associated with chronic alcoholism leads to a decrease in muscle mass and physical strength. Risk of injury is much higher during periods of acute intoxication.

Illicit drugs
The use of unclean or used needles for IV drug use risks the development of bacteraemia and seeding of infection in bone (osteomyelitis) or joints (septic arthritis). The need for long courses of antibiotics in patients with difficult vascular access proves challenging in this cohort.

Employment
Find out whether the patient is in employment, and what they do. Repetitive tasks lead to overuse and strain injuries. Additionally, severe MSK disease is disabling and may prevent someone from continuing in their line of employment.

Physical activity
Enquire whether the patient is active in their daily life, and whether they take any exercise. A sedentary lifestyle significantly reduces muscle and bone strength. Reduced mobility from MSK disease greatly impacts on cardiovascular and respiratory health.

Table 11.9 *Non-musculoskeletal manifestations of MSK disease*

Disease	Non-MSK consequence
Rheumatoid arthritis	Splinter haemorrhages
	Scleritis
	Anaemia
	Rheumatoid skin nodules (especially elbows)
	Lung fibrosis
	Pericardial effusions
	Splenomegaly (Felty's syndrome)
Psoriatic arthritis	Nail pitting
	Onycholysis
	Scleritis
SLE	Periungual telangiectasia
	Splinter haemorrhages
	Mouth ulcers
	Facial butterfly rash
	Lung fibrosis
	Splenomegaly
	Hepatomegaly
Dermatomyositis	Gottron's papules

Hobbies

Some sports, such as tennis or running, cause overuse injuries.

Social circumstances

Patients requiring walking aids or using wheelchairs require adequate space to mobilise and the installation of ramps, rails and specialised beds or bathing equipment in order to maintain independence and dignity through their disease. Ask if they live in a house or a flat, if there are stairs in and to get to their accommodation and if there is a lift if they live above the ground floor. If a patient does not own their property, permission is needed from the legal owner before modifications can be made.

Functional capacity

Establish functional capacity and how this has changed in recent months to years. Ask if symptoms have affected:

- their daily life
- ability to work
- enjoyment of interests and hobbies.

The provision of adapted equipment, including cutlery / crockery, beds and walking aids greatly improves a patient's ability to function independently.

11.4.4 Family history

Ask about:

- rheumatological disease, especially that of early onset as these are sometimes hereditary
- congenital deformities.

11.4.5 Systems review

Many rheumatological diseases manifest signs and symptoms outside of the MSK system, and these often present before the onset of focal MSK symptoms (**Table 11.9**).

11.5 Signs of musculoskeletal disease

11.5.1 Hand and nail changes

Deformities

- A number of joint deformities (**Figure 11.2**) occur within the hands which are specific to either rheumatoid arthritis or osteoarthritis (**Table 11.10**)
- Other deformities include:
  - ☐ Dupuytren's contracture – fixed flexion of

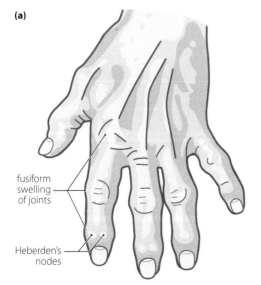

(a)

fusiform swelling of joints

Heberden's nodes

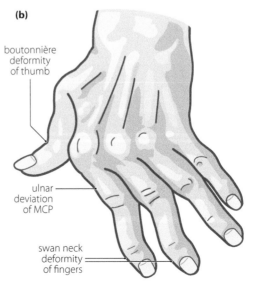

(b)

boutonnière deformity of thumb

ulnar deviation of MCP

swan neck deformity of fingers

Figure 11.2 Hand changes with (a) osteoarthritis and (b) rheumatoid arthritis.

Rheumatoid arthritis		**Osteoarthritis**	
Swan neck deformity	DIP hyperflexion with PIP hyperextension	Bouchard's nodes	Bony swelling of PIPs
Z thumb	Hyperextension of interphalangeal joint with fixed flexion and subluxation of MCP	Heberden's nodes	Bony swelling of DIPs
Boutonnière deformity	PIP flexion with DIP hyperextension		
Finger ulnar deviation	Deviation of fingers towards ulnar aspect of wrist		

Table 11.10 *Hand deformities associated with rheumatoid arthritis and osteoarthritis*

PIP = proximal interphalangeal joint; DIP = distal interphalangeal joint; MCP = metacarpophalangeal joint

one or more metacarpophalangeal joints (MCPs) caused by abnormal thickening of the palmar fascia
☐ sausage-shaped fingers associated with psoriatic arthritis
☐ gouty tophi – fleshy, nodular, yellow growths that form on joints with chronic gout.

Muscle wasting
Muscle wasting occurs as a result of:
■ chronic joint disease and immobility
■ motor neuron lesion
■ nerve entrapment syndrome
■ wasting of the thenar eminence is typically seen with carpal tunnel syndrome.

Nail changes
Nail changes are common with rheumatological diseases and are often typical of the underlying condition:

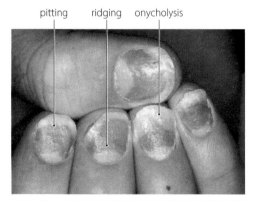

pitting   ridging   onycholysis

Figure 11.3 Nail changes associated with psoriasis.

■ Psoriatic arthritis is associated with nail pitting and ridging, thickening (hyperkeratosis), discolouration, and separation from the nail bed (onycholysis) (**Figure 11.3**).
■ Telangiectases around the nail are seen with SLE and scleroderma.
■ Rheumatological causes for splinter haemorrhages include SLE and rheumatoid arthritis.

11.5.2 Eyes

Dry eyes are associated with Sjögren's syndrome. Red and painful eyes (scleritis) occur with the seronegative spondyloarthropathies and rheumatoid arthritis. Conjunctival pallor is a sign of anaemia of chronic disease from long-standing rheumatological illness.

11.5.3 Mouth

Mouth ulcers are common and usually benign. However, they are also associated with reactive arthritis and SLE.

11.5.4 Skin

Hair and scalp
Alopecia (hair loss) and short broken hairs occur with SLE. Psoriatic plaques are often seen on the scalp, particularly on the hairline and behind the ears.

Face

There are three classical facial appearances seen in rheumatological diseases:

- A tight-skinned face with a 'salt-and-pepper' complexion is seen with scleroderma
- SLE is associated with a butterfly rash across the nose and cheeks
- A purple rash (heliotrope rash) develops around the eyes with dermatomyositis.

Shoulders

A red rash in a shawl-like distribution is seen in dermatomyositis. It is needed alongside muscular inflammation to confirm the diagnosis.

Elbows

Rheumatoid nodules are seen in the elbows and are easily missed. These are subcutaneous, firm and immobile. A similar swelling is caused by gout.

General

Psoriatic plaques can be small and appear anywhere on the body. Always take a good look across all of the skin; this often requires the patient to undress. Raised, painful, red-blue shin lesions called erythema nodosum occur with many diseases including sarcoidosis, inflammatory bowel disease and drug reactions. Patchy loss of pigmentation (vitiligo) is linked to a wide variety of autoimmune and inflammatory diseases. Gottron's papules are red, scaly and raised lesions that develop over the extensor surfaces of finger joints, elbows and knees with dermatomyositis.

11.5.5 Muscles

As with the small muscles of the hands, larger skeletal muscles waste away due to:

- inactivity of a diseased or deformed joint
- poor innervation from a motor neuron injury
- chronic inflammation of skeletal muscle, as with dermatomyositis and polymyositis; typically these conditions cause a proximal muscle inflammation and wasting.

11.5.6 Changes in posture

Ankylosing spondylitis causes an exaggerated kyphosis and loss of normal lumbar lordosis,

leading to a characteristic 'question mark' posture (**Figure 11.4**). A cushingoid appearance suggests recurrent courses of steroids for frequently flaring rheumatological disease.

11.5.7 Non-musculoskeletal signs

There are signs of rheumatological conditions outside of the MSK system that should not be missed. They indicate severe or advanced disease due to the involvement of additional organs.

Thorax

- Fine inspiratory crackles are heard when pulmonary fibrosis secondary to rheumatoid arthritis, SLE and other connective tissue diseases occurs
- Pericardial effusions associated with connective tissue diseases are auscultated as a pericardial rub.

Abdomen

- Rheumatoid arthritis and SLE cause palpable splenomegaly
- SLE also causes hepatomegaly.

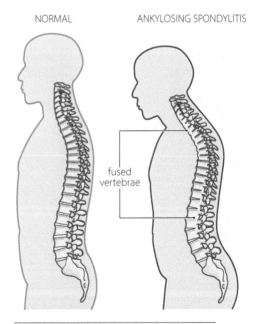

NORMAL   ANKYLOSING SPONDYLITIS

fused vertebrae

Figure 11.4 The 'question mark' posture of ankylosing spondylitis.

11.6 The musculoskeletal examination

Like all examinations, a consistent and thorough approach is required (**Table 11.11**). The MSK system examination begins with a screening examination of the gait, arms, legs and spine (GALS) before focusing on areas of interest or concern. The more detailed joint-specific examinations follow the general rule of look, feel, move, function (if appropriate) and special tests.

> The mnemonic **'DWARFS'** – **D**eformities, **W**asting, **A**symmetry, **R**ashes, **F**asciculations and **S**cars – is a useful memory aid when inspecting for musculoskeletal abnormalities.

11.6.1 'ID CHECK'

This is detailed in *Section 3.2*.
The patient should be in their underwear and standing up if possible.

11.6.2 Endobedogram

Have a good look at the patient:

■ Are they in discomfort?
■ Is their resting posture normal and are they able to maintain it?
■ Do they have any obvious deformities?
■ Can you see any mobility aids, wheelchairs or orthotic devices?
■ Do they have any medications with them?

11.6.3 GALS

Screening questions

Ask the patient:
■ "Do you have any pain in your back, joints or muscles?"
■ "Can you dress yourself without problems?"
■ "Can you walk up and down stairs on your own?"

Inspection

Ask the patient to stand in the anatomical position and look at them from the front, side and back (**Figure 11.5**):

Front
■ Assess muscle bulk and symmetry of the shoulders, hips and quadriceps

Table 11.11 *Overview of MSK examination*	
Element	**Details**
Screening questions	Ask about general MSK function
Inspection	Observe for 'DWARFS' (see highlighted box for explanation) front, side and back
Gait	Observe and assess gait and turning ability
Arms	Assess movement and screen for joint disease in upper limbs
Legs	Assess movement and screen for joint disease in lower limbs
Spine	Assess shape and movement of spine
Review	Note abnormal area and focus on for further examination
Look	Inspect selected joint for abnormalities
Feel	Palpate joint for tenderness, heat or swelling
Move	Assess active and passive movement of joint
Special tests	Perform special tests according to joint being examined

(a) 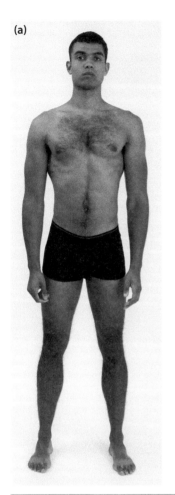   **(b)** 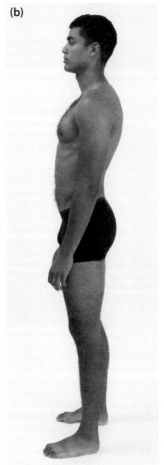   **(c)**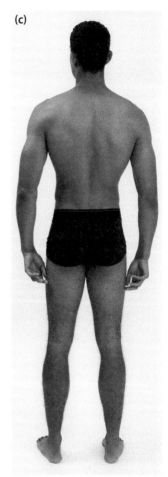

Figure 11.5 GALS inspection for 'DWARFS' from (a) front; (b) side; (c) back.

- Note the alignment of the knees and any swelling or deformities
- Check for foot deformity.

Side

- Look at the spine and note normal or abnormal curvature
- Check for knee hyperextension
- Assess foot arches – low arches = pes planus, high arches = pes cavus.

Back

- Assess muscle bulk and symmetry of the shoulder, hips and gluteal muscles
- Note the alignment of the spine and iliac crests
- Check for swelling behind the knees (such as a Baker's cyst).

Gait

Ask the patient to walk across the room and back. Assess for abnormal gaits (**Table 11.12**) and comment on:

- smoothness
- step height (high in foot drop)
- ataxia
- ease of turning.

Arms

Ask the patient to perform a routine of manoeuvres:

1. "Place your hands behind your head" – this tests shoulder abduction, external rotation and elbow flexion (**Figure 11.6**).
2. "Hold your hands out, with the palms down

Table 11.12 *Abnormal gaits*

Type of gait	Description	Cause
Antalgic	Limping	Pain from injury or joint disease
Circumductive	Circular movement of hips giving appearance of leg 'swinging around' hip	Hemiplegia
Waddling	Straight-legged gait with legs turned out	Congenital hip dysplasia
High-stepping	Abnormally pronounced hip flexion leading to high raising of the knee	Foot drop
Scissoring	Slightly crouching with thighs and knees hitting and/or crossing during gait	Cerebral palsy

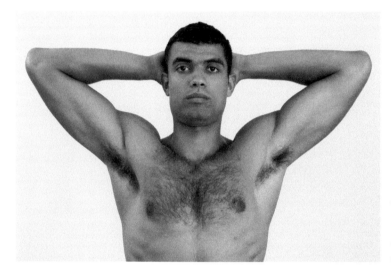

Figure 11.6 Testing shoulder abduction, external rotation and elbow flexion.

and fingers spread" – this allows inspection for joint swelling, muscle bulk and other deformities.

3. "Turn your hands over" – this tests supination and allows inspection of thenar and hypothenar eminences.
4. "Make fists and squeeze my fingers" – this tests grip strength.
5. "Touch each finger to your thumbs in turn" – this tests precision grip.

Gently squeeze across the MCP joints for any tenderness indicating joint inflammation.

Legs

Ask the patient to lie on the couch and perform the following manoeuvres:

1. Passively fully flex and extend the knee, whilst feeling over the patella for crepitus. Repeat for the opposite leg.
2. Whilst holding the knee flexed at 90°, passively rotate the hip internally and externally, observing for tenderness. Repeat on the opposite leg (**Figure 11.7**).
3. Perform a patellar tap on both knees (**Figure 11.8**).
4. Inspect the feet for joint swelling, deformities and callosities.
5. Gently squeeze across the metatarso-phalangeal joints for any tenderness indicating joint inflammation.

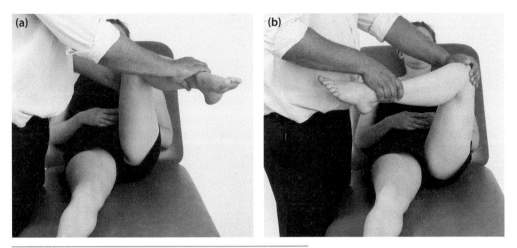

Figure 11.7 Assessing (a) internal and (b) external hip rotation.

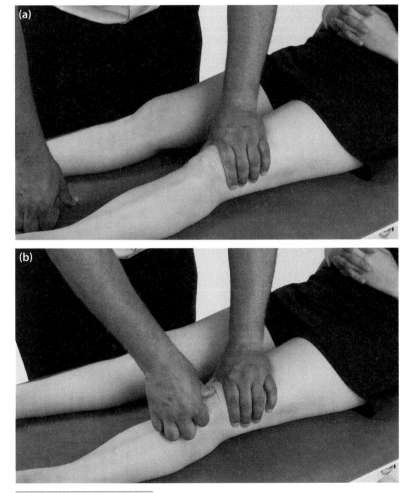

Figure 11.8 The patellar tap.

> **The patellar tap:**
> - Slide your left hand along the thigh to the patella (**Figure 11.8a**).
> - Keep your left hand in position and firmly press down on the patella with the fingers of your right hand (**Figure 11.8b**).
> - If a large effusion is present, you will feel the patella tapping against the femur.

Spine

Inspect the spine from the back for scoliosis and from the side for abnormal lordosis and kyphosis (**Figure 11.9**).

Assess cervical spine lateral flexion: "Tilt your head to touch your ear to each shoulder" (**Figure 11.10**).

Assess lumbar flexion by placing two fingers over consecutive lumbar vertebrae. Ask the patient to bend forward then stand back up. Your fingers should move apart during lumbar flexion and come together during lumbar extension.

11.6.4 Finishing off

After completion of the GALS screen, continue to a more dedicated examination of the affected joints.

11.6.5 Hand examination

Look

Inspect the dorsal and ventral aspects of the hands, the forearms and elbows for the changes described previously.

Feel

- Using the back of your hands, assess the temperature over the forearms, wrists and MCP joints
- Palpate the bulk of the thenar and hypothenar eminences
- Palpate the palm for thickening associated with Dupuytren's contracture
- Assess the radial and ulnar pulse
- Assess sensation of the radial, median and ulnar nerves
- Palpate each MCP, interphalangeal and carpometacarpal joint for deformity, heat and tenderness.

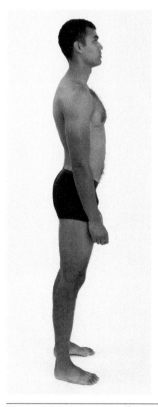

Figure 11.9 Inspection of the spine.

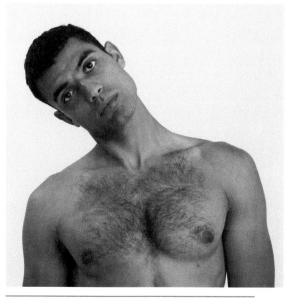

Figure 11.10 Assessing cervical spine lateral flexion.

Move

Tell the patient:

- "Spread your fingers" – testing finger extension
- "Make a fist" – testing finger flexion
- "Put your palms together and raise your elbows" (prayer sign) – testing wrist extension
- "Put the backs of your hands together and raise your elbows" (reverse prayer sign) – testing wrist flexion.

Test motor function:

- Radial nerve – wrist extension against resistance
- Ulnar nerve – finger abduction against resistance
- Median nerve – thumb abduction against resistance.

Function

Tell the patient:

- "Squeeze my fingers with your hands" – testing power grip
- "Make a ring with your finger and thumb and don't let me break it" – testing pincer grip
- "Pick up a pencil from the table" – testing coordination and fine movement.

Special tests

Tinel's test

Tap repeatedly over the carpal tunnel. Paraesthesia over the radial nerve sensory distribution suggests median nerve compression.

Phalen's test

Ask the patient to perform the reverse prayer hand position for 60 seconds. Paraesthesia over the radial nerve sensory distribution is also suggestive of median nerve compression.

11.6.6 Spine examination

Look

Inspect the spine from the front, side and back as in the GALS screen.

Feel

Palpate the following for tenderness and assess their alignment:

- spinal processes
- sacroiliac joints
- paraspinal muscles.

Move

Cervical spine

Tell the patient:

- "Touch your chin to your chest" – testing flexion
- "Tilt your head backwards" – testing extension
- "Touch your ear to your shoulder" – testing lateral flexion
- "Turn your head to your shoulder" – testing rotation.

If the patient is unable to perform the full movement, gently assess passive movement, noting any stiffness or tenderness.

Thoracic spine

Assess rotation by asking the patient to fold their arms and turn their chest from side to side.

Lumbar spine

Tell the patient:

- "Bend forwards to touch your toes" – testing flexion
- "Lean backwards" – testing extension
- "Run your hand down your leg as far as you can" – testing lateral flexion.

Special tests

Schober's test

- Find the level of both posterior superior iliac spines (PSIS) (**Figure 11.11**)
- Mark the skin 10cm above and 5cm below this level (i.e. 15cm apart)
- Ask the patient to lean forward as far as possible
- Measure the distance between the two marks.

Normally, the marks should move to ≥20cm apart. Marks <20cm apart indicate reduced lumbar flexion, as seen with ankylosing spondylitis.

Sciatic stretch test

- Ask the patient to lie down on the couch
- Whilst holding the ankle and keeping the leg straight, passively raise the leg and flex the hip
- When at maximal hip flexion, dorsiflex the foot
- Pain in the posterior thigh and buttock indicates sciatic nerve irritation.

Femoral stretch test

- Ask the patient to lie face down on the couch

(a) 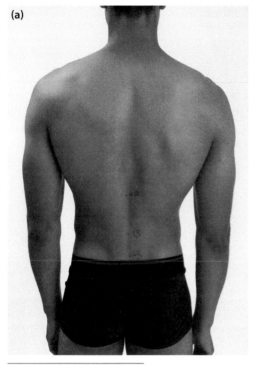   **(b)**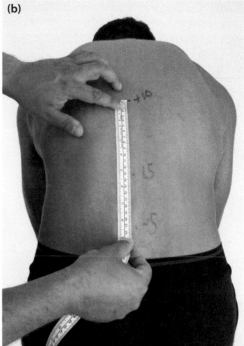

Figure 11.11 Schober's test.

- Flex the knee, extend the hip then plantarflex the foot
- Pain in the groin and thigh indicates femoral nerve irritation.

11.6.7 Hip examination

Look
- Inspect the hips, buttocks and lumbar spine from the front, side and back for 'DWARFS'
- Assess the patient's gait.

Feel
- Palpate over hips and greater trochanter for pain and evidence of inflammation.
- Measure the true and apparent length of each leg, noting if one leg is longer than the other.

> **True leg length** = distance from anterior superior iliac spine to medial malleolus
> **Apparent leg length** = distance from umbilicus to medial malleolus

Move
Active movements
- Ask the patient to bring their knee in to their body to assess hip flexion.

Passive movements
- Push the patient's knee towards their chest and note the degree of hip flexion
- With the knee bent, gently rotate the foot outwards and assess range of internal hip rotation
- Then gently rotate the foot inwards to assess external hip rotation
- With the leg straight, gently abduct the leg whilst keeping a hand on the contralateral hip to assess hip abduction
- Gently pull the leg across the other to assess hip adduction
- Ask the patient to roll over on the couch and lift each leg to assess hip extension.

Special tests
Trendelenburg's test
- With the patient standing, kneel down and place a hand on each side of their pelvis
- Ask them to raise one leg
- Observe which of your hands moves up or down
- Normally, the side with the raised leg should rise up
- If the side with the raised leg drops, this indicates a weakness of hip abductors on the contralateral side (i.e. the 'sound side sags').

11.6.8 Knee examination

Look
- Inspect the knees from the front, side and back for deformity, swelling (especially in the popliteal cavity) and muscle wasting.
- Assess the patient's gait as you would in the GALS examination.

Feel
Feel the temperature of the knees and palpate the quadriceps for tenderness.
Flex the knee to 90° then palpate the:
- patella for position and pain
- joint lines for pain and irregularity
- popliteal fossae for swelling.

Perform a patellar tap (as per GALS screen).
Perform the sweep test:
- Slide your left hand along the thigh to the patella; at the same time, slide your right hand along the medial side of the knee
- Release both hands then slide one along the lateral side of the knee
- A ripple or bulge appearing at the medial side indicates the presence of an effusion.

Move

Active movements
- Ask the patient to bend and straighten their knee to assess flexion and extension.

Passive movements
- Passively flex and extend the knee, noting the range of movement and any crepitus within the joint
- With the legs relaxed, pick each up by the heels and observe for hyperextension of the knees.

Special tests
Anterior and posterior drawer test
- Flex the knee to 90° with the foot flat on the couch (**Figure 11.12**)
- Place your hands around the knee with your thumbs aligned along the proximal tibia
- With the patient relaxed, gently pull the tibia forwards; excessive movement indicates anterior cruciate ligament insufficiency
- Then gently push the tibia backwards; excessive movement here indicates posterior cruciate ligament insufficiency.

Collateral ligaments
- Extend the knee fully whilst the patient is sitting on the couch
- Place a hand on the medial side of the knee and gently push laterally; if the joint margin opens out, this indicates weakness of the lateral collateral ligament (**Figure 11.13a**)
- Move your hand to the lateral side of the knee and gently push medially; abnormal joint opening here indicates medial collateral ligament weakness (**Figure 11.13b**).

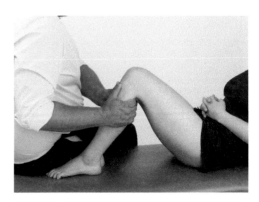

Figure 11.12 Anterior and posterior drawer test.

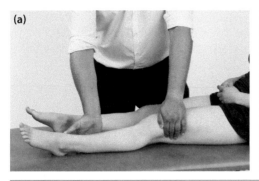
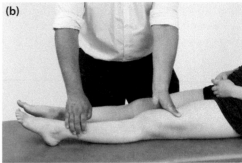

Figure 11.13 Testing the (a) lateral and (b) medial collateral ligaments.

11.7 Common investigations

There are many tests used to investigate, diagnose and monitor MSK disease.

11.7.1 Radiography

Plain X-rays can be taken of almost any bony part of the body to visualise fractures and assess joint damage. Usually two views are taken (e.g. anterior and lateral) so that the location of the fracture within the 3-dimensional design of the bone is found.

11.7.2 CT

CT scans are used to confirm fractures that are suspected but not seen on X-ray (especially hip fractures). When combined with positron emission tomography (CT-PET), metabolically active areas, such as those affected with acute flares of rheumatological disease, are visualised.

11.7.3 MRI

An MRI scan gives detailed views of soft tissues which are not easily differentiated on CT. It also detects changes such as bone oedema which is associated with osteomyelitis, thus reducing the need for tissue biopsy.

11.7.4 Ultrasound

US examination of swollen joints confirms the presence of fluid indicating active inflammation (synovitis).

11.7.5 Blood tests

As well as testing for auto-antibodies associated with rheumatological disease, serum blood tests are used for monitoring:
- markers of active inflammation
- evidence of medication side-effects (e.g. liver and bone marrow impairment)
- evidence of infection in immunosuppressed patients.

11.7.6 Joint aspiration

Joint fluid is analysed for:
- microscopy and culture to confirm or exclude septic arthritis
- polarised light microscopy for crystal arthropathies
- the presence of negatively birefringent crystals is diagnostic of gout
- positively birefringent crystals are seen with pseudogout.

11.7.7 Tissue biopsy

When diagnosis is unclear or the confirmation is necessary to commit a patient to a long-term treatment, a tissue biopsy is required. This involves physically removing a sample of tissue, preserving it, staining it with various markers and analysing it under a light or electron microscope. Examples of tissues used include:

- blood vessels (e.g. temporal arteries)
- muscle
- lymph nodes
- kidneys.

11.8 System summary

MSK diseases are common. Their early detection and treatment delay or prevent deterioration to disability and help patients maintain independence and a pain-free quality of life. Many MSK diseases have multiple systemic manifestations and present insidiously, with links being found only in hindsight; understanding these signs and their significance is crucial to enable early diagnosis and prevent diseases progressing to irreversible disability.

11.9 Answers to starter questions

1. The easy answer is all three. The two mainstays of treatment in rheumatoid arthritis are managing painful symptoms and limiting the burden of disease. Long-term and repeated medical review in the rheumatology clinic are needed to instigate and monitor these managements, especially in observing for side-effects or deciding to escalate treatment regimens. Surgical interventions range from release procedures for nerve entrapments such as carpal tunnel syndrome to joint replacement for severely damaged joints. Ongoing comprehensive occupational therapy input is vital in preserving patient independence with rheumatological disease. This ranges from dexterity aids such as adapted pens and cutlery to walking aids and stairlifts, and adapted baths and beds.

2. Maintaining eye contact is a key component of good communication. It engages patients, focuses your attention and builds rapport. Rheumatologists are true generalists; they deal with diseases that affect every system in the body and it is not uncommon for patients destined for the Rheumatology clinic to be referred to other specialties first with a seemingly random cluster of symptoms. By looking someone in the eye you might just notice something that leads to an earlier diagnosis of rheumatological disease and allows for early treatment before disabling changes occur.

3. The chronic inflammation between vertebrae that occurs with ankylosing spondylitis leads to back stiffness and ossification of the intervertebral discs (giving a 'bamboo spine' appearance on spinal X-rays). Patients with ankylosing spondylitis classically develop a 'question mark' posture with loss of lumbar lordosis, fixed kyphosis and a compensated extension of the cervical spine (**Figure 11.4**). This posture limits further neck extension, leading to potential difficulty watching fireworks.

4. Many rheumatological conditions and their treatments are associated with the development of fibrotic lung disease. The diagnosis of these requires specialised high resolution CT scans coupled with spirometry, and these patients should be managed and monitored under a Respiratory specialist alongside the care they receive in a Rheumatology clinic. In patients who develop kyphoscoliotic changes from rheumatological disease, their ability to adequately ventilate is reduced, due to the effective restriction on thoracic expansion. This is particularly problematic at night where the respiratory muscles lose tone, leading to nocturnal hypoventilation. Patients often require non-invasive ventilation at night to compensate.

Chapter 12
Psychiatry

Starter questions

1. Should all patients with depression take antidepressants?
2. Are psychiatric disorders due to chemical imbalances?
3. Why might a patient with an eating disorder have an abnormal ECG?
4. Should suicidal people call for an ambulance?

Answers to questions are to be found in *Section 12.7*.

12.1 Introduction

Exploring someone's psychological state requires careful and practised enquiry, whilst respecting social and personal boundaries. Unlike other specialties, there are only a few quantitative and objective measurements available to the psychiatrist when evaluating mental health, and almost all the information required to treat the patient comes from interpreting how the patient looks, speaks and acts. Therefore the doctor must be perceptive, persistent, and aware of what the patient does and doesn't say.

Psychiatric patients present a unique challenge in clinical treatment, as there is no single treatment that works for everyone all of the time. Psychiatric disorders are rarely cured, so psychiatrists work toward keeping their patients in the best health they can manage. Some patients do not believe they are unwell, so they must be treated against their wishes. Doctors must be patient and try to develop a trusting relationship with their patients, as far as they are able.

Case 12 A change in mood

Presentation

Amanda Thomas is a 53-year-old woman. Her daughter has brought her to her GP's surgery as she is concerned that her mother is 'having a nervous breakdown'.

'Nervous breakdown' is not a medical diagnosis, but a commonly used lay term. Patients usually use the term to denote that their mental health symptoms have exceeded the coping strategies that they use to deal with them, and that they have reached a crisis point.

Initial interpretation

Changes in mood and personality are due to psychological, social or biological processes. The medical history and examination is the key method of detecting the root causes. The differential diagnosis cannot be determined without further exploration.

History

Amanda is withdrawn and doesn't offer much information in the consultation. Her daughter describes a severe deterioration in her mother's mood over the last 6 months. She has stopped doing activities she previously enjoyed, such as volunteer work, and now rarely leaves the house. She cries often and is unable to explain why. She no longer interacts with her family or friends. She used to enjoy reading, but now watches television all day or sits alone in the living room. She reports poor sleep during the night, and often falls asleep during the day. Her appetite is poor and she eats very little. Despite her family's best efforts, she refuses to talk about these changes, and becomes angry when they pursue the subject.

Interpretation of history

Amanda is exhibiting features of depression, including anhedonia (not taking pleasure in things), irritability, insomnia and withdrawal from social activities. Depression is either reactive (often called exogenous) due to psychosocial stressors, or endogenous in nature. Finally, it is possible that her symptoms are due to an undiagnosed biological condition. Hypothyroidism, hypo- and hypercortisolism, and CNS diseases mimic the symptoms of depression.

Further history

Exploration of Amanda's symptoms is limited by her lack of engagement in conversation. She speaks rarely, and answers the GP's questions with a quiet 'yes', 'no', or 'don't know'. She denies having auditory hallucinations, and the doctor is unable to detect any delusional beliefs. She also denies any thoughts about suicide, but her daughter volunteers that Amanda has spoken about wanting to be with her husband Joe, who died 7 years earlier. It emerges that Amanda experienced a bout of severe depression in her 20s, and postnatal depression after the birth of her daughter. She does not have any medical problems and takes no medication nor recreational drugs.

Examination

Amanda is withdrawn and does not move very much throughout the consultation. She looks unkempt, with creased clothing and unwashed hair. She does not make eye contact, but looks at the floor. Her voice is quiet and monotonous. A full neurological examination is normal, although she engages poorly with testing of power and coordination. Her blood pressure and heart rate are both normal.

Interpretation of findings

Considering Amanda's symptoms, signs and past psychiatric history, a diagnosis of recurrent depression is likely. The absence of any hallmark neurological or endocrine abnormalities supports this diagnosis. The desire to join her deceased husband is a particularly concerning feature, and may indicate suicidal thoughts.

Case 12.1 *continued*

Investigations

Amanda is referred to a rapid access mental health practitioner, who evaluates the intensity and impact of her depressive features using several validated scores. These results, along with the presence of several biological features of depression, such as poor appetite and sleep disturbance, indicate that Amanda has severe depression, without evidence of psychosis.

Diagnosis

Severe depression must be treated carefully, as attempted or completed suicide remains a real risk. Each patient must be individually evaluated,

and those thought to be at high risk of self-harm are cared for as inpatients. Outpatients are monitored by community mental health teams. Amanda's psychiatric team decides to commence oral antidepressant therapy with fluoxetine (a selective serotonin reuptake inhibitor). After 2 weeks of treatment, there is no appreciable change in her symptomatology, so the dose is increased. At 6 weeks, Amanda's mood has improved slightly, and she is able to engage with cognitive behavioural therapy (CBT) with her community psychiatric nurse. After 3 months, she has become more optimistic in her mood, and slowly begins to participate in the voluntary work she previously enjoyed.

12.2 System overview

The specialties of psychiatry and neurology are closely related. The lobes of the brain, their function, and the consequence of their dysfunction are explored in *Section 9.2.1*.

12.2.1 Neurobiology

Neurons are the cells that make up the central nervous system (CNS). Changes in polarity within a neuron generate an electrical impulse that travels the length of the cell. Each neuron terminates in a synapse, a specialised structure at the terminal point of a neuron which enables it to connect to adjacent neurons.

Synapses

Synapses release neurotransmitters that cross the synaptic cleft (the space between the presynaptic and postsynaptic neurons) and activate membrane receptors on the postsynaptic membrane (**Figure 12.1**). This generates an action potential (a change in electrical charge) in the next neuron, which transmits electrical impulses along its length, and so on. Most psychotropic medications (medications that affect a patient's mental state) act upon CNS synapses,

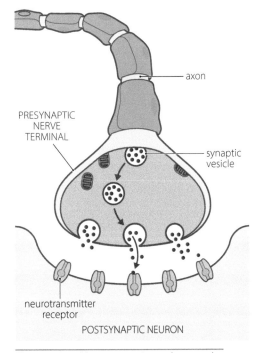

Figure 12.1 Neurotransmitter release at the synapse.

by either blocking or enhancing the effect of neurotransmitters on the postsynaptic membrane.

Neurotransmitters

Neurons release different neurotransmitters, and each postsynaptic membrane expresses several kinds of receptor (**Table 12.1**).

After binding with the postsynaptic receptors, neurotransmitters are eliminated through one of the following processes:

- They are deactivated by specific enzymes – e.g. acetylcholine is degraded by acetylcholinesterase in the postsynaptic membrane
- They are channelled back into the presynaptic membrane ('reuptake') – e.g. serotonin undergoes reuptake after binding to serotonin receptors
- They diffuse out of the synaptic cleft to be absorbed by glial cells – e.g. dopamine.

Selective serotonin reuptake inhibitors (SSRIs) are one of the most widely prescribed medications in the UK. They enhance the effect of serotonin at the postsynaptic membrane, thereby acting as an antidepressant.

12.2.2 Classification

The diagnostic hierarchy of disorders (**Figure 12.2**) is a psychiatric classification tool. A lower order diagnosis should not be made unless a higher order diagnosis has been ruled out. This recognises that higher order diagnoses incorporate features of a lesser order diagnosis. For example, an organic disease (a disease caused by abnormal physiology or anatomy), such as

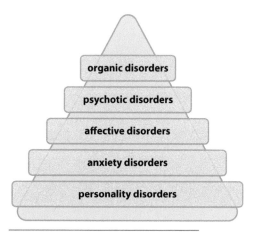

Figure 12.2 The diagnostic hierarchy of psychiatric disorders.

Table 12.1 Classes of neurotransmitters within the CNS, with their clinical significance		
Class	**Neurotransmitter**	**Clinical significance**
Acetylcholine	Acetylcholine (ACh)	Degeneration of ACh activity in the CNS is implicated in Alzheimer's dementia
Amines	Noradrenaline (NA)	Decreased NA and serotonin activity is implicated in depression
	Serotonin	
	Dopamine	Responsible for pleasure and reward in the CNS
		Stimulant recreational drugs trigger massive dopamine release
		Schizophrenia medication blocks dopamine activity
Amino acids	Glutamate	Glutamate abnormalities are implicated in stroke, Parkinson's disease and Huntington's disease
	Gamma-aminobutyric acid (GABA)	Has an inhibitory effect on CNS activity
		Many anticonvulsant medications enhance GABA to prevent seizures
		They are thought to act via a similar mechanism in regulating affective disorders

a brain tumour, may cause psychotic features that could be inappropriately diagnosed as schizophrenia.

12.2.3 Psychology

Psychology is the science of the mind and how it expresses itself in behaviour. It comprises many aspects of human existence (**Figure 12.3**). Clinical psychologists work with patients to identify the driving forces and effects of their symptoms, and create a treatment appropriate for each individual. Clinical psychology is more appropriate for patients who have a good insight into their condition and have a desire to change. Patients with psychosis, such as those with severe mood disorders or schizophrenia, are usually unable to engage with the therapeutic process.

The most common forms of psychotherapy are psychodynamic therapy and cognitive behavioural therapy (CBT). The clinical psychologist chooses each modality carefully on a case-by-case basis, as not all treatments work for each patient.

Psychodynamic psychotherapy

This approach stems from the psychoanalytical movement of the late 19th and early 20th centuries. It is based on the idea that distressing psychological symptoms stem from unconscious motivations, fears and desires, often originating in childhood. The therapist helps the patient uncover and explore these unconscious phenomena.

Cognitive behavioural therapy

CBT is one of the most widely used psychological interventions. It identifies and modulates or eliminates recurrent thoughts that trigger distressing moods and behaviours. It helps develop coping strategies and avoid maladaptive coping strategies, such as recreational drug abuse or self-harm. It requires a high level of engagement from the patient, but has good

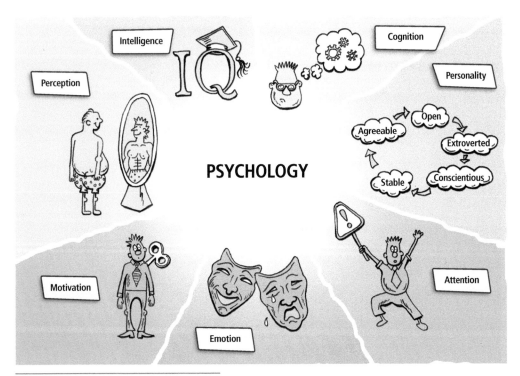

Figure 12.3 Key study areas in psychology.

outcomes, especially for patients with personality disorders, depression and anxiety disorders.

Group psychotherapy

This brings people together to discuss their experiences with a certain condition. The therapist guides the discussion and used psychodynamic techniques to treat attendees as a group.

> **Group therapy was initially developed to treat Second World War soldiers with post-traumatic stress disorder (PTSD).** It is now mostly known for treating patients with addiction issues, such as Alcoholics Anonymous.

12.2.4 Ethical issues

Some patients do not have insight into their condition. This is problematic if they do not believe that they are ill or require treatment. If a patient was judged to be a risk to themselves, either through self-harm, self-neglect, or engaging in high risk behaviour, then they are treated in their best interests. There are two ways of doing this in the UK.

Deprivation of Liberty Safeguards

A Deprivation of Liberty Safeguard (DoLS) permits treatment of a patient in their best interest under the Mental Capacity Act (2005). It can only be used if the patient lacks capacity to make their own decisions about treatment. They may or may not have a mental disorder. It is most commonly used for patients with an organic disorder, such as dementia or delirium.

> **Depriving a patient of their liberty is not merely preventing them from leaving.** Preventing a patient from making decisions, using physical or chemical restraint (sedatives), and keeping someone under continuous observation all qualify as deprivations of liberty.

Capacity

Demonstrating that a patient does not have capacity is a legal requirement of DoLS. A patient is always assumed to have capacity unless proven otherwise. Capacity is the ability to make informed and reasoned decisions about your own health and treatment.

Patients must fulfil four criteria to have capacity:

- The patient can take in information about their condition
- The patient can retain this information and repeat it
- The patient can analyse this information to make a decision
- The patient can express their decision.

Capacity to make a decision is specific to that decision at that time. Capacity may change over time and must be reassessed whenever circumstances change. Lacking capacity for one decision does not mean the patient lacks capacity for another decision.

> Patients who have capacity have the right to make decisions about their own healthcare, even if these are thought to be harmful. This only pertains to refusal of treatment, such as chemotherapy or heart attack medication. A patient with capacity cannot demand a treatment that their doctor does not want to give.

Detention under the Mental Health Act

This is commonly known as 'being sectioned', named after the different Sections of the Act that are used. It is exclusively used to detain patients with mental disorders in hospital for assessment or treatment, or for their own (or other people's) safety. These patients may have capacity in that they can absorb and weigh up information, but still refuse treatment, usually on the basis that have no insight into their condition (see *Section 12.5.8*) or do not want to get better (severe depression).

12.3 Features of psychiatric disease

12.3.1 Glossary

The terminology surrounding mental disorders can be confusing. The glossary shown in **Table 12.2** explains the common psychiatric terms used in everyday practice.

> **Depression is one of the commonest reasons to consult a GP in the UK.** Other common psychiatric disorders in primary care are anxiety, eating disorders and dementia.

12.3.2 Change in mood

Patients with affective (mood) disorders have low mood, elevated mood, or cycle between the two extremes.

Low mood

This is a feature of depression and dysthymia.

Depression

Depression is a common mental health disorder, with 10% of people experiencing it during their lifetime. It may be mild, moderate or severe. Diagnosis is based on the presence of core and additional features (**Figure 12.4**). The symptoms must be present for two weeks to meet the diagnostic criteria.

When assessing for the associated features of depression, use the acronym 'SLEEP CAVES' (**Table 12.3**).

Dysthymia

This is a chronically low mood that does not meet the criteria for depression. It usually lasts many years or can even be lifelong. Patients with dysthymia describe themselves as having a 'depressed personality' or always being miserable. Dysthymia is a major risk factor for depression.

> **Postnatal depression is the occurrence of depressive symptoms within a year of childbirth.** It affects 1 in 10 mothers. It has severe repercussions within the family and interferes with mother–baby bonding.

Elevated mood

This takes the form of mania – an extremely heightened and euphoric mood – or hypomania, which is less extreme.

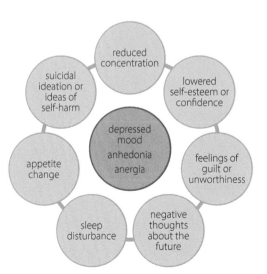

severity of depression	number of symptoms
mild	2 core, 2 additional
moderate	2 core, 3 additional
severe	3 core, 4 additional
severe with psychotic symptoms	3 core, 4 additional plus abnormalities of thought content

Figure 12.4 The diagnostic criteria for depression. Symptoms should be present for 2 weeks.

Table 12.2 *Glossary of psychiatric terms*

Term	Definition
Affect	The professional's observation of the patient's mood. In depression a flat affect is common: minimal animation and variation in tone during speech, and little expression of emotional or feeling. Patients with a normal affect are euthymic.
Akathisia	Extreme psychomotor agitation, usually accompanied by pacing the room, seen in mania, as a side-effect to psychotropic medication, or in drug or alcohol withdrawal.
Anhedonia	The inability to take pleasure in anything.
Cyclothymia	A milder form of bipolar affective disorder (BAD), incorporating hypomanic and mild depressive episodes.
Delusion	A fixed and concrete belief that is demonstrably false.
Depersonalisation	Unpleasant feeling that one's thoughts or feelings are not one's own.
Derealisation	Feeling that one's surroundings are not real or are somehow artificial or 'staged'.
Disinhibition	This is the inappropriate, over-friendly or flirting speech and behaviour of a patient with mania.
Dysthymia	Chronic low mood over months or years, not amounting to depression.
Hallucination	A perception of a thing / person / phenomenon that does not exist.
Illusion	A misinterpretation of a sight / sound / smell / sensation that feeds into a delusional belief.
Mood	The patient's experience of their emotional state over time.
Organic	Disease due to physical, pathological changes that are observed on examination or investigation, such as a scan or a blood test. Organic brain syndromes are delirium, dementia, encephalitis and encephalopathy.
Parkinsonism	A side-effect of antipsychotic medication due to dopamine blockade. Manifests as: bilateral pill-rolling hand tremor, festinate gait and tardive dyskinesia (persistent lip-smacking or chewing movements).
Perception	How the patient interprets the world around them.
Poverty of speech	Minimal conversation, seen in depression and a negative symptom of schizophrenia.
Pressure of speech	Rapid and verbose speech that is difficult to interrupt, a common feature of mania.
Psychomotor agitation	The inability to sit still, seen in mania, including fidgeting, rocking, shaking of legs and hand-wringing.
Psychomotor retardation	Minimal movement and body language, seen in depression and schizophrenia.
Psychosis	The inability to differentiate what is real and what is unreal, i.e. hallucinations, delusions, illusions.
Tone	In relation to speech, it is the normal variation in pitch and tone during conversation. Patients with depression or negative symptoms of schizophrenia have monotonous speech.

Table 12.3	Use **SLEEP CAVES** to enquire about the associated features of depression	
Feature	**As a feature of depression**	**Questions to ask the patient**
Sleep	Insomnia presents as either: ■ difficulty falling asleep ■ early morning wakening at 4–5 am Hypersomnia is a rarer feature	"How are you sleeping right now?" "Are you sleeping through the night?"
Libido	Loss of interest in sex	"When people are feeling low they can lose interest in everything, including sex. Is this something you recognise?"
Energy	Apathy, anergia and demotivation	"How are your energy levels?"
Enjoyment	Lack of enthusiasm for and pleasure in hobbies and interests	"Do you still enjoy doing things you used to do?" "What do you do to relax and have fun now?"
Depressive **P**sychosis	Rare, and only in severe depression	"Do you have a conviction or belief that no one else seems to share?" "Is anything strange or inexplicable happening to you?"
Concentration	Loss of concentration at work or school, difficulty following conversations or plots of books	"How are you managing at work / school?" "Are you having trouble focusing?"
Appetite	Appetite is usually poor, although a few patients experience increased appetite ('comfort eating')	"Are you managing to eat?" "Are you losing weight?"
Variation during day	Depressive symptoms are usually worse in the morning, and alleviate slightly at night	"Is your mood worse at particular times of day?"
Self-**E**steem	Poor self-esteem, feeling worthless, even guilty	"How do you feel about yourself?"
Suicidality / self-harm	Vague or specific intentions / plans to end their life Compulsion to hurt themselves, e.g. by cutting or burning themselves	"When things get very bad, some people think that ending their life is the only way out. Have you ever felt like this?" "Have you ever had thoughts about hurting yourself?"

Mania

This an elevated mood associated with overactivity, pressured speech and grandiose ideas or plans. Manic patients have short attention spans and become irritable if asked to slow down or reflect on their thoughts and actions.

Mania is a feature of bipolar affective disorder (BAD) and stimulant recreational drugs.

Bipolar affective disorder. BAD is characterised by recurrent manic episodes which may or may not be interspersed with depressive episodes.

The features of mania can be recalled using the mnemonic 'CASING' (**Table 12.4**).

Table 12.4 *Use* **CASING** *to enquire about the associated features of mania*

	Explanation	Common examples
Concentration	Decreased attention span and easily distractible	The patient struggles to follow the thread of a conversation and jumps quickly between topics
Activity	Patients display psychomotor agitation	During a consultation the manic patient can't sit still in a chair, and has to pace around the room
Sleep	Minimal and fragmented sleep	Manic patients may go several days without any sleep at all
Inhibition and risk	General disinhibition in their speech and behaviour, or engaging in high risk behaviour	The patient spends huge sums of money on shopping sprees, or develops abnormal hypersexuality
Noise	Speech is loud and chaotic, and gestures and movements are exaggerated	The patient continually breaks off speaking to shout or sing
Grandiosity	Suddenly inflated self-esteem and grandiose plans	The patient believes they are a genius and are going to establish a multi-million property empire

Drug-induced mania. Some recreational drugs produce a profound euphoria with some of the hallmarks of mania. Common drugs are:

- cocaine
- MDMA/ecstasy
- GHB (gamma-hydroxybutyric acid)
- methamphetamines.

Drug-induced mania is transient as it is followed by an unpleasant 'coming down' sensation that may lead to depression.

> **Recreational drugs ('street drugs') have a bewildering array of nicknames, which change from year to year and place to place.** If you don't recognise a drug by its street name, clarify it with the patient. You need to know what they have taken in order to treat them properly.

Hypomania

This has many of the same features as mania, but not the severity. It occurs in BAD and cyclothymia. It is, by definition, never associated with psychosis. Bipolar type II is a less severe form of BAD

characterised by episodes of hypomania and depression.

Cyclothymia

This is a mild form of bipolar disorder characterised by episodes of hypomania (not amounting to a manic episode) and mild depression. It is a risk factor for developing BAD. It is a chronic condition and often goes undiagnosed.

12.3.3 Psychosis

Psychosis is a serious abnormality in thinking, perception or behaviour. Patients with psychosis are unable to make distinctions between what is real and what is unreal, experiencing the following symptoms:

- Hallucinations
- Disorganised thinking
- Delusions
- Negative symptoms.

Hallucinations

These are sensory perceptions that have no real cause. They are related to any of the sensory modalities, and can therefore be auditory, visual, olfactory, gustatory or somatoform. Hallucinations are not exclusive to schizophrenia, and occur in other psychiatric conditions (**Table 12.5**).

Disorganised thinking

Disorganised thought processes manifest as disorganised speech patterns and content. The patient displays chaotic and incomprehensible speech, rapidly shifting topics and moving onto conversational tangents.

Delusions

A delusion is an unshakeable belief held by the patient that is evidently false to other people. Like hallucinations, delusions occur in several disorders (**Table 12.6**).

Table 12.5 *Types of hallucinations with their associated condition*		
Type of hallucination	**Description**	**Associated conditions**
Auditory	Usually takes the form of conversation	Schizophrenia
▪ Thought broadcast	▪ Patient hears their own thoughts being spoken aloud	
▪ 2nd person	▪ Patient hears a voice speaking directly to them	
▪ 3rd person	▪ Patient hears a voice or voices talking about them	
Visual	Can be people or objects, either in isolation or as part of an entire hallucinatory 'scene'	Schizophrenia Alcohol withdrawal Drug psychosis Parkinson's disease Dementia with Lewy bodies Temporal lobe epilepsy
Olfactory	Usually unpleasant smells. A patient with nihilistic delusions in association with depressive psychosis may smell their own 'dead' body rotting. A schizophrenic with persecutory delusions may smell poison in their food	Depression Schizophrenia Temporal lobe epilepsy
Gustatory	Usually occurs with olfactory hallucinations	Schizophrenia Temporal lobe epilepsy
Somatoform	Usually relates to skin sensation	
▪ Formication	▪ Sensation of insects crawling under the skin	▪ Schizophrenia ▪ Alcohol withdrawal ▪ Stimulant recreational drugs ('cocaine bugs')
▪ Passivity phenomena	▪ Sensation that someone else is controlling their body parts, including touching / stroking them	▪ Schizophrenia
▪ Visceral	▪ Sensation that their inner organs are being manipulated	▪ Schizophrenia

Table 12.6 *Types of delusions with their associated conditions*

Delusion	Description	Associated conditions
Thought control	Thought withdrawal: someone is stealing their thoughts Thought insertion: someone is putting thoughts into their mind	Schizophrenia
Religious delusions	Belief that they are communicating with God, or the devil, or are on a religious mission	Schizophrenia Mania
Delusions of grandeur	Belief that they are important, or somehow 'chosen'	Mania Hypomania
Nihilistic delusion	Overwhelmingly negative belief, such as that they are already dead, have no money or are being punished for a perceived wrongdoing	Depressive psychosis
Persecutory delusion	Paranoid belief that they are being persecuted or monitored in some way, e.g. *"my neighbours are trying to kill me"*	Schizophrenia
Delusion of reference	Belief that coincidences, items on television, radio or in newspapers are direct communication to them	Schizophrenia

Negative symptoms

Delusions, thought disorders and hallucinations are new symptoms brought on by schizophrenia, so are called positive symptoms. Negative symptoms refers to the absence of feelings and behaviours normally present in a person in good mental health (**Table 12.7**).

> **Students often feel frightened or intimidated by patients with psychosis, fearing they may be violent.** In fact, most psychotic patients are frightened and vulnerable people. Students are never left with patients who are judged to have a propensity to violence.

Causes of psychosis

The commonest psychotic psychiatric disorder is schizophrenia, which affects around 1 in 100 individuals worldwide.

Usually the first sign of schizophrenia is that the patient experiences dramatic problems in their ability to look after themselves and continue to work or study. They are often brought to the doctor by a concerned friend or relative. Psychotic symptoms are also found in the following conditions:

- Drug-induced psychosis, due to either recreational drugs such as LSD, cannabis or amphetamines, or prescribed medications, such as steroids
- Postpartum psychosis, a rare condition experienced by some mothers following childbirth
- Mania
- Severe depression.

12.3.4 Anxiety

These are conditions characterised by chronic anxiety or fear. Patients often experience intermittent panic attacks, which consist of some or all of the following:

- Palpitations
- Hyperventilation and dyspnoea
- Sweating
- Chest pain
- Peripheral paraesthesia
- Presyncope (but not syncope)

Table 12.7 *The negative symptoms of schizophrenia can be recalled as the 8 As*

Features	Definition
Apathy	Lack of interest in activities the patient previously enjoyed
Absent emotional responses	Patient has a flat or blunted affect, and does not exhibit emotional reactions to good or bad news
Alogia	Little interest in conversation, reduced or even absent speech (mutism)
Avolition	Withdrawal from social activities and interactions, and a lack of interest in the world around them
Attention deficits	The patient struggles to concentrate on tasks that require little effort, such as following films or even conversation
Anhedonia	Also a symptom of depression; the patient is unable to experience pleasure or enjoyment
Anorgasmia and decreased libido	The patient has little or no interest in sex or loving relationships
Anergia	The patient has no energy or motivation to exert themselves in any way

- A strong belief that they are dying
- Derealisation and depersonalisation (see **Table 12.2**).

Generalised anxiety disorder

Patients with this condition have severe anxiety symptoms that are not tied to a specific phenomenon. It is sometimes called 'free-floating anxiety' as it is not anchored to a recognised trigger.

Post-traumatic stress disorder

PTSD is a prolonged psychological condition that follows a traumatic life event. It is characterised by:
- intrusive and distressing flashbacks to the event
- sleep disorders
- avoidance of situations that remind the patient of the initial event
- anxiety attacks.

Obsessive–compulsive disorder

This is a chronic condition characterised by the following:
- Obsessive and intrusive thoughts. These are thoughts that the patient is unable to block or distract themselves from, and cause anxiety and distress. Common obsessive thoughts usually involve some kind of harm befalling the patient or their loved ones unless the patient performs certain tasks.
- Compulsions to perform repetitive tasks or rituals, which usually provide transient relief from obsessive thoughts. Common rituals include washing, counting, tapping and checking that doors are locked and appliances switched off.
- Obsessive–compulsive disorder (OCD) is often accompanied by depression.

> **OCD has taken on a 'lay' meaning of 'extra caution' or 'perfectionism'.** This misuse of the term is upsetting for patients with OCD, as it suggests that their condition is a personality trait, rather than a disabling illness. The key difference between OCD and perfectionism is that OCD sufferers obtain no pleasure or satisfaction from performing rituals, such as constant house cleaning, just a brief release.

Phobias

These are anxiety disorders in which the symptoms of fear and panic are linked to a specific situation. Phobias are considered severe if they negatively impact on the patient's daily life. For example, patients with agoraphobia struggle to leave their home without severe anxiety symptoms. Patients with hospital or needle phobias stay away from seeking medical help, even when they become ill.

12.3.5 Self-harm

This takes the form of cutting, burning or self-poisoning (e.g. taking an overdose), or self-neglect, such as not taking prescribed medication. It is a maladaptive coping strategy, often done to provide temporary relief from intolerable psychological distress. It may be used to communicate their mental disorder to other people, such as family or doctors. It is a feature of depression but is also associated with personality disorders, especially emotionally unstable personality disorder.

Personality disorders

These are deeply ingrained and inflexible personality traits and behaviours that interfere with biopsychosocial wellbeing, in the absence of other psychiatric diagnoses. The subtypes are listed in **Table 12.8**.

> **Emotionally unstable personality disorder**
> was formally called 'borderline personality disorder', as it was thought to be on the borderline of schizophrenia. This term was officially abandoned as it implied that it did not amount to a 'real' mental disorder.

12.3.6 Disordered eating

These are extremely complex disorders revolving around an abnormal fixation on food and body self-perception.

Anorexia nervosa

The patient with anorexia has an intentionally low bodyweight and a morbid fear of appearing obese. There is an association with body dysmorphia, an obsessional belief that part of the body appearance is abnormal or unattractive.

Patients often exercise obsessively and refuse food perceived to be fattening, even to the point of collapse or even organ failure and death. It is associated with malnutrition, osteoporosis, and amenorrhoea in women.

Bulimia nervosa

The patient with bulimia experiences episodes of overeating (bingeing), followed by self-induced vomiting (purging). They often abuse drugs that assist weight loss, such as laxatives, diuretics and thyroxine.

12.3.7 Confusion

This is a clouding of the mental processes. Patients with severe depression often exhibit a 'pseudodementia', having problems with recall, concentration and registration. Patients with anxiety experience short-term memory problems and impaired concentration. Mental 'fogginess' is a common side-effect of psychotropic medication, and is usually transient.

Patients with a formal thought disorder appear confused to others, due to their changes in affect and personality, odd speech patterns and bizarre delusions.

The two organic disorders that cause confusion are delirium and dementia.

Delirium

Delirium is a temporary and reversible impairment in cognitive function, which lasts minutes, hours or days. Patients with poor 'brain reserve', such as the elderly, patients with dementia, and patients with a pre-existing organic brain syndrome, are at higher risk of delirium.

Delirium is either hypoactive or hyperactive.

■ Hypoactive delirium: psychological withdrawal, poor communication and minimal speech, emotional blunting and occasionally decreased conscious level
■ Hyperactive delirium: agitation, irritability, fear, emotional lability, excessive movement and activity, shouting out and disinhibited behaviour.

Delirium is common in medical inpatients, regardless of the presenting condition. The common causes of delirium can be recalled using the mnemonic 'A HIP DAME' (**Table 12.9**).

Table 12.8 *The main personality disorders with their common features*

Type	Common attributes
Emotionally unstable personality disorder	Chronic feelings of emptiness or numbness
	Inability to form lasting relationships, prone to forming intense and short-lasting relationships
	Impulsive actions, including self-harm
	Strong and unstable emotional reactions to life events
Paranoid personality disorder	Long-standing feeling of paranoia
	Suspicious of other people and their motivations
	Pervading sense of danger or oncoming harm
Schizoid personality disorder	Many milder forms of the 'negative' features of schizophrenia
	Generally uninterested in the world or social interactions
Dissocial / antisocial personality disorder	Inability to feel empathy for others
	Minimal evidence of internal 'conscience'
	Impulsive, often criminal, behaviour
Dependent personality disorder	Long-standing dependence on others
	Minimal independence
	Require constant approval and validation from others
Anankastic personality disorder	Some milder traits of OCD
	Need to be in control
	Constant, often distressing need for perfectionism in self and others
Avoidant personality disorder	Highly anxious and socially inhibited
	Poor self-esteem
	Extremely sensitive to perceived disapproval
	Fear of being humiliated or rejected
Histrionic personality disorder	Attention-seeking behaviours and emotions
	Exaggerated behaviours and emotional reactions
	Extroverted, sometimes inappropriately seductive or disinhibited behaviour

As with any drug, alcohol withdrawal occurs when intake is stopped suddenly after a long period of excess. The symptoms are sweating, agitation, tremor and delirium. If untreated, a small proportion develop seizures, hallucinations or even death.

Delirium may be due to several of these factors, rather than one in isolation.

Dementia

Dementia is an irreversible and progressive decline in cognitive function. Types of dementia are shown in **Table 16.5**.

Table 12.9 *The causes of delirium are remembered using* **A HIP DAME**

Cause	Details	Specific treatment
Alcohol	Acute intoxication	None
	Acute alcohol withdrawal	Benzodiazepines
Hypoxia	Even mild hypoxia impairs cognitive function	Oxygen therapy
Infection	Any infection of any source has the potential to induce delirium in high risk patients; for example, a simple UTI causes delirium in a large proportion of elderly patients	Antibiotics
	Encephalitis is a viral infection of the CNS that causes delirium alongside other neurological symptoms	Antivirals, e.g. aciclovir
Psychosis	Acute psychosis in the context of schizophrenia or mania presents as delirium	Psychotropic medication
Drugs	Recreational drugs cause dissociative states, mania or hypomania, psychosis and confusion	None
Autoimmune	Autoimmune encephalitis is an extremely rare cause of prolonged delirium	Immunosuppression
Metabolic	Metabolic causes include acute electrolyte derangement, especially: ■ hypo- / hypernatraemia ■ hypo- / hypercalcaemia	Correction of electrolyte abnormality
	Hepatic encephalopathy is one of the hallmarks of acute decompensation of liver disease (see *Section 6.5.3*)	Regular laxatives
	Uraemic encephalopathy occurs in severe kidney disease	Renal dialysis
	Some endocrinopathies precipitate delirium. Causes include: ■ hypoglycaemia ■ severe hyperthyroidism (thyrotoxicosis) ■ severe hypothyroidism (myxoedemic coma) ■ severe hypocortisolism (Addisonian crisis)	Correction of hormone abnormality Dextrose infusion for hypoglycaemia
Epileptic	Patients who have just experienced a seizure (the post-ictal phase) may have a hypoactive or hyperactive delirium	Anticonvulsants
	Non-convulsive status is a state of ongoing epileptic activity without any physical signs of epilepsy; it is diagnosed on EEG	

12.4 The psychiatric history

Establishing a professional rapport is challenging when a patient does not follow the usual norms and conventions of social interaction. Patients may talk excessively or not at all, or deviate repeatedly from the thread of the discussion to talk about unrelated or inconsequential matters. Sticking to a rigid structure is tricky and counterproductive, leading to frustration for you and irritability or confusion for the patient. Be flexible in how you approach the history-taking, so that you cover the main topics in a more natural way, whilst maintaining the rapport.

The psychiatric history is slightly different to the standard medical history.

12.4.1 Presenting complaint

As with a standard history, this is the symptom that led to the patient seeking medical help.

12.4.2 History of presenting complaint

Explore the presenting complaint, and establish timeframes. Depending on the patient's symptoms, screen for common symptoms of depression (**Table 12.2**), anxiety, OCD, schizophrenia or eating disorders. In addition to psychiatric symptoms, evaluate for physical symptoms that are often associated with psychiatric illness.

> When psychological and physical symptoms co-occur, you must take a careful history to determine whether the patient has a biological illness that causes psychological effects, or vice versa. For example, severe hypothyroidism causes fatigue, poor appetite, weight gain and excessive sleeping; but these may also be features of depression.

12.4.3 Past medical / psychiatric history

As well as exploring any previous physical diseases, determine whether this is the patient's first presentation with mental health issues. Most psychiatric diseases are either chronic or recurrent. Ask which treatments – both chemical and non-chemical – the patient has tried before, and whether they have needed treatment in a hospital.

A patient with limited insight into their condition often denies previous episodes. This is common with schizophrenia. If the patient believes that they are not ill, ask them whether there have been times when other people or doctors believed them to be ill, even if they did not agree.

12.4.4 Drug history

Document the patient's medications and ask about compliance; patients with psychiatric illness often have chaotic social lives and find concordance with medication difficult.

Psychiatric medications often induce neurological symptoms, such as antipsychotic-induced parkinsonism, and some neurological medications produce psychiatric conditions. Dopamine agonists, used in parkinsonian diseases, cause significant personality and behavioural changes in a small proportion of patients, including compulsive shopping, excessive gambling or hyper-sexuality.

The common medications used to treat psychiatric disorders are listed in **Table 12.10.**

12.4.5 Family history

Schizophrenia, depression and bipolar affective disorder have genetic components, so ask about members of the patient's family. Anxiety and phobia disorders often cluster in families, due to a combination of nature and nurture.

12.4.6 Personal history

This is a lengthy section that requires a 'deep dive' into the patient's life and upbringing in order to identify salient predisposing and precipitating triggers for mental illness, as well as its consequences (**Table 12.11**).

Table 12.10 *Common medications used in psychiatry, their indications and common side-effects. Typical antipsychotics were first generation drugs, and have been largely superseded by atypical antipsychotics, which have a more favourable side-effect profile.*

Drug type	Class	Action	Examples	Common side-effects
SSRIs	Antidepressant	Potentiate the action of serotonin in CNS neurotransmission	Fluoxetine Paroxetine Citalopram	Hyponatraemia Prolonged QTc
Serotonin–noradrenaline reuptake inhibitors (SNRI)	Antidepressant	Potentiate the action of serotonin and noradrenaline in CNS neurotransmission	Venlafaxine Duloxetine	Discontinuation syndrome Decreased libido and anorgasmia
Tricyclic antidepressants (TCA)	Antidepressant	Potentiate the action of serotonin and noradrenaline in CNS neurotransmission	Amitriptyline *(also used for neuropathic pain)* Dosulepin Imipramine	Blurred vision Dry mouth Dangerous in overdose
Benzodiazepines	Anxiolytic Sedative Treatment of alcohol withdrawal	Enhance action at cerebral GABA receptors	Diazepam Lorazepam Midazolam Temazepam	Drowsiness Falls in elderly patients
Typical antipsychotics	Antipsychotic	Block cerebral dopamine pathways	Haloperidol Chlorpromazine	Parkinsonism Sedation Akathisia
Atypical antipsychotics	Antipsychotic	Block cerebral dopamine pathways	Olanzapine Quetiapine	Less severe parkinsonism Dyskinesia Weight gain
Anticonvulsants	Mood stabiliser	Affect cerebral GABA and glutamate pathways	Sodium valproate Lamotrigine Carbamazepine	Mental clouding Nausea Hyponatraemia
Lithium	Mood stabiliser	Unknown		Diabetes insipidus Dangerous in overdose Lithium toxicity
Acetylcholinesterase inhibitors	Improve symptoms of dementia	Acetylcholinesterase inhibitor	Donepezil Galantamine Rivastigmine	QTc prolongation

Table 12.11 *The components of the personal history*

	Question	Interpretation
Birth history	Did you have a normal delivery?	Complicated and instrumental deliveries have been implicated in the aetiology of schizophrenia
Developmental history	Did you achieve normal developmental milestones as a child?	Developmental delays are associated with adult psychiatric illness
Childhood history	What was your childhood like?	Symptoms of childhood neurosis, such as bed-wetting and separation anxiety, are linked to adult anxiety disorders
	What was your family like?	Did they have a loving family? Childhood abuse and neglect are strongly associated with mental health issues including depression and anxiety
	Were there any major adversities or upheavals during childhood?	Major adverse life events, e.g. bereavement or parental divorce, predispose to psychological conditions
Academic history	Did you perform well or poorly at school?	This helps determine the patient's education level
	Was there a history of bad behaviour or truancy?	This identifies personality traits that predispose to psychiatric illness
	Were you bullied?	Bullying can lead to anxiety, depression and, in severe cases, PTSD
Occupational history	What jobs have you had?	The occupational history identifies behaviour over time. For example, has the patient been repeatedly fired from jobs, or do they struggle to hold down a job?
Psychosexual history	Are you married or in a relationship?	Sexual orientation, gender identity, and marital status have strong influences on mental health
		Determine whether there was ever domestic violence or sexual abuse
Family history	Do you have children?	If so, ask about their health, whether they live with the patient, with a relative / ex-partner or in social care
		Difficulty in maintaining a stable family environment is a feature of many psychiatric illnesses
Religious history	Would you consider yourself religious?	Delusional beliefs often have a religious element, such as believing oneself to be sent from God, on a religious mission or possessed by another power
Forensic history	Have you ever been in trouble with the law?	Criminality and imprisonment may be aetiologies or consequences of psychiatric diseases
Premorbid personality	How would you describe your normal self, before you became unwell?	This provides insight into how the patient sees themself, and their expectations of treatment

As the section title implies, the questions asked here are extremely personal and require a good rapport for the patient to be able to be honest.

12.4.7 Social history

Patients' social circumstances both greatly affect, and are greatly affected by, mental illness.

Drugs, alcohol and smoking

Drug and alcohol abuse are much more common in patients with psychiatric illnesses. Many use drugs and alcohol to alleviate distressing symptoms of depression, anxiety, PTSD or schizophrenia ('self-medicating'). Recreational drugs often mimic psychiatric disorders. Smoking is more prevalent in psychiatric patients. Therefore respiratory, cardiovascular, and liver diseases are much more common amongst psychiatric patients.

Current occupation and financial situation

Patients with mental health disorders often find maintaining work difficult. Many require long periods of sick leave, which causes further anxiety. They may find it difficult to interact with others, or have poor schooling due to psychosocial problems at school age. Many patients struggle to make ends meet, and rely on state welfare and social care, and have a social worker.

Alternatively, some patients with mental health issues maintain extremely complex and high-demand jobs. In these patients, determine how they are continuing to manage and whether any changes could be made at work to accommodate their illness.

Social support

Who is there for this patient? Who is with them at home? Do they have a supportive social network? These questions help you establish how to treat the patient, such as an inpatient or outpatient basis, and whether difficult social circumstances are perpetuating their disorder.

12.4.8 Determine risk

This includes risk to themselves and risk to others.

Risk to self

Is the patient at risk of self-harm? Is there a history of self-injury or overdoses? These issues are often difficult to determine, but the following questions help:

- "When people feel down and depressed, they can feel that life is no longer worth living. Have you ever felt like this?"
- "Have you ever made plans to end your life?"

Making plans of suicide, writing suicide notes, or putting one's affairs in order, such as making a will, are extremely strong predictive factors for suicide and place the patient at high risk.

Risk to others

Patients who experience auditory hallucinations instructing them to hurt someone, or who have a delusional belief that they must hurt someone, require urgent admission to hospital and further assessment and treatment. Often, a patient's compulsion to hurt someone might be based on a 'rational' argument, such as believing the person to be possessed by the devil or an enemy in disguise.

- "Have you ever felt compelled to hurt someone else, even if you don't want to?"

12.5 The mental state examination

The mental state examination (MSE) is unique in that much of it is carried out alongside the psychiatric history, rather than after it. As the clinician engages with the patient to elicit a history, they are also noting how the patient appears, how they speak, how they respond to verbal and non-verbal cues such as smiles, jokes and facial expressions, and their impressions

about the patient's thought processes. Common findings of the MSE are listed in **Table 12.12**.

12.5.1 Appearance

Observe a patient's appearance as they enter the consultation area. Look for clues about the patient's lifestyle and ability to look after themselves.

Table 12.12 *The common findings in the MSE for the main psychiatric disorders*

MSE	Mania / hypomania	Depression	Anxiety	Schizophrenia
Appearance	Bizarrely dressed Unkempt	Self-neglect Self-harm	Agitated Fearful Tearful	Self-neglect Suspicious
Behaviour	Disinhibited Psychomotor agitation	Psychomotor retardation Poor rapport	Restless	Psychomotor retardation, catatonic (negative symptoms) Agitated, evasive (positive symptoms)
Speech	Loud Pressure of speech	Monotonous Poverty of speech	Normal tone Fast rate	Angry, accusatory, suspicious
Affect	Elevated Euphoric Irritable	Flat	Anxious	Blunted Incongruous Agitated
Thoughts	Flight of ideas Tangential	Suicidality Poverty of thought	Strong focus on anxiety triggers if known Paranoia	Delusions Loosening of associations Thought blocking
Perceptions	Delusion of grandeur	Nihilistic delusion if depressive psychosis	Normal	Hallucinations Illusions
Cognition	Poor concentration and recall	Poor concentration and recall	Usually good, may have poor concentration	Impairment in all domains of MMSE Refusing to engage in MMSE
Insight	Limited / non-existent	Good	Good	Limited / non-existent

- Are they dressed appropriately for the consultation? Patients with mania or schizophrenia may wear bizarre clothes or elaborate costumes. Disinhibited patients often dress provocatively or overtly sexually.
- Is there evidence of an underlying medical condition? Are they using a wheelchair or a walking aid?
- Do they appear to be looking after themselves, or is there evidence of self-neglect? Patients with depression often lose interest in their personal appearance, and have unwashed hair and clothes, are unshaven or have poor personal hygiene.
- Is there any visible self-harm, such as burns or cutting? This signifies depression or a personality disorder.
- Do they appear a normal weight and well nourished? Patients with anorexia often have very low body weight. Patients with severe depression may lose their appetite and lose weight, or alternatively eat to excess, leading to weight gain.

■ Is there a smell of alcohol, tobacco or marijuana? Are there injection sites along the veins of their arms, indicating drug abuse?

> **Trichotillomania is an anxiety condition associated with OCD.** Patient feel a compulsion to pull out strands of hair – usually from the head. This results in bald patches that are quite noticeable during the MSE.

12.5.2 Behaviour

Observe the patient's non-verbal communication and body language during your consultation.

■ Can you establish a rapport? Does the patient look you in the eye and respond to your comments verbally and non-verbally? Patients with depression and schizophrenia are apathetic and are difficult to engage in conversation.

■ What is the patient's attitude towards you? Are they suspicious and hostile, indicating paranoid thoughts?

■ What is their level of psychological arousal: are they calm? Patients experiencing auditory hallucinations or paranoid delusions are agitated, aggressive or fearful.

■ What is their psychomotor function? Are their movements and responses slow and sluggish, in keeping with depression? Are they restless and fidgety, in keeping with hypomania?

■ Are they tearful or tense? Are there outward signs of anxiety?

■ Are there any notable movement disorders or signs of neurological disease?

12.5.3 Speech

Normal fluent speech varies in volume, tone, rate and fluency during conversation. Listen to how the patient speaks (not what they are saying; this is covered in *Section 12.5.5*).

■ What is the volume and tone of speech? Manic patients speak loudly, and depressed patients have soft, monotonous speech. Patients with psychosis may have an angry or accusatory tone.

■ What is the rate of speech? Patients with mania or psychosis have pressurised speech patterns and it is difficult for the interviewer to get a word in. Depressed patients speak slowly with long pauses.

■ Is their speech fluent and varied, or slow and monotonous?

12.5.4 Mood and affect

Mood is how the patient perceives their own emotion to be. Affect is your objective and observable perception of the patient's emotional state.

Mood

If the topic of the patient's current mood has not been discussed in the patient history, ask about it now. Useful questions include:

■ "How would you describe your mood right now?"

■ "How have you been feeling lately?"

Affect

Note your impression of the patient's affect. A patient with normal affect responds easily to verbal and non-verbal cues, shows variation in their facial expression as they talk and listen during conversation, makes eye contact, and shows interest in what you are saying. Common types of affect are:

■ euthymic – normal mood
■ agitated – a feature of psychosis, mania and anxiety
■ apprehensive / anxious
■ irritable – indicating mania / hypomania or psychosis
■ depressed / low
■ euphoric – seen in mania
■ suspicious / paranoid.

Range of affect describes the emotional variety expressed during the consultation (**Figure 12.5**). The range of affect can be:

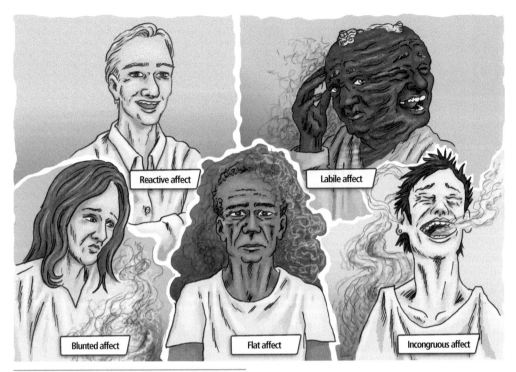

Figure 12.5 Descriptive terms for range of affect.

- **reactive**: this is a normal range of emotions displayed through the consultation that are congruent with what is being discussed.
- **labile**: this is a rapid change of emotions from one extreme to the other, such as moving from laughter to tears. It is seen in rapid cycling BAD and in some neurological conditions, including brain injury, multiple sclerosis and motor neurone disease.
- **flat**: the patient has minimal emotional reaction. It is associated with depression.
- **blunted**: the emotional range is markedly reduced and the emotions expressed are very mild in intensity. It is seen with the negative symptoms of schizophrenia.
- **incongruous**: the emotional reactions do not fit the subject being discussed. The patient is happy when discussing something sad, or vice versa. It is a sign of possible psychosis.

> **Sometimes mood and affect don't 'match'.** A patient might state that they are very depressed, but have good eye contact, a reactive affect, and appear euthymic. Recording these observations helps define the risk for the patient.

12.5.5 Thought

Patient speech content is used as a surrogate for their thoughts, on the basis that speech is 'vocalised thought'. Analyse what the patient is saying during the consultation, and note the content and stream of their thoughts.

Content

Note what the patient talks about.

- Is the patient preoccupied with one particular topic? Patients with eating disorders are preoccupied with their weight. Patients with specific anxiety disorders – PTSD, OCD and phobias – continually refer back to their anxiety triggers.

- Are their thoughts mostly depressive? Have they ever thought about suicide?
- Do they have delusions (**Table 12.5**)?

> **Delusions are concrete beliefs for patients, as real as the room they are sitting in.** Using logic and reason to explain to patients that their delusion is not real is never successful, and will induce paranoia and mistrust. Instead, be sympathetic.

Stream

- Note how the patient's thoughts flow during the consultation. Thought disorders interrupt the natural stream of thought (**Table 12.13**).

12.5.6 Perception

This is how the patient interprets the world around them. Disorders of perception are hallucinations and illusions. Hallucinations are sensory perceptions that have no basis in reality (**Table 12.5**).

Illusions

Whilst hallucinations are perceptions created in the absence of sensory information, illusions are misperceptions of actual sensory information, such as sounds, sights and smells. An example would be a patient hearing traffic on the road outside and interpreting that as voices whispering about them. Illusions usually support a patient's delusion.

12.5.7 Cognition

This is an assessment of the patient's intellectual processes. The Mini-Mental State Examination (MMSE) is used as it tests the domains of concentration, recall, and orientation in place and time. A cognitive assessment informs decisions about whether the patient lacks capacity, and therefore has a medico-legal significance.

The MMSE is a diagnostic tool for dementia and delirium. A score of ≤24 suggests cognitive impairment. The insidious onset of dementia means that patients make adaptations to compensate for their failing cognition, unintentionally 'masking' their diagnosis. The MMSE brings their condition to light.

It is a struggle to complete the MMSE if the patient:

- is agitated or paranoid
- is manic / hypomanic and can't sustain interest
- is severely depressed or has schizophrenia with marked poverty of speech and thought

Table 12.13 *The types of thought disorders and their associated conditions*		
Thought disorder	**Definition**	**Associated condition**
Poverty of thought	Diminished flow of thought, poverty of speech, slow thinking processes, struggling to concentrate	Depression Negative features of schizophrenia
Pressure of thought	Rapid flow of ideas, pressure of speech	Mania Hypomania
Loosening of associations ('knight's move thinking')	Moving abruptly between unassociated topics with no apparent pattern, using non sequiturs and rapid and baffling subject changes	Schizophrenia
Flight of ideas	Tangential speech, frequently changing topic of conversation via tenuous links	Mania Hypomania
Thought blocking	Patient suddenly stops speaking and is unable to pick up the thread of the conversation again	Schizophrenia

Table 12.14 *The common investigations used in psychiatry*

Investigation	Rationale
Blood tests:	
Thyroid function	Thyrotoxicosis and severe hypothyroidism mimic mania and depression, respectively
Folate and B12	Deficiencies in both cause toxic changes in the CNS resulting in dementia
Full blood count	Screen for anaemia or an infectious cause of the symptoms
	Monitoring for drug effect; lithium and clozapine cause agranulocytosis as a rare side-effect (total depletion of white blood cells)
Liver function tests	If hepatic encephalopathy is thought to be the reason for their psychiatric symptoms
Biochemistry	Hypercalcaemia causes depression and confusion
	Hyper- and hyponatraemia cause delirium
	Severe renal failure causes uraemic encephalopathy
	SSRIs occasionally cause hyponatraemia via syndrome of inappropriate secretion of ADH (see **Table 13.2**)
CT head / MRI head	New symptoms may herald a structural brain lesion, such as a tumour or a small bleed
	It is primarily used in new delirium or dementia, or personality changes
	Patients with classic signs of depression, schizophrenia, anxiety or eating disorders do not need brain imaging
EEG	Temporal lobe epilepsy produces symptoms and signs that look very much like acute psychosis
	The patient will start acting strangely, exhibit formal thought disorder or bizarre ideas
	EEG detects any epileptic activity
Urine toxicology	This differentiates between a recreational drug-induced and a psychiatric condition
	When meeting a patient for the first time with an acute psychosis, confusion or mania, and you cannot obtain a medical history
LP	Acute personality changes, confusion or psychosis are occasional presenting symptoms of viral encephalitis – especially if the patient is also febrile or has raised inflammatory markers
	Antibodies against certain synaptic receptors cause autoimmune encephalitis, e.g. anti-voltage gated potassium channels and anti-NMDA (*N*-methyl-D-aspartate) antibodies; these antibodies are detected in either the CSF or on blood tests
ECG	SSRIs and acetylcholinesterase inhibitors rarely cause prolongation of the QT interval, so ECG is obtained before and after initiating treatment

■ has a formal thought disorder.
In these cases it is better to make a note of their struggle to focus as part of your assessment, rather than doggedly persist in completing the MMSE.

12.5.8 Insight

This refers to the patient's ability to comprehend and appreciate their illness. Patients with affective and anxiety disorders have good insight, whereas patients with psychosis have little insight.

Determine whether the patient understands their own psychological health.

- Does the patient believe that they are ill?
- Does the patient want to be treated?

Determining whether the patient has insight helps decide on their treatment. Patients with no insight often refuse treatment as they perceive it as unneeded; these patients require sectioning under the Mental Health Act to treat them in their best interest.

12.5.9 Finishing off

Thank the patient for their time and their honesty.

12.6 Common investigations

The diagnostic hierarchy (**Figure 12.2**) mandates that organic conditions are ruled out before psychiatric diagnoses are considered (**Table 12.14**). This is to prevent disease such as delirium, dementia, brain lesions and encephalitis being inappropriately treated with psychotropic medication. All of these conditions mimic features of certain psychiatric disorders, so clinical history and MSE are not sufficient in their diagnosis.

12.7 Answers to starter questions

1. In psychiatry not all treatments work for all people. Some people respond to low doses of a medication, whilst others require high doses of multiple medications. Psychological therapies are very effective for some patients, whilst others find them no help at all. Choosing the right treatment for the individual patient is an important skill, although many patients try a few treatments before finding one that works for them.

2. There is no evidence that patients with mental health conditions have an alteration in their brain chemistry, because there is no way of measuring neurotransmitters in the CNS. We know that modulating the effects of neurotransmitters has profound effects on psychiatric conditions, but we don't know if this is because we are correcting an imbalance or diminishing the symptoms by artificially increasing neurotransmitter effects.

3. Patients who repeatedly vomit – whether self-induced or due to another illness – deplete their body's potassium and sodium content due to gastric losses. Inappropriate use of laxatives compounds the intestinal loss of electrolytes by inducing diarrhoea. Finally, the abuse of diuretics leads to renal electrolyte losses. Hyponatraemia causes impaired consciousness and seizures. Hypokalaemia leads to dangerous ECG changes, including ST depression, T wave inversion, prolonged QT interval and the presence of a U wave after the T wave. Severe hypokalaemia leads to fatal arrhythmias and sudden cardiac death, which is the cause of nearly a third of all deaths in anorexia nervosa.

4. Most people experiencing suicidal ideation do not take their own life. A suicide crisis, when the patient makes firm plans to kill themselves, or feels unable to stop themselves, is an emergency. It is crucial that the patient is moved to a place of safety, where they can be closely observed and do not pose a risk to themselves. Patients with known psychiatric disorders who experience a suicide crisis call mental health crisis teams, who arrange urgent assessment. For patients without access to such teams, the emergency department is the safest place for them to be.

Chapter 13
Endocrine system

Starter questions

1. Why do endocrine doctors like looking at patients' old photos?
2. Why can most endocrine problems be treated with tablets except diabetes?
3. Why might patients with chronic diabetes struggle to attend their outpatient clinic appointments?
4. Who is responsible for a diabetic patient's care?
5. Why might someone with pituitary disease keep bumping into things?

Answers to questions are to be found in *Section 13.9.*

13.1 Introduction

The endocrine system can be compared with the nervous system: it regulates the entire body via systemic pathways. Whilst the nervous system uses electrical messages via neurons, the endocrine system uses hormones via the bloodstream. Hormones are molecules that bind to receptors on target organs and modulate their function.

The endocrine system controls metabolism, physiological homeostasis, and normal growth and development from infancy to adulthood.

Therefore endocrine deregulation results in body-wide illness that incorporates all aspects of metabolism: energy levels, appetite, bowel habit, weight, sleep, growth, heart rate and blood pressure and even mood. Nearly all endocrine disorders are treated by blocking or suppressing overactive endocrine glands, or replacing deficient hormones via medication. This typically results in a very rapid improvement in the patient's symptoms and quality of life.

Case 13.1 Fatigue

Presentation

Michelle is 33 years old. She has attended the GP due to debilitating tiredness, which is beginning to affect her day-to-day life.

Initial interpretation

Generalised fatigue is a very common presentation in primary care. Organic causes include cardiovascular, respiratory, haematological, neurological and endocrine dysfunction, so the differential diagnosis is wide. We need to explore her history, co-morbidities and psychosocial conditions.

History

Michelle describes herself as very energetic until the last six months. She is a full-time mum to three children, and is starting to find it difficult to keep up with them. She often naps during the day. She lives with her husband, who is supportive and concerned for her. She has stopped going swimming regularly, which she used to enjoy, because she doesn't have the energy.

Interpretation of history

Michelle is describing severe fatigue which has disrupted her daily activities. Considering her age, heart failure is extremely unlikely to be the cause of her symptoms. Respiratory conditions such as asthma, COPD and pulmonary fibrosis cause profound fatigue in association with breathlessness, but she has not volunteered any respiratory symptoms thus far.

Anaemia causes fatigue, and is not uncommon in women with heavy periods. A menstrual history and blood test for haemoglobin will help make this diagnosis. A rarer cause of iron-deficiency anaemia in young people is coeliac disease, due to poor iron absorption.

Endocrine causes of fatigue include diabetes mellitus, hypothyroidism and adrenal insufficiency. Diabetes is associated with extreme thirst, weight loss and excessive urination. Hypothyroidism causes a general slowing of the metabolism, and

is associated with weight gain, feeling cold and constipation. Adrenal insufficiency is associated with nausea, hypovolaemia and general malaise.

Finally, chronic fatigue syndrome is a medical illness of unknown aetiology. It is characterised by long-term fatigue that is not relieved by rest, generalised body pains and impairment in memory and concentration.

Further history

Michelle describes herself as being 'fit and happy' before these symptoms began. Her only past medical history is the skin complaint vitiligo. She describes her periods as regular and light. She has not noticed any bowel disturbance, and eats a normal diet. She denies excessive thirst or urination. She is losing weight, which she ascribes to having a poor appetite. She often feels nauseated, and if she tries to make herself eat she occasionally vomits.

She does not have any neurological symptoms, but does often feel light-headed when she stands up from sitting. She does not have any aches or pains. She does not feel depressed.

Examination

Michelle has a tanned complexion, with occasional spots of vitiligo on her hands. There is no conjunctival pallor. Her blood pressure is 110/80mmHg, but this falls to 90/50 when she stands up. Her heart rate is 60 beats per minute and regular. Cardiac, abdominal and respiratory examinations are normal.

There are no thyroid masses. Her neurological examination is normal.

Interpretation of findings

Michelle has six months of fatigue and tiredness, associated with nausea, poor appetite and weight loss. She has postural hypotension. She does not have pallor; rather, she has a darker complexion. She has a history of vitiligo – an autoimmune condition – and patients often have more than one autoimmune disease.

Having clinically excluded anaemia, cardiac

and respiratory disease, and depression, the likely diagnoses are hypothyroidism or adrenal insufficiency. These conditions are readily diagnosed on blood testing.

Investigations

As expected, Michelle's full blood count is normal: she is not anaemic. Her thyroid function tests are normal. A measurement of her early morning cortisol is low at 171mmol/L. Her doctor arranges an adrenocorticotrophic hormone (ACTH) test to discover if her adrenal glands appropriately secrete cortisol in response to ACTH. The results are:

- Serum cortisol before ACTH
  injection   190mmol/L
- Serum cortisol 30 minutes after
  ACTH injection   212mmol/L
- Serum cortisol 60 minutes after
  ACTH injection   200mmol/L.

Diagnosis

The serum cortisol should at least double in healthy individuals following an ACTH test. The

failure of her adrenal glands to respond to ACTH means that her low cortisol is due to adrenal insufficiency, rather than ACTH insufficiency (which is a pituitary problem).

Further blood tests reveal the presence of anti-adrenal antibodies, confirming the diagnosis of autoimmune adrenal disease, leading to adrenal insufficiency. This condition is called Addison's disease. Patients with adrenal insufficiency usually have extremely elevated levels of ACTH, which reflects the pituitary's efforts to stimulate cortisol release from the adrenals; it is high ACTH levels which cause the darkening of the skin, as seen in Michelle's case. Adrenal insufficiency promotes salt loss, and to a lesser degree, water loss from the kidney, leading to hyponatraemia and hypovolaemia. The hypovolaemia is responsible for Michelle's postural hypotension.

Treatment with regular cortisol medication (called hydrocortisone) allows patients to live a normal life, and ameliorates all symptoms.

13.2 System overview

The endocrine system is composed of several hormonal axes. A hormonal axis is a group of hormones and endocrine glands that perform one particular metabolic function. A hormonal axis comprises one or two 'releasing hormones' that are secreted by one endocrine gland. These releasing hormones then act upon another endocrine gland to produce a target hormone, that acts upon metabolic processes in the body. The releasing hormones have no systemic effect on metabolic pathways; they serve only to stimulate the production of target hormones.

Target hormones inhibit further release of their own releasing hormones, thus regulating their own circulating levels and maintaining homeostasis.

Dysregulation of these individual axes results in systemic metabolic disturbances. Major hormonal imbalances are due to tumour or hyperplasia of a gland, autoimmune disease or ectopic hormone production (**Table 13.1**).

13.2.1 Hypothalamus

The hypothalamus is in the forebrain. It is the link between the neurological system and the endocrine system. It receives incoming data from the nervous system and secretes releasing hormones which act upon the pituitary (**Figure 13.1**).

Table 13.1 *Major hormonal imbalances and their causes*

Hormone	Cause of increased levels	Cause of decreased levels
Triiodothyroxine, thyroxine (T_3, T_4)	Goitre Graves' disease Thyroiditis	Hashimoto's Post-thyroidectomy Pituitary failure
Cortisol	Cushing's disease ACTH-producing pituitary tumour Exogenous steroid therapy ACTH-producing neuroendocrine tumour	Adrenal insufficiency, e.g. Addison's disease Inborn errors of cortisol production Pituitary failure Sudden withdrawal of long-term steroid treatment
Aldosterone	Adrenal adenoma (Conn's syndrome) Excessive renin production ■ renin-secreting tumour ■ renal artery stenosis	Adrenal insufficiency Inborn errors of aldosterone production Chronic renal failure, especially diabetic nephropathy
Parathyroid hormone (PTH)	Parathyroid hyperplasia Parathyroid cancer	Post-thyroidectomy
Catecholamines	Phaeochromocytoma	Adrenalectomy
Antidiuretic hormone (ADH)	Syndrome of inappropriate ADH production ■ excess ADH from pituitary ■ ectopic ADH from neuroendocrine tumour ■ drug-induced ■ idiopathic	Diabetes insipidus
Gonadotrophins	Gonadotrophin-producing pituitary tumour Menopause	Pituitary failure Elevated prolactin
Growth hormone (GH)	Pituitary tumour (acromegaly)	Pituitary failure Chromosomal abnormalities Genetic mutations

13.2.2 Pituitary gland

The anterior pituitary releases five hormones (**Table 13.2**). It responds to releasing hormones from the hypothalamus, and receives negative feedback from circulating hormones.

The posterior pituitary secretes two hormones:
■ antidiuretic hormone (ADH), which causes water reabsorption in the kidney
■ oxytocin, which stimulates lactation and uterine contractions in women.

Pituitary apoplexy occurs when the vascular supply to the pituitary is compromised. This 'switches off' all hormonal axes in the body. The patient takes hormonal supplements in order to maintain normal endocrine function.

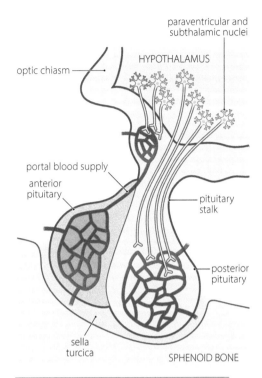

paraventricular and
subthalamic nuclei

HYPOTHALAMUS

optic chiasm

portal blood supply

anterior
pituitary

pituitary
stalk

posterior
pituitary

sella
turcica

SPHENOID BONE

Figure 13.1 The gross anatomy of the pituitary gland, demonstrating its position within the sphenoid bone, its connection to the hypothalamus, and its close proximity to the optic chiasm.

13.2.3 Adrenal glands

The adrenal glands produce three main hormones: cortisol, aldosterone and catecholamines (**Table 13.3**).

Cortisol

The hypothalamic–pituitary–adrenocortical axis controls cardiovascular and metabolic homeostasis (**Figure 13.2**). Cortisol is a major catabolic hormone, meaning that it helps break down large molecules (such as glucose) into smaller molecules to release energy. Cushing's *disease* is a pituitary disorder wherein excessive ACTH is secreted, which is non-responsive to the negative feedback effects of high circulating cortisol levels (hypercortisolaemia).

Cushing's *syndrome* is the collection of signs and symptoms associated with excess cortisol, and results from:

- Cushing's disease
- iatrogenic use of exogenous steroids for chronic inflammatory disease
- excessive cortisol secretion from an adrenal tumour.

In these latter two scenarios, the serum ACTH is low, reflecting negative feedback of hypercortisolaemia upon the pituitary.

Table 13.2 *Anterior pituitary hormones and their hypothalamic releasing hormones*		
Pituitary hormone	**Responsible hypothalamic hormone**	**Action**
Thyroid-stimulating hormone (TSH)	Thyrotrophin-releasing hormone (TRH)	Triggers triiodothyroxine and thyroxine release from thyroid
Adrenocorticotrophic hormone (ACTH)	Corticotrophin-releasing hormone (CRH)	Triggers cortisol release from the adrenals
Growth hormone (GH)	Growth hormone-releasing hormone (GHRH)	Increases muscle mass Increases bone mineralisation Increases serum glucose
Prolactin	Thyrotrophin-releasing hormone (TRH) Inhibited by dopamine	Promotes lactation during pregnancy Suppresses GnRH
Gonadotrophins ■ follicle-stimulating hormone (FSH) ■ luteinising hormone (LH)	Gonadotrophin-releasing hormone (GnRH)	Sex steroid production and gamete maturation

Table 13.3 *Hormones released from the adrenal glands and their effects*

Hormones	Releasing mechanism	Effects
Cortisol	ACTH	Increases serum glucose
		Anti-inflammatory
		Sodium retention
		Suppresses digestion
Aldosterone	Angiotensin via the renin–angiotensin system	Regulates blood pressure via sodium and water retention
		Increases potassium loss
Catecholamines	Psychological stress	Works in concert with the sympathetic nervous system to:
	Sympathetic nervous system activation	■ increase heart rate
		■ increase BP
		■ increase serum glucose
		■ trigger 'fight or flight' response

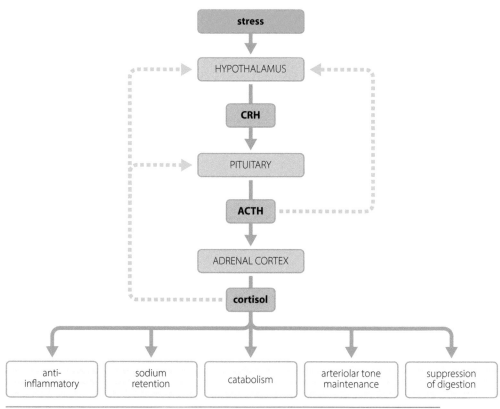

Figure 13.2 The hypothalamic–pituitary–adrenocortical axis. Cortisol from the adrenal gland provides most of the negative feedback at the pituitary. ACTH, adrenocorticotrophic hormone; CRH, corticotrophin-releasing hormone.

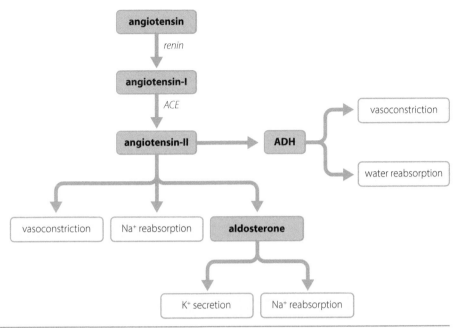

Figure 13.3 The renin–angiotensin–aldosterone system of BP homeostasis. Renin is secreted by the nephron in response to decreased renal blood flow, which is interpreted as systemic hypotension.

Hypocortisolism is usually due to Addison's disease, an autoimmune destruction of the adrenal glands. This is primary adrenal insufficiency. Rarer causes of hypocortisolism are:
■ secondary adrenal insufficiency, due to pituitary failure to release ACTH
■ tertiary adrenal insufficiency, due to hypothalamic failure to release corticotrophin-releasing hormone.

Aldosterone

Aldosterone is secreted by the adrenal gland in response to renal hormones, such as angiotensin and renin (**Figure 13.3**). These renal hormones also trigger the release of ADH from the pituitary, which causes vasoconstriction and water retention.

High aldosterone levels (hyperaldosteronism) result in excessive salt and water retention, causing hypertension, and excessive potassium loss, causing hypokalaemia. Conn's syndrome is a common type of hyperaldosteronism, and is due to a benign adenoma of the adrenal gland.

Hypoaldosteronism is usually due to renal disease, and failure to release renal hormones, such as angiotensin.

Catecholamines

The main catecholamines are adrenaline and noradrenaline. These hormones work with the sympathetic nervous system to raise the heart rate, blood pressure and metabolic rate. A phaeochromocytoma is a catecholamine-producing tumour of the adrenals. The features are tachycardia, hypertension, tremor and panic attacks.

Phaeochromocytoma is difficult to diagnose, as the intermittent symptoms of massive catecholamine release are identical to panic attacks. It is very common for patients who are ultimately diagnosed with phaeochromocytoma to be treated for months or years with anxiolytics before receiving the correct diagnosis.

13.2.4 Thyroid gland

The thyroid gland sits in the anterior neck. It releases the thyroid hormones triiodothyronine (T_3) and thyroxine (T_4) in response to thyroid-stimulating hormone (TSH) from the pituitary

(**Figure 13.4**). These hormones regulate metabolic activity (**Table 13.4**). Both hyperthyroidism and hypothyroidism are associated with goitre – a palpable thyroid swelling in the neck.

Hyperthyroidism

This is due to excessive thyroid secretion of T_3 and T_4. Measurements of serum TSH are characteristically low, reflecting the negative feedback of thyroid hormones upon the pituitary. A rarer cause of hyperthyroidism is a pituitary tumour secreting excess TSH. The features of hyperthyroidism are in keeping with a raised metabolic rate and sympathetic activation.

The severest form of hyperthyroidism is a thyroid storm, which is characterised by pyrexia, tachyarrhythmias, heart failure and agitation.

Table 13.4 *Comparing the effects of hyper- and hypothyroidism*	
Hypothyroidism	**Hyperthyroidism**
Fatigue	Agitation and tremor
Feeling cold	Feeling hot, excessive sweating
Bradycardia	Tachycardia
Weight gain	Weight loss
Menorrhagia	Oligo- / amenorrhoea
Constipation	Diarrhoea

Causes

Graves' disease. This is autoimmune stimulation of TSH receptors in the thyroid. In addition to the generic features of hyperthyroidism, it causes pedal oedema and a goitre. It also causes Graves' eye disease, due to swelling of the retro-orbital tissues. This leads to exophthalmos (protrusion of the eyes) and ophthalmoplegia (impaired eye movements).

Toxic multinodular goitre. This is a simple goitre with many nodules that secrete excessive T_3 and T_4. More rarely, patients develop a solitary toxic nodule.

Thyroiditis. Inflammation of the thyroid is a result of viral infection, postpartum or drug-induced. Thyroid function usually returns to normal after days or weeks.

Hypothyroidism

This is due to impaired secretion of T_3 and T_4. TSH levels are characteristically high, reflecting the pituitary's efforts to stimulate the thyroid.

The severest form of hypothyroidism is myxoedema coma: hypothermia, acute delirium and bradyarrhythmias.

Causes

Hashimoto's thyroiditis. This is autoimmune destruction of the thyroid gland.

Iatrogenic. Patients who have previously undergone thyroidectomy for a large goitre or severe hyperthyroidism require lifelong thyroxine replacement therapy.

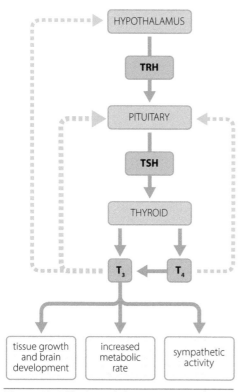

Figure 13.4 The hypothalamic–pituitary–thyroid axis. Most of the action and negative feedback is mediated by triiodothyronine (T_3), formed from peripheral conversion of thyroxine (T_4). TRH, thyrotrophin-releasing hormone; TSH, thyroid-stimulating hormone.

Iodine deficiency. This is the commonest cause worldwide, but rare in developed countries.
Postpartum thyroiditis. This affects 5% of women following childbirth. Most women return to normal thyroid function but 30% remain hypothyroid lifelong.

13.2.5 Parathyroid gland

There are four pea-sized parathyroid glands embedded within the thyroid gland. They are responsible for calcium and bone homeostasis (**Figure 13.5**). They secrete parathyroid hormone (PTH), which increases serum calcium via four pathways:
- Increased resorption in the kidney
- Increased absorption from the gut
- Increased hydroxylation of inactive vitamin D to its active form, which augments intestinal absorption of calcium
- Release of calcium from bone via osteoclast activity.

PTH is suppressed by elevated serum calcium via negative feedback. Hyperparathyroidism causes hypercalcaemia, and hypoparathyroidism causes hypocalcaemia.

Calcitonin is a hormone released by the thyroid in response to hypercalcaemia. It inhibits osteoclast activity and favours calcium movement into bone.

> The effects of hyperparathyroidism are remembered by 'stones, bones, groans and psychological moans'.
> **Stones**: Chronic hypercalcaemia leads to calcium renal stone formation
> **Bones**: Excessive bone remodelling causes bone pain
> **Groans**: Hypercalcaemia causes severe constipation and abdominal pain
> **Psychological moans**: Hypercalcaemia causes depressive symptoms

13.2.6 Gonads

The hypothalamic–pituitary–gonadal axis is responsible for the production of steroid sex hormones (**Figure 13.6**):

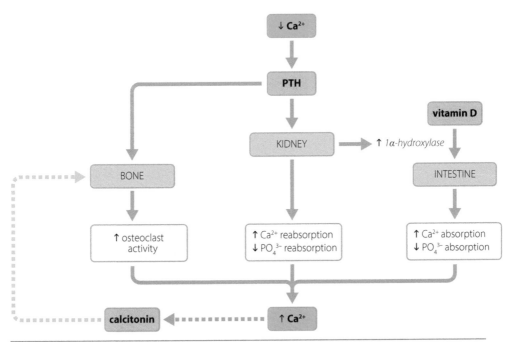

Figure 13.5 Calcium regulation. Parathyroid hormone (PTH) is released in response to hypocalcaemia and acts in conjunction with vitamin D to raise the calcium level. Calcitonin antagonises the action of PTH. PO_4^{3-}, phosphate ion.

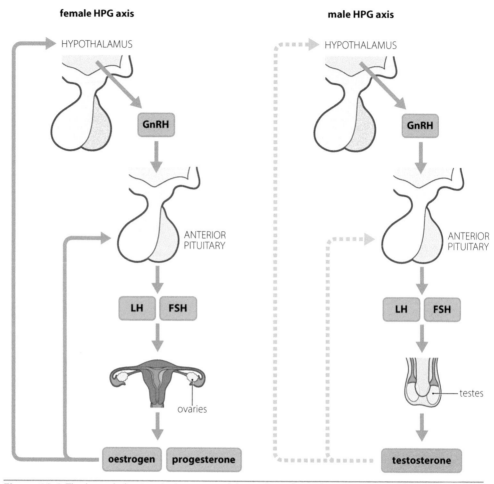

Figure 13.6 The hypothalamic–pituitary–gonadal axis. Gonadotrophins are released from the pituitary in response to gonadotrophin-releasing hormone from the hypothalamus. Sex steroids provide negative feedback at the pituitary.

■ Androgens such as testosterone
■ Oestrogens
■ Progesterone.

In men, androgens develop testes formation, maintain muscle mass and aid spermatogenesis. In women, androgens are the molecular precursor to oestrogens. Oestrogen and progesterone are responsible for regulating the menstrual cycle, developing secondary sex characteristics and maintaining pregnancy.

13.2.7 Pancreas

The pancreas produces insulin, which increases liver storage of glucose as glycogen, and facilitates

intracellular glucose metabolism. Diabetes mellitus incorporates two disease processes: type 1 and type 2 diabetes. Both diseases are associated with hyperglycaemia. There are many long-term effects of chronic hyperglycaemia (**Table 13.5**).

Type 1 diabetes mellitus

Autoimmune destruction of the pancreas impairs insulin secretion. The patient is unable to lower glucose levels by storing it as glycogen, or metabolise glucose for energy. Despite significant hyperglycaemia, the patient exhibits signs of starvation: weight loss, fatigue and muscle breakdown.

Table 13.5 *Long-term complications of diabetes mellitus*

System	Pathology	Common associations
Neurological	Autonomic failure	Postural hypotension Resting tachycardia
	Peripheral neuropathy	Foot injury Neuropathic pain in feet
Ophthalmic	Diabetic retinopathy	Vision loss
	Cataracts	
Renal	Diabetic nephropathy	Progressive renal failure
Cardiovascular	Coronary heart disease	Angina, heart attack
	Peripheral vascular disease	Ulcers Ischaemic limbs
	Microvascular damage	Erectile dysfunction
Immunological	Immunosuppression	Urinary tract infections Fungal skin infections
GI	Gastroparesis	Abdominal pain, vomiting

Type 2 diabetes mellitus

This is due to insulin resistance. Despite elevated levels of serum insulin, the patient is insensitive to its effects. The result is chronic hyperglycaemia. Whilst there is a genetic component in its aetiology, the strongest risk factor is obesity.

13.3 Symptoms of endocrine disease

The key symptoms are: fatigue, change in weight, thirst, decreased libido, subfertility, palpitations, menstrual disorders and change in bowel habit.

13.3.1 Fatigue

Feeling constantly tired is a common symptom in the general population, but can be a sign of many physiological and pathological processes. Patients describe anergia: a constant lack of energy. The endocrine causes are:

- Addison's disease, due to insufficient cortisol
- hypothyroidism, due to insufficient thyroid hormones
- diabetes type 1 and 2, due to an inability to metabolise glucose.

Cardiovascular causes

Congestive cardiac failure is associated with decreased cardiac output, which in turn causes chronic tiredness.

Respiratory causes

Severe lung diseases, such as COPD and pulmonary fibrosis, are associated with constant fatigue.

Haematological causes

Fatigue is the commonest presenting symptom of chronic anaemia.

Neurological causes

Chronic fatigue syndrome (also known as myalgic encephalomyelitis, ME) is a disease of unknown aetiology that causes chronic fatigue, muscle and joint pain and serious impairment of day-to-day function. It is a diagnosis of exclusion, as organic conditions (which respond to treatment and may cause serious morbidity if left undiagnosed) must be checked for first.

13.3.2 Change in weight

Endocrine dysfunction causes changes in weight and adiposity due to the effects of hormones on the metabolic pathways in the body. Endocrine dysregulation increases or reduces the basal metabolic rate, and the patient finds that they cannot control or prevent weight loss or gain. Thyroid hormone and cortisol have the most profound effect on the metabolic rate.

Weight loss

Unintentional weight loss is usually recognised by the patient when their clothes no longer fit. The commonest causes are divided into endocrine, gastrointestinal and psychological.

Endocrine

Hyperthyroidism. The elevated metabolic rate of hyperthyroidism causes weight loss despite a normal appetite.

Hypocortisolism. Weight loss in adrenal insufficiency is due to chronic nausea and decreased appetite (**Figure 13.7**).

> **Adrenal insufficiency causes excessive sodium loss.** Patients therefore often experience salt cravings, which must be asked about in the history.

Type 1 diabetes mellitus. Due to the inability to metabolise glucose, patients with type 1 diabetes rapidly lose weight.

Gastrointestinal

Chronic GI disorders impair digestion and result in weight loss. Causes include:

- inflammatory bowel disease
- achalasia
- malabsorption syndromes, such as coeliac disease.

Psychological

Depression and anorexia nervosa are common psychiatric causes of poor oral intake and weight loss.

Weight gain

The commonest cause of weight gain is consuming more calories than are expended in exercise. Obesity levels due to poor diet and insufficient exercise are rising worldwide, and are responsible for the massive increase in the global prevalence of type 2 diabetes.

Pathological causes of weight gain are divided into endocrine, cardiovascular, gastrointestinal and psychological.

Endocrine

Hypothyroidism. A low basal metabolic rate results in weight gain.

Cushing's disease. Hypercortisolaemia leads to increased adipose tissue, amongst many other features (**Figure 13.8**).

Type 2 diabetes mellitus. Increased body fat is a risk factor for type 2 diabetes. Weight loss is often difficult, but results in increased insulin sensitivity and reduces the need for medication. Sufficient weight loss often negates the need for any diabetic medication at all.

> **If an obese patient is experiencing difficulties with weight loss, the cause nearly always lies in their lifestyle choices**, including diet, exercise and alcohol consumption. If a patient is experiencing rapid unexplained weight gain, cannot lose weight despite lifestyle modifications, or is experiencing other metabolic disturbances, then they should be screened for endocrine disorders.

Cardiovascular

Generalised oedema secondary to heart failure results in generalised weight gain. This weight gain is all 'water weight' due to significant fluid retention, rather than adipose tissue.

Gastrointestinal

Chronic liver disease results in ascites, which greatly increases the total body weight.

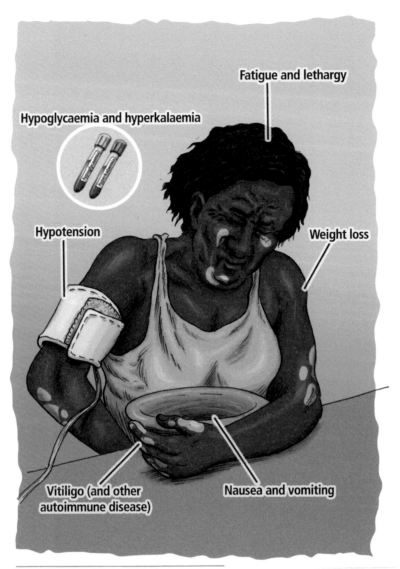

Figure 13.7 The hypocortisolaemic patient.

Psychological

People who binge eat in relation to psychological distress have an increased BMI.

13.3.3 Thirst

Polyuria is excessive urination. Polydipsia is excessive thirst. Polydipsia is usually a result of polyuria.

Endocrine causes

Diabetes mellitus

The combination of polyuria and polydipsia is the commonest mode of presentation to doctors with a new diagnosis of diabetes (both type 1 and 2). Diabetes causes hyperglycaemia. When serum glucose levels are sufficiently elevated, the kidney is unable to resorb water in the nephron, resulting in an osmotic diuresis.

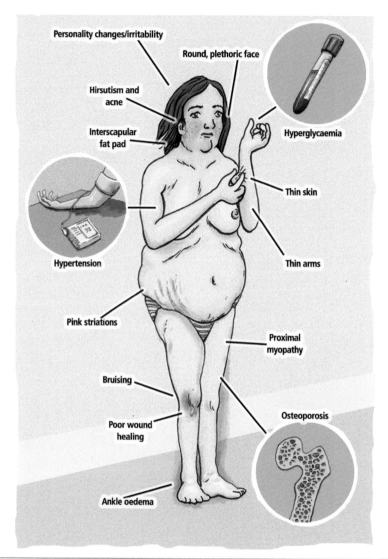

Personality changes/irritability

Round, plethoric face

Hirsutism and acne

Interscapular fat pad

Hyperglycaemia

Thin skin

Hypertension

Thin arms

Pink striations

Proximal myopathy

Bruising

Osteoporosis

Poor wound healing

Ankle oedema

Figure 13.8 The hypercortisolaemic patient. Due to its strong historical correlation with Cushing's disease, this phenotype is often referred to as a 'cushingoid appearance'.

Diabetes insipidus

This is a rare condition in which the body either does not produce ADH, or is insensitive to its effects. Without the ability to retain pure water, the patient becomes dehydrated and hypernatraemic, leading to thirst and passing large amounts of dilute urine.

Hypercalcaemia

Elevated serum calcium leads to profound dehydration, as calcium induces polyuria in the kidney. It is the result of:

■ excessive PTH release from hyperplastic parathyroids (primary hyperparathyroidism)
■ excessive calcium release from bone disease, such as a bone tumour.

Other causes

Patients who are taking excessive doses of diuretic medications develop polyuria, which in turn causes polydipsia. These patients also develop hyponatraemia, as diuretics cause both sodium and water loss from the kidney.

Psychogenic polydipsia is a rare psychiatric condition. Patients have a compulsive desire to drink excessive amounts of water, often exceeding the safe level of 4L/day. It results in dilutional hyponatraemia.

13.3.4 Decreased libido

Dysregulation of the hypothalamic–pituitary–gonadal axis results in decreased production of sex hormones (hypogonadism). Decreased levels of sex hormones affect both fertility levels and libido (sex drive), whether the cause is primary or secondary hypogonadism.

Primary hypogonadism

This is due to testicular or ovarian failure and is rare. Circulating levels of sex hormones (oestrogen, progesterone and testosterone) are low. Levels of gonadotrophins (FSH and LH) are elevated, as the pituitary has no negative feedback.

Congenital causes include genetic abnormalities or errors of metabolism. Acquired causes are usually due to damage to the gonads via surgery, radio- or chemotherapy, or trauma.

Secondary hypogonadism

This is also called hypogonadotrophic hypogonadism, as it is it due to pituitary failure to release gonadotrophins. Both gonadotrophins and sex hormones are low.

Other causes

Decreased libido is a common symptom of depression. Some medications, such as antidepressants, decrease the libido.

13.3.5 Subfertility

Subfertility manifests as difficulty or inability for a woman to become pregnant. In males, it indicates a problem with the number, morphology or characteristics of their spermatozoa, or with the seminal fluid. Endocrine causes of subfertility include:

- pituitary failure, leading to decreased FSH and LH levels; this interferes with ova production in women and sperm production in men
- PCOS (affecting women only)
- prolactin excess (in men and women).

These (and other) causes of female subfertility are discussed in *Section 8.7.1*.

13.3.6 Palpitations

Palpitations are caused by tachycardia, bradycardia and arrhythmia. Hyperthyroidism is the commonest endocrine cause of tachycardia, and causes constant or intermittent bouts of sinus tachycardia, atrial fibrillation or atrial flutter. Conversely, hypothyroidism causes bradycardia, which is perceived by the patient as slow palpitations.

13.3.7 Menstrual disorders

Endocrine causes have a profound effect on the menstrual cycle, which is governed by hormones. The commonest menstrual abnormality due to endocrine disease is oligo- /amenorrhoea. Causes include:

- PCOS
- hyperthyroidism
- pregnancy
- prolactin excess.

Menorrhagia is associated with hypothyroidism. Hypercortisolism is associated with both forms of menstrual irregularity.

Differential diagnoses of menstrual disorders are explored in *Section 8.5.1*.

13.3.8 Change in bowel habit

This is when a patient's bowel habit changes from being normal to a more unpredictable pattern, which is either diarrhoea, constipation or alternating between the two. Endocrine causes of constipation are:

- hypercalcaemia
- hypothyroidism.

Endocrine causes of diarrhoea are:

- adrenal insufficiency
- hyperthyroidism.

Differential diagnoses of constipation and diarrhoea are explored in *Section 6.3.3*.

13.4 Endocrine history

The endocrine history must investigate the patient's presenting problems, and screen for any coexisting endocrine dysfunction.

13.4.1 Past medical history

Autoimmune disorders occur in isolation, or in 'clusters' in one patient. If there is a suggestion of one autoimmune disease, ask about others, including:

- Addison's disease
- type 1 diabetes mellitus
- autoimmune thyroid disease
- primary biliary cirrhosis, primary sclerosing cholangitis and autoimmune hepatitis
- vitiligo (autoimmune skin pigment loss)
- alopecia areata (autoimmune hair loss)
- rheumatoid arthritis.

Multiple endocrine neoplasia is a genetic condition associated with tumours and overactivity of several endocrine glands, so ask about all endocrine symptoms.

Resistant hypertension, i.e. not responding to several different antihypertensive medications, often has an endocrine cause, such as hypercortisolism, phaeochromocytoma, hyperthyroidism or hyperaldosteronism.

Ask about the patient's puberty and menstruation, as congenital endocrine disorders lead to delayed or precocious puberty.

13.4.2 Drug history

Ask about medications that affect the main hormonal axes. Many patients taking long-term steroid therapy (such as prednisolone or hydrocortisone) for inflammatory conditions have iatrogenic hypocortisolism, where exogenous steroid causes complete suppression of pituitary ACTH release. Common inflammatory conditions requiring chronic or recurrent courses of steroid treatment include rheumatoid arthritis,

> **The commonest insulin therapy regime is the 'basal-bolus' regime.** The patient takes a long-acting (basal) insulin once a day, which mimics the pancreas's background, low-level insulin secretion, and a 'bolus' of short-acting insulin with every meal, to mimic the sudden insulin spike from the pancreas whilst eating.

Table 13.6 *Classes and actions of diabetic medications for type 2 diabetes*

Class	Examples	Mechanism	Side-effects
Biguanides	Metformin	Increases insulin sensitivity Reduces gluconeogenesis in the liver	Nausea and diarrhoea
Sulphonylureas	Gliclazide Glimepiride	Stimulates pancreatic insulin release	Hypoglycaemia Weight gain
Dipeptidyl peptidase-4 inhibitor	Sitagliptin Linagliptin	Inhibits glucagon release and stimulates insulin release	Arthralgia Hypoglycaemia Heart failure
Glucagon-like peptide-1 receptor agonist	Exenatide Liraglutide	Stimulates pancreatic insulin release	Nausea Pancreatitis
Sodium/glucose cotransporter 2 inhibitors	Canagliflozin Dapagliflozin	Promotes renal excretion of glucose	Increased risk of urinary tract and candidal infections Hypoglycaemia

polymyalgia rheumatica and COPD. These patients must never abruptly stop their steroid therapy, as it induces an Addisonian crisis (see **Table 13.10**).

Diabetic regimes are individualised for each patient, so record the exact doses and timings of insulin therapy. Type 1 diabetics only take insulin, whereas type 2 diabetics take oral insulin-sensitising agents, insulin-stimulating agents, injectable insulin, or a mixture (**Table 13.6**).

Establish whether they are taking medications which interfere with normal endocrine function (**Table 13.7**).

Table 13.7 *Medications that affect endocrine regulation*

Drug	Role	Effect
Amiodarone	Anti-arrhythmic	Causes either hypo- or hyperthyroidism
Diuretics	Reduces circulating volume Antihypertensive	Excessive urinary electrolyte loss, causing hypokalaemia and hyponatraemia
Anticonvulsants	Prevents seizures	Many anticonvulsants induce syndrome of inappropriate antidiuretic hormone (SIADH)
SSRIs	Antidepressant	May cause SIADH
Oral contraceptive pill	Contraception	Suppresses ovulation Suppresses menstruation
Lithium	Mood stabiliser	Induces diabetes insipidus via ADH insensitivity at the nephron

Table 13.8 *Endocrine systems review*

System	Symptoms	Endocrine causes
Respiratory	Cough Haemoptysis	Neuroendocrine lung tumour secreting hormones such as parathyroid hormone, ACTH and ADH
Cardiovascular	Chest pain	Type 1 and 2 DM accelerate coronary vascular disease
Gastrointestinal	Constipation / abdominal pain	Hypercalcaemia
	Weight gain	Untreated type 2 diabetes Hypothyroidism
	Weight loss	Hyperthyroidism Untreated type 1 diabetes
Genitourinary	Impotence	Type 1 and 2 DM accelerate microvascular disease leading to erectile dysfunction
	Polyuria	Hyperglycaemia Diabetes insipidus
	Renal stones	Hypercalcaemia
Neurological	Peripheral neuropathy Vision problems / retinopathy	Diabetes (type 1 and 2)

13.4.3 Social history

Ask about smoking, as neuroendocrine lung cancers secrete hormones, including ACTH, PTH and ADH.

Excessive alcohol usually causes chronic inflammation and impairment of the pancreas, affecting insulin secretion.

13.4.4 Family history

Ask about autoimmune diseases, which are often familial. Type 2 diabetes has a strong genetic component, and type 1 diabetes has a milder genetic component.

13.4.5 Systems review

A full systems review is shown in **Table 13.8**.

13.5 Signs of endocrine disease

13.5.1 Skin changes

The common skin changes and their causes are listed in **Table 13.9**.

13.5.2 Abnormal blood pressure

Patients with adrenal insufficiency are hypotensive, reflecting their hyponatraemic state and resulting hypovolaemia. They also have a postural drop in blood pressure: the BP decreases suddenly when changing from lying down to standing. This postural drop is associated with transient light-headedness, and is due to the fact that the patient does not have sufficient circulating blood volume.

Severe hypothyroidism also causes hypotension.

Certain endocrine disorders cause elevated blood pressure by increasing the circulating volume or causing peripheral vasoconstriction. Causes of endocrine-induced hypertension are:

- hypercortisolism (e.g. Cushing's disease)
- hyperthyroidism

Table 13.9 *Skin changes associated with endocrine disorders*		
Skin condition	**Features**	**Association**
Granuloma annulare	Papules on the limbs and extremities in shape of ring	Diabetes
Necrobiosis lipoidica diabeticorum	Waxy erythematous eruption, usually on the shins	
Ulceration	May be vascular or neuropathic in aetiology	
Hirsutism	Appearance of dark body hair on the face, torso or limbs	PCOS Androgen excess
Tanned complexion	Darkening of the skin	Adrenal insufficiency
Bruising	Spontaneous, or bruising to trivial injury	Hypercortisolism
Striae	Thick purple stripes, usually on abdomen	
Pretibial myxoedema	Waxy discolouration and thickening of skin in lower limbs	Graves' disease
Coarsening of skin on face	Often associated with loss of the outer third of the eyebrows	Hypothyroidism
Excess sweating	Hyperhidrosis	Acromegaly

- acromegaly
- hyperaldosteronism (e.g. Conn's disease)
- phaeochromocytoma (due to increased levels of catecholamines).

13.5.3 Abnormal heart rates

Hyperthyroidism and phaeochromocytoma increase sympathetic tone of the heart, leading to sinus tachycardia, atrial fibrillation and atrial flutter. Hypothyroidism causes bradycardia.

13.5.4 Blood sugar changes

Cortisol and adrenaline are catabolic hormones. When excreted in excess, they induce hyperglycaemia and insulin resistance; in effect, they cause type 2 diabetes. Exogenous steroids similarly cause type 2 diabetes.

Adrenal insufficiency causes hypoglycaemia, as do rare tumours of the pancreas which secrete insulin (insulinomas). However, hypoglycaemia is most commonly seen in the context of known diabetics, if they:

- intentionally or accidentally take too much insulin
- take their normal insulin but skip a meal.

Hyperglycaemic emergencies

Severe hyperglycaemia leads to dangerous abnormalities in fluid status and internal biochemistry. In type 1 diabetes, the inability to metabolise glucose forces the body to derive energy from the breakdown of fat. Fat metabolism results in ketones, which are highly acidic chemicals. As ketones are produced, the patient develops diabetic ketoacidosis (DKA).

Type 2 diabetics rarely develop DKA, as they still have residual insulin production and insulin sensitivity. Instead, untreated hyperglycaemia leads to a hyperosmolar hyperglycaemic state (HHS). In HHS, the blood becomes viscous and prone to venous thromboembolism. The glucose-saturated kidney is unable to retain water, and the patient develops a dangerous hypovolaemia, losing up to 9 or 10 litres of their circulating volume.

Both DKA and HHS are fatal without treatment. Other endocrine emergencies are explored in **Table 13.10**.

13.5.5 Dehydration

Dehydration is seen in poorly controlled type 1 or type 2 diabetes mellitus, due to polyuria. Affected patients experience polydipsia as a result, but are rarely able to keep up with their renal fluid losses.

Adrenal insufficiency impairs the kidney's ability to retain salt and water, and results in dehydration.

Diabetes insipidus is associated with large renal losses of free water, which often results in dehydration and hypernatraemia, due to concentration of salt in the blood.

Hypercalcaemia decreases renal sensitivity to ADH, inducing transient diabetes insipidus.

13.5.6 Tremor

Tremor is commonly seen in hyperthyroidism and phaeochromocytoma. It is usually a fine action tremor. Different forms of tremor are explored in *Section 9.5.3*.

13.5.7 Tetany

Tetany is due to hyperexcitability of peripheral nerves in hypocalcaemic states. The clinical signs are:

1. **Chvostek's sign**: tapping over the angle of the jaw results in twitching of the ipsilateral facial muscles.
2. **Trousseau's sign**: occlusion of the brachial artery (for example, by inflating a blood pressure cuff) results in spasm of the muscles in the hand and forearm.

These signs are abolished when normal calcium levels are restored.

13.5.8 Muscle weakness

Endocrine myopathy refers to muscle weakness due to hormonal disease. It mainly affects the proximal muscle groups. Endocrine myopathy is caused by:

Table 13.10 *The endocrine emergencies*

Emergency	Cause	Features
Myxoedema coma	Profound hypothyroidism	Hypotension Hypothermia Delirium, leading to psychosis, leading to coma
Thyroid storm	Profound hyperthyroidism	Hypertension Tachycardia Hyper-pyrexia
Acute adrenal insufficiency (aka Addisonian crisis)	Severe and sudden hypocortisolism	Hypotension Hypoglycaemia Hyperkalaemia
DKA	Uncontrolled hyperglycaemia in type 1 diabetics	Dehydration Polyuria Thirst
HHS	Uncontrolled hyperglycaemia in type 2 diabetics	Dehydration Polyuria Thirst Delirium, drowsiness
Hypoglycaemia	Usually excessive insulin administration	Sweating Pallor Confusion Slurred speech Coma Abdominal pain

- hypocalcaemia
- hypercortisolism (including exogenous steroid therapy)
- hyperthyroidism.

13.5.9 Abnormal reflexes

Hyperthyroidism causes hyper-reflexia, manifesting as an exaggerated reflex response to the tendon hammer.

Hypothyroidism causes slow-relaxing reflexes: the reflex is normal but the muscle takes a few seconds to return to its normal resting state.

Both types of reflexes are best seen when performing the ankle jerk reflex test.

13.5.10 Ophthalmoplegia

Weakness of the extra-ocular muscles is seen in Graves' disease. The patient also experiences exophthalmos (**Figure 13.9**). Abnormalities of

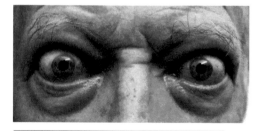

Figure 13.9 Retro-orbital swelling in Graves' disease, causing exophthalmos.

eye movements cause diplopia, which is either persistent, or in certain directions of gaze.

13.5.11 Peripheral vascular disease

Chronic hyperglycaemia is a major contributing factor to peripheral vascular disease. Patients with poorly controlled diabetes mellitus develop neuropathic ulcers and often require amputation of toes, feet or even the whole lower leg. The additional problem of peripheral neuropathy means that diabetic patients are often unaware if they suffer small injuries to their feet. Even trivial injuries can develop into severe infections.

13.6 Thyroid examination

The following sequence follows the order of the examination itself (**Table 13.11**).

13.6.1 'ID CHECK'

This is detailed in *Section 3.2*.
The patient should be sitting in a chair. You will need a glass of water for the patient to sip as part of the examination.

13.6.2 Endobedogram

Have a good look at the patient:
- Are they still, or are they restless or agitated, indicating hyperthyroidism?
- Are they dressed appropriately, or do they seem overtly cold or hot?

Table 13.11 *The sequence of the thyroid examination*

Stage	Question
Inspection	Is there a thyroid mass?
	Is the patient agitated or still?
	Are there any peripheral signs of thyroid disease?
	Is there thyroid eye disease?
Palpation	Is there a mass? Is it mobile?
	What is the heart rate?
	Is there lymphadenopathy?
Auscultation	Is there a thyroid bruit?
Other	Is there a proximal myopathy?
	Are the reflexes abnormal?

- Is there a visible thyroid swelling?
- Are they underweight or overweight?

13.6.3 Inspection

Hands

Examine their hands for signs of hyperthyroidism:
- Sweating
- Palmar erythema
- Fine tremor
- Thyroid acropachy: this is swelling of the fingers and nail clubbing associated with Graves' disease (**Figure 13.10**).

> **A fine tremor of hyperthyroidism may not be noticeable at first.** Try placing a piece of paper on their outstretched hand and see whether it remains still or begins to tremble.

Radial pulse

Note the rate and rhythm of the radial pulse. Is there a bradycardia or a tachycardia, or even an arrhythmia? These are all signs of endocrine disease.

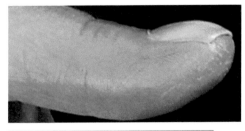

Figure 13.10 Thyroid acropachy leading to convex nails.

Neck

Examine the neck for:

- goitre
- anterior scar of a previous thyroidectomy.

If the patient has a noticeable anterior neck mass, ask them to take a sip of water. The thyroid is attached to the swallowing muscles, and a mass of thyroid origin will move up and down as they swallow. This differentiates it from other causes of neck lumps, such as lymphadenopathy or a swollen salivary gland.

Face

Examine the face for signs of hypothyroidism:

- Coarse, dry skin
- Loss of the outer third of the eyebrows.

Eyes

Move behind the patient and ask them to tilt their head back slightly (**Figure 13.11**). Look for bulging of the eyes (exophthalmos).

Check for ophthalmoplegia by sitting in front of the patient and asking them to follow your finger in each direction of gaze. Ask them whether they experience any diplopia.

Check for lid lag, which is a sign of exophthalmos. Ask the patient to follow your finger as you move it quickly from above to below their face. In lid lag, the downward movement of the upper eyelid will lag behind the downward movement of the eye, revealing the white of their eye above the iris.

13.6.4 Palpation

Stand behind the patient once more.

Thyroid

Palpate the thyroid gently, feeling for any masses. If a mass is felt, ask the patient to take another sip of water to detect whether it moves with swallowing. Estimate the size of the mass, and whether it feels smooth, indicating a single goitre, or bumpy, indicating a multinodular goitre.

Lymph nodes

Enlarged lymph nodes are associated with thyroid cancer. Palpate for lymphadenopathy in the:

- anterior cervical chain
- posterior cervical chain
- supraclavicular fossae
- submental chain.

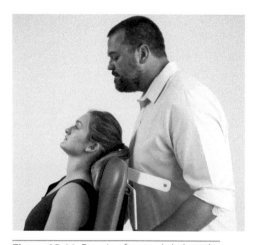

Figure 13.11 Examine for exophthalmos by standing behind the patient and asking them to tilt their head back slightly.

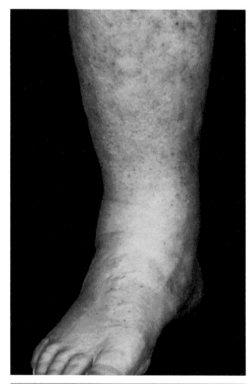

Figure 13.12 Pretibial myxoedema in association with Graves' disease.

13.6.5 Percussion

Detect for retrosternal extension of a thyroid mass by percussing over the superior border of the sternum, starting at the sternal notch. Listen for a dull percussion note, and, if detected, percuss gradually down the sternum to detect its size.

> **Do not percuss over the thyroid gland itself.**
> This is extremely uncomfortable and frightening for patients.

13.6.6 Auscultation

Auscultate the left and right lobe of the thyroid gland with the diaphragm of the stethoscope. Listen for a bruit, indicating turbulent blood flow through a thyroid mass. If you hear a bruit, ensure you have not mistaken a carotid bruit (due to carotid stenosis) for a thyroid bruit. Carotid bruits are only heard over the carotid itself, which is much more lateral to the thyroid gland.

13.6.7 Other tests

Proximal muscle strength
Ask the patient to hold their elbows in abduction and test their shoulder girdle muscular strength.

Next, ask them to cross their arms across their chest and stand up from a sitting position, to assess proximal lower limb strength.

Examine lower leg
Check the anterior shins for pretibial myxoedema, which is a sign of Graves' disease (**Figure 13.12**). Despite the name, pretibial myxoedema is not related to myxoedema coma (due to profound hypothyroidism).

Reflexes
Check the knee or ankle jerk for signs of exaggerated or slow-relaxing reflexes.

13.7 Diabetic examination

The following sequence follows the order of the examination itself (**Table 13.12**).

Table 13.12 *The sequence of the diabetic examination*

Stage	Question
Inspection	Is the patient underweight or overweight?
	Are there any amputations?
	Is there evidence of repeat capillary blood glucose testing?
	Is there peripheral vascular disease?
Palpation	Are the peripheral pulses palpable?
	Is there a peripheral neuropathy?
Fundoscopy	Is there evidence of diabetic retinopathy?
	Are there cataracts?

13.7.1 'ID CHECK'

This is detailed in *Section 3.2*.

13.7.2 Endobedogram

Have a good look at the patient:
- Are they overweight, more in keeping with type 2 diabetes?
- Are they underweight, more in keeping with type 1 diabetes?
- Do they have insulin pens or glucose testing kits nearby?

> **Whilst patients with type 1 diabetes can be underweight or overweight, they are nearly always underweight in the first stages of the disease, around the time of their diagnosis.**
> This reflects their 'starved' state due to their inability to metabolise glucose.

13.7.3 Inspection

Hands
Examine the fingertips for the small pinpricks of repeated capillary blood glucose testing.

Skin
Look for the skin eruptions associated with diabetes (**Table 13.9**).

Ophthalmoscopy
Examine the retina bilaterally for diabetic retinopathy (see *Section 10.6.4*).

Lower limbs
Assess the lower limbs for signs of peripheral vascular disease and peripheral neuropathy, both of which are common complications of poorly controlled diabetes.

Peripheral vascular examination
A peripheral arterial examination is covered in *Section 4.7*.

In addition to venous and arterial ulcers, look for neuropathic ulcers. These ulcers are the result of a small injury which cannot heal. They are often on the sole of the foot, which is more likely to become damaged as it comes in contact with the floor. This means that they go unnoticed by the patient for some time.

Peripheral neurological examination
This examination is covered in *Section 9.6*.

Examine the ankle joint for Charcot's arthropathy. This is a progressive destruction and degeneration of a weight-bearing joint due to microvascular and neuropathic disease. The joint is swollen, irregular and has limited range of movement.

In diabetic peripheral neuropathy, sensory loss is the primary deficit. Motor weakness only occurs in severe disease. Vibration is the first sensory modality to be affected, and precedes fine touch and pain loss by many years.

Fine touch is assessed by the use of a microfilament, which is designed to apply gentle pressure without breaking the skin; never use a sharp object such as a neurotip to assess the diabetic foot, as this may cause breaks in the skin, which often have dire long-term consequences for such patients, such as neuropathic ulcers.

13.8 Common investigations

Investigations include blood tests, imaging and hormone challenge tests.

13.8.1 Blood tests

Early morning cortisol
Cortisol levels show a diurnal pattern, reflecting the body's changing metabolic needs during the day. Cortisol is at its lowest in the early morning, and this time is used as a benchmark to detect hypocortisolism.

HbA1c
Glycosylated haemoglobin (HbA1c) is a measurement of a patient's serum glucose over time. It is useful for monitoring long-term diabetic control. An elevated HbA1c implies that on average, a patient has elevated serum glucose, and therefore needs optimisation of therapy.

Serum osmolality
Osmolality refers to how concentrated a fluid is. In hyperglycaemic states, the increased glucose concentration increases the serum osmolality; this is what drives the symptom of unquenchable thirst.

In diabetes insipidus, the lack of ADH results in the excretion of a large volume of dilute (in other words, hypo-osmolar) urine, leading to an increased serum osmolality. In this instance, comparison of the serum and urine osmolality is essential to making the diagnosis.

13.8.2 MRI brain

Magnetic resonance imaging produces the most anatomically detailed images of brain tissue, such as the pituitary gland. It reveals pituitary growth, and whether an enlarged pituitary gland is pressing upon the optic chiasm.

13.8.3 Hormone challenge tests

There are two hormonal challenge tests used to diagnose endocrine dysfunction:

Dexamethasone suppression test

This is to diagnose Cushing's disease. The patient's serum cortisol is measured before and after the administration of dexamethasone, a corticosteroid that mimics cortisol. In normal populations, dexamethasone has a negative feedback effect on pituitary ACTH, and therefore suppresses endogenous cortisol. In patients with Cushing's disease, the pituitary secretes excessive ACTH and is immune to negative feedback, so the cortisol level remains constant.

ACTH challenge test

This is a test for hypocortisolism. Serum cortisol is measured before and after synthetic ACTH ('synacthen') administration. If cortisol levels fail to double, then the adrenal glands are insensitive to ACTH, diagnosing adrenal insufficiency. If the hypocortisolaemic patient's cortisol levels double or more, then the hypocortisolism is due to pituitary failure to secrete ACTH.

Oral glucose tolerance test

The oral glucose tolerance test (OGTT) is used to diagnose diabetes mellitus and acromegaly. It measures how the patient handles a bolus of glucose, which is drunk in a sugar solution.

Diabetes mellitus

In healthy patients, the OGTT will not cause any noticeable changes in serum glucose. Patients with impaired glucose tolerance – often called 'prediabetes' as it is usually the precursor to diabetes mellitus – have an elevated serum glucose following the test.

Acromegaly

It is not possible to measure serum growth hormone (GH) accurately as it is released in a pulsatile manner throughout the day. A surrogate test is for insulin-like growth factor 1 (IGF-1), which is a hormone stimulated by GH. In healthy patients, the OGTT should suppress IGF-1 levels; failure of IGF-1 levels to fall following the OGTT indicates autonomous GH release from the pituitary.

13.9 Answers to starter questions

1. Acromegaly is a disease caused by excessive growth hormone (GH) release from the pituitary, resulting in enlargement of the hands, feet, jaw, forehead and nose. These changes occur slowly, and often go unappreciated by the patient. Examination of old photographs of the patient helps doctors evaluate whether the face has changed over the years, in keeping with a diagnosis of acromegaly.

1. Insulin is deactivated by stomach enzymes, so cannot be taken orally. Patients with type 1 diabetes give themselves subcutaneous insulin injections, but insulin can also be given intravenously in hospitals. Some diabetics have an insulin pump, which administers a continuous insulin infusion during the day, and larger boluses when they eat meals. This reduces the need for constant injections, and mimics the action of a normal pancreas.

2. Patients with chronic diabetes can become quite disabled. Poor glycaemic control leads to multiple end-organ damage such as diabetic retinopathy (causing vision impairment), peripheral vascular disease (leading to painful ulceration and amputation of the lower extremities) and stroke, which causes further disability.

   For a patient with multiple complications of chronic diabetes, leaving the house to go on a hospital visit requires careful organisation of carers, disabled access transport and walking aids / wheelchairs.

3. Patients with diabetes require the care of a large multidisciplinary team in order to maintain their health. The team includes a diabetes consultant, a diabetes specialist nurse, a podiatrist in order to maintain good foot health, regular eye screening with an ophthalmologist, and a dietitian. The GP is responsible for maintaining links with this vast interprofessional network, and ensuring the patient receives holistic, joined-up care.

4. If the pituitary increases in size, due to adenomatous or malignant growth, it compresses

the nearest adjacent cranial structure, which is the optic chiasm. Compression of the optic chiasm results in a bilateral temporal hemianopia, so that the patient can only see directly in front of them, and not out of the 'corner of their eye'. This visual field defect usually comes to the patient's attention because they start walking into things to their immediate left and right.

Chapter 14
Paediatrics

Starter questions

1. Should all babies with larger-than-normal heads be referred for a paediatric review?
2. Why do doctors care so much about nappy changing?
3. Does a parent always need to give permission for a child's treatment?
4. Should parents worry if their child does not play with others?

Answers to questions are to be found in *Section 14.8*.

14.1 Introduction

Paediatric medicine is a broad specialty, treating children from birth through to adulthood. General paediatrics encompasses all body systems and their development through childhood. A paediatrician cannot always ask their patient what is wrong, and when they can, they do not always get an answer. A paediatrician's greatest tools to diagnosis are through observation, collateral history and detailed examination of the unwell child.

Case 14.1 Failure to thrive

Presentation

Abdi Sadiq is 6 weeks old. His parents bring him to the Emergency Department because he is unwell and not feeding. His mother has noticed that his breathing had become faster.

Initial interpretation

An unwell child is frightening for a parent. A 6-week-old has little physiological reserve and may become unwell over a short period of time. From this information it is impossible to predict the underlying diagnosis and the differential is wide:

- Respiratory problems, such as pneumonia or aspiration
- Cardiac problems, such as heart failure
- Acute renal failure with fluid overload and acidosis
- Metabolic and mitochondrial disorders
- GI disease such as gastroenteritis, constipation or intussusception
- Neurological disease with raised intracranial pressure.

Case 14.1 *continued*

History

Abdi was born at 39 weeks and 5 days and is the first child in his family. His mother was diagnosed with gestational diabetes but this was well controlled with insulin throughout. He grew within the normal limits and was born via a normal vaginal delivery. His neonatal examination was normal and he was discharged from hospital at 2 days old.

He had been feeding well up until the last 2 days. His mother noted that he was opening his eyes less than usual and that his breathing rate was increased. She called an ambulance when she noticed he was making wheezing noises over the last few hours. He has become pale and floppy. She has not noted any vomiting, diarrhoea or fevers.

Interpretation of history

A floppy baby is always a concern and should be seen as quickly as possible. Wheeze is a high-pitched sound caused by obstruction of the bronchioles, the main causes being bronchospasm or pulmonary oedema. As such, respiratory or cardiac disease is likely.

It should be noted that normal growth and anomaly scans during pregnancy do not always mean that a child will have no problems at birth.

Gestational diabetes is usually associated with growth defects such as a large (macrosomic) or small (microsomic) baby. It has also been associated with incomplete lung maturation with reduced surfactant production, leading to respiratory distress syndrome. Surfactant has its greatest role in providing surface tension to keep alveoli open after a baby's first breath, so this would present much earlier than 6 weeks.

Whatever the problem, the diagnosis is not clear and the management for these differentials varies considerably. The child must be examined to correlate the clinical signs.

Examination

Abdi is clearly in respiratory distress; his respiratory rate is 55, oxygen saturations are 73% on room air, and his heart rate is 190 beats per minute. He is lethargic and noted to have sternal and intercostal recession. His eyes are slightly yellow. On auscultation of his chest there is wheeze and he is noted to have a loud pansystolic murmur throughout. His liver is enlarged and can be felt at 3cm below the costal margin.

Interpretation of findings

Abdi is in biventricular cardiac failure. He has evidence of left-sided heart failure with pulmonary oedema – he is in respiratory distress and has wheeze throughout his chest. Right-sided failure is supported by him having hepatomegaly. He has a loud pansystolic murmur, making a congenital cardiac defect highly likely.

Causes of acyanotic heart defects include:
- ventricular septal defects
- patent ductus arteriosus
- pulmonary stenosis
- atrial septal defects
- coarctation of the aorta
- aortic stenosis.

Of these, ventricular septal defects are most common and fit best with Abdi's clinical picture (**Table 14.1**). However, the management of these conditions varies greatly and the diagnosis must be confirmed on direct echocardiographic imaging of the suspected defect.

Investigations

Abdi is given high flow oxygen. A chest radiograph confirms pulmonary oedema and he is treated with intravenous diuretics. He responds well and his oxygen saturations rise as his respiratory rate declines. When stable, an echocardiogram is performed and confirms a large ventricular septal defect.

Diagnosis

Abdi Sadiq has a ventricular septal defect (VSD). These account for 32% of congenital heart defects. Without correction, these lead to a left-to-right shunt causing damage to the pulmonary blood flow, leading to irreversible vascular

Case 14.1 *continued*

Table 14.1 *Acyanotic congenital cardiac defects*

Name	Cardiac failure	Murmur
Ventricular septal defect	Yes	Pansystolic
Patent ductus arteriosus	Very late	Continuous 'machinery' murmur
Pulmonary stenosis	Rare	Ejection systolic radiating to the back
Atrial septal defect	Yes	Ejection systolic and 'rumbling' mid-diastolic
Coarctation of the aorta	Yes	Ejection systolic murmur best heard between scapulae
Aortic stenosis	Yes	Ejection systolic radiating to the neck

damage and pulmonary hypertension. Some VSDs close spontaneously but surgical correction is required if there are severe symptoms causing failure to thrive or evidence of pulmonary hypertension. Abdi needs ongoing diuretic therapy and referral to a paediatric cardiothoracic surgeon.

14.2 Overview

Paediatric medicine is a broad specialty encompassing the care of children from birth through to adulthood. Most body systems are immature at birth. To reach adulthood, a child must physically grow, their physiology mature and their intellect develop. The success of this process is intimately reliant on environmental and genetic factors.

Paediatric medicine is a generalised term encompassing the entirety of childhood medicine. As with adult medicine, care can be specialised according to body system or disease type (e.g. paediatric cardiology, gastroenterology or oncology) or by age (e.g. neonatology or adolescent medicine). To cover history-taking and examination skills for all subspecialties is beyond the scope of this chapter. The aim is to introduce the main themes of paediatric disease and a sound approach towards examining a child.

14.2.1 Terminology

Children are grouped by their age:
- Neonate: birth to 30 days
- Infant: 1 month to 2 years
- Young child: 2–6 years
- Child: 6–12 years
- Adolescent: 12–18 years.

This terminology helps to link children to particular expected stages of development. A child within a certain age group may have a higher chance of developing a particular problem than a child of a different group.

14.2.2 Challenges

Communication

Arguably, the biggest challenge in paediatric medicine is communication. To be able to appreciate and understand a symptom and explain it to a doctor requires a high level of intelligence which comes with age. Either through age or learning disability, many children are unable to give a history. As such, collateral history from a parent or carer (and sometimes multiple people) is vital in investigating and diagnosing childhood illness.

Most children are naturally nervous or even

frightened of new people. It takes a level of trust for a child to answer probing questions or to allow somebody to touch and examine them.

Consent

To be able to give valid consent to any part of medical treatment (in the UK), one must be able to understand information about the treatment or investigation, retain that information, weigh it up to reach a decision and then communicate it. These steps are difficult and most children are unable to complete them. As such, consent for examination and investigation must be taken from a legal guardian, usually the parents.

Parents / caregivers

Often, all the information and consent relies on the parents or caregivers of the child. This responsibility should not be underestimated:

- A parent cannot know every single experience a child has or what they are truly feeling.
- Being parent to an unwell child is frightening and stressful. Often a parent needs more reassurance and soothing than the child!

Some symptoms and problems may be embarrassing to a child, especially adolescents, and they may withhold or deny certain information whilst their parents are present. This is particularly challenging with regard to sexual activity and intimate health.

Vulnerability

Children are vulnerable people. Any health professional working with children must always be alert and trained to recognise signs of, and raise concerns about, potential abuse.

14.2.3 Top tips

Paediatrics is an art that takes practice:

- Take your time.
- Be prepared to improvise.
- Listen to the parents or caregivers – they are experts in their children. They help soothe their child and often notice signs before you do.
- Watch the child. Notice how they play, behave and move. They often show you a problem despite not being able to tell you.
- Seeing a doctor and being examined, especially when unwell, can be a frightening experience for children. A kind and non-intimidating demeanour is vital. Toys and a promise of stickers help to allay many fears.
- Remember that an unwell child is usually accompanied by a frightened parent or caregiver. They will need support too.

14.3 Paediatric presentations

As with adults, children present with diseases in any organ system – too many to explore in this chapter. Some of the commonest symptoms are stridor, difficulty breathing, rash, abdominal pain and joint pain. The underlying cause is benign in the majority of cases but each has a potentially life-threatening differential that must first be confidently excluded.

14.3.1 Stridor

Stridor is a harsh inspiratory wheeze indicating obstructed airflow through the upper airways (**Figure 14.1**).

Inhaled foreign body

Children often put small objects in their mouths and accidentally inhale them. This is most common between the ages of 6 months and 4 years. The inhalation event is often unwitnessed. These objects may require bronchoscopic removal.

Respiratory

Croup

Croup is a viral infection, usually parainfluenza or influenza, that causes tracheal swelling and is associated with a hoarse voice and 'barking' cough. It is usually self-limiting after one or two days but may require treatment with oral steroids if it continues beyond this.

Tracheitis

Tracheitis is a bacterial infection, usually *Staphylococcus aureus*, causing tracheal

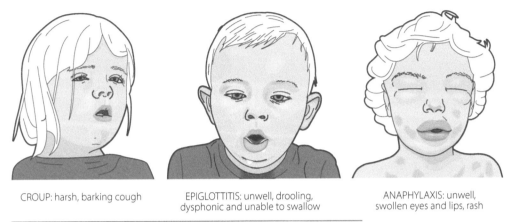

| CROUP: harsh, barking cough | EPIGLOTTITIS: unwell, drooling, dysphonic and unable to swallow | ANAPHYLAXIS: unwell, swollen eyes and lips, rash |

Figure 14.1 Typical appearance of children with different causes of stridor.

inflammation. It is often a complication of more benign viral infections. It requires rapid treatment with antibiotics.

Epiglottitis

Epiglottitis is inflammation and swelling of the epiglottis from infection, usually *Haemophilus influenzae*. It is a medical emergency as it rapidly progresses to total airway obstruction. Treatment is with intravenous antibiotics and ensuring early airway protection (i.e. endotracheal intubation).

For epiglottitis, think of the 'Ds':
- **D**rooling saliva
- **D**ysphonia (abnormal voice sound)
- **D**ysphagia (difficulty swallowing)
- **D**O NOT EXAMINE THE PHARYNX – this risks laryngospasm. Only an experienced anaesthetist who is capable of rapid intubation should examine.

Anaphylaxis

Anaphylaxis is a systemic allergic reaction that causes widespread histamine release. Stridor is caused by upper airway oedema. Treatment is with rapid adrenaline administration, antihistamines and inhaled bronchodilators. As with epiglottitis, one should have a low threshold for early endotracheal intubation to protect the airway. If the precipitant is inside the body (e.g. an

ingested nut or insect sting), it will need physical removal.

14.3.2 Breathlessness

Breathlessness is frightening for both children and their parents. As with adults there are multiple causes, ranging in severity from relatively benign to life-threatening.

Respiratory

Bronchiolitis

This is self-limiting bronchiolar inflammation causing breathlessness and wheeze. It is usually caused by respiratory syncytial virus and is much more common in winter.

Pneumonia

Pneumonia is a bacterial lower respiratory tract infection identified by consolidative changes on chest radiography. It can lead to sepsis and respiratory failure if not treated with antibiotics.

Asthma

Asthma is a chronic reversible airway inflammation from bronchospasm, usually in response to an irritant such as dust, cold weather, pet fur or pollen. It is more common in children with atopic conditions such as hayfever or eczema. Treatment is with inhaled or nebulised bronchodilators and corticosteroids. Severe exacerbations of asthma are life-threatening and sometimes require invasive ventilation.

Metabolic

Acidosis

Acidaemia stimulates centrally-mediated hyperventilation in an effort to exhale carbon dioxide, thus raising serum pH. Causes include:

- metabolic acidosis in severe infection and sepsis
- diabetic ketoacidosis.

> "Kussmaul's respiration" describes the increased deep, rapid and gasping breathing pattern specific to diabetic ketoacidosis.

Cardiovascular

Centrally driven breathlessness is stimulated by the circulation of poorly oxygenated blood due to:

- pulmonary oedema in cardiac failure
- arteriovenous shunting in congenital malformations.

14.3.3 Rash

A rash is usually differentiated by its appearance, distribution over the body and associated symptoms (**Table 14.2**).

Allergy

Allergic rashes are typically urticarial. They develop soon after exposure to an allergen (e.g. pollen, insect venom, ingested food). Always ensure there is no sign of anaphylaxis developing.

Vasculitis

Vasculitic rashes are purpuric and typically cover the limbs and back. They are associated with underlying cutaneous capillary immunological inflammation.

Infection

Viral

Viral exanthematous rashes are the most common rashes in children. Associated viral infections include:

- measles
- mumps
- rubella
- parvovirus B19
- human herpesviruses 6 and 7.

Chickenpox is a very common childhood illness. Whilst unpleasant and itchy, there are usually no long-lasting effects to the child. The chickenpox rash has four phases (**Figure 14.2):**

- Macule
- Papule
- Fluid-filled vesicle
- Burst vesicle with crusting.

Meningitis

Bacterial meningitis is a life-threatening infection. The child will be systemically unwell or septic and may be confused or drowsy. Classic physical signs and symptoms include photophobia, neck stiffness and a petechial rash. The rash develops

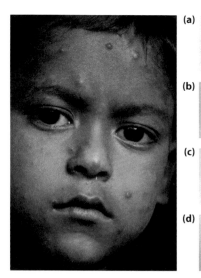

Figure 14.2 Stages of chickenpox rash: (a) macular rash; (b) papular rash; (c) vesicle formation; (d) vesicle rupture and crusting.

Table 14.2 Paediatric rashes	
Type	**Appearance**
Urticaria	Raised, itchy red bumps in patches
Vasculitis	Palpable and purpuric
Exanthematous	Widespread red spots over body
Petechial	Non-blanching red–pink colouration developing to gangrene

in the extremities and rapidly progresses, leading to digital and limb ischaemia. The glass test, where pressure is placed over the rash through a transparent object such as a glass, helps to distinguish a petechial from a non-petechial rash. A non-petechial rash will disappear (blanch) with pressure whereas a petechial rash will not (non-blanching).

14.3.4 Abdominal pain

Abdominal pain is a common complaint in children. The examples below describe the classical ways in which different causes of abdominal pain present. However, be mindful that these are not the *only* way these pathologies present.

Gastrointestinal
Appendicitis
Appendicitis typically causes a constant severe ache that starts at the umbilicus and migrates towards the right iliac fossa.

Gastroenteritis
Abdominal pain is more generalised (i.e. across most or all of the abdomen) with gastroenteritis and is associated with diarrhoea and/or vomiting. This occurs with or without a fever.

Constipation
Constipation causes a central, colicky (intermittent and griping) pain associated with passing hard stool or being unable to pass any stool. Constipation in children is often associated with vomiting.

Urological
Lower urinary tract infection
Lower urinary tract infections cause a constant lower abdominal pain that is associated with dysuria or haematuria.

Pyelonephritis
Pyelonephritis causes a dull ache in the flank. Children with pyelonephritis are often unwell and have fevers or even sepsis.

Renal calculi
Stones within the renal tract cause a sharp pain that radiates from "loin to groin". It is associated with fevers and vomiting and often haematuria.

Mesenteric adenitis
Compared to that of an adult, a child's immune system is immature and often over-reacts to infection. Sometimes, an infection in a different part of the body causes the abdominal lymph nodes to enlarge. The swelling is painful and causes a non-specific abdominal pain that does not quite fit with any of the above descriptions. This process is called mesenteric adenitis. It is a diagnosis of exclusion as there are more serious causes to confidently rule out; it is typically mistaken for appendicitis. It is a temporary condition and resolves once the infection elsewhere is cleared.

Neurological
The abdominal organs and viscera have a large and complex network of nerves. Much like in the brain, some people develop abdominal migraines.

14.3.5 Joint pain / limping

It is common for children to report pain in their joints and limbs, particularly around times of growth. However, the cause of the pain is often attributed to 'growing pains' whereas there may be a more serious underlying condition.

Transient synovitis
Transient synovitis is a self-limiting irritation of the synovial membrane. The cause is unknown but it is most commonly seen following a viral illness. It typically affects large joints such as the hips ('irritable hip') or knees.

Musculoskeletal
Developmental abnormality
Congenital joint abnormalities are often not apparent until a child is crawling or walking. Congenital hip dysplasia is caused by underdeveloped and shallow acetabulum, leading to recurrent hip dislocations.

Osteomyelitis
Osteomyelitis is an infection within the bones, usually through haematological spread of infection from elsewhere in the body. It is an emergency and requires urgent antibiotic treatment. These intravenous antibiotics usually continue for prolonged periods (i.e. six weeks or more).

Septic arthritis

Septic arthritis is an infection within a joint and is a surgical emergency. It requires urgent surgical washout and antibiotic treatment.

Perthes' disease

Perthes' disease describes an idiopathic avascular necrosis of the femoral heads. It usually occurs bilaterally. Typically, it affects boys around the age of 8 years.

Haematological

Leukaemia

Leukaemia is an uncontrolled overproduction of white blood cells within the bone marrow. It leads to reduced immunity and causes bony pain through the pressure effect of overfilled bone marrow. Erosion of bony tissue occurs from tumour growth. This damages the highly innervated periosteum, causing severe pain.

Haemoglobinopathy

Deformed red blood cells from haemoglobinopathies get stuck within capillaries, causing blockages. The occlusions cause infarction within bone tissue (and many other tissues) causing pain. If severe and ongoing, this leads to death of bone cells (avascular necrosis).

Trauma

Children's bones are particularly fragile and prone to bony injuries, especially whilst the bones are still growing. Children tend to fall over more than adults and are often fearless to risk, which contributes to more bony injuries!

Non-accidental injury

Non-accidental injury describes injuries arising from physical abuse. One must correlate the injury with the described mechanism. Be alert to warning signs such as bruises from finger marks (especially in a place the child cannot reach themselves), withdrawn or fearful behaviour, or a caregiver who avoids questioning. Spiral fractures of long bones usually occur via a 'yanking' mechanism where the limb is suddenly pulled.

> When suspecting non-accidental injuries, always ask for help when examining the child and ensure the child is safe at all times.
> Look in the nose, ears and mouth and around the eyes for evidence of bleeding. This might suggest the child has been shaken.

14.4 The paediatric history

14.4.1 Past medical history

A paediatric past medical history may be minimal or vast. It is important to note any major diagnoses or whether the child is under investigation for another problem unrelated to the current presentation. Often, a cluster of seemingly unrelated symptoms occur which later transpire to relate to one unifying problem.

Pregnancy

Ask the following:
- Were there any complications during the pregnancy?
- Did the child develop normally during gestation?
- Did the mother have any medical problems or take any medications during the pregnancy (and whilst breastfeeding)? If so, what?

Birth

- How was the child born (normal vaginal, instrumental, caesarean section)?
- Were any problems encountered during the delivery?
- Was the child born prematurely?
- What was the child's weight at birth?

Neonatal

- Were there any problems following birth?
- Did the child need to be admitted to the Special Care Baby Unit (SCBU) or Neonatal Intensive Care Unit (NICU)? If so, what for?

14.4.2 Medications

A clear medication history is important. Ask about recent courses of antibiotics, OTC medications and herbal remedies.

Medication doses vary depending on the age or weight of the child, so be very clear about the dosage of any medications taken. A child's skin is much more porous than that of an adult so ask about the amount (usually in 'fingertips') of medicated creams or lotions being used; similarly, establishing the amount of puffs taken of an inhaler is important.

If a medication-related illness is suspected, ask the parents if there are any other medications in the house and if the child could or would be able to find them.

Ask about any allergies or sensitivities the child may have (including asthma, hay fever or eczema).

14.4.3 Immunisations

Ask whether the child is up to date with their vaccinations (**Table 14.3**) and if there was a reaction to any of them. For infants, these are recorded in their Red Book.

14.4.4 Social history

A detailed social history is vitally important in the paediatric history. Problems at home or school, especially in early childhood, significantly impact a child's development. The following headings detail the key questions to cover. If a potential problem is identified it should be enquired into further. Be mindful that this can be sensitive or embarrassing for parents / caregivers, so ask sensitively and avoid accusations.

Home

- What type of accommodation does the child live in?
- Who cares for the child and what is their occupation?
- Who else lives with the child?
- Is anyone else in the house unwell or do they require any special support?
- Does anyone smoke in or around the house?
- Are there any pets at home?

Table 14.3 *Overview of UK national vaccination programme (from autumn 2019)*

Age	Vaccination
8 weeks	6-in-1 (diphtheria, hepatitis B, *Haemophilus influenzae* type b [Hib], polio, tetanus, pertussis)
	Pneumococcal (PCV)
	Meningococcal type B (MenB)
	Rotavirus
12 weeks	6-in-1 (second dose)
	Rotavirus (second dose)
16 weeks	6-in-1 (third dose)
	Pneumococcal (second dose)
	MenB (second dose)
One year	Hib, Meningococcal type C (MenC)
	Pneumococcal (third dose)
	Measles, mumps and rubella (MMR)
	MenB (third dose)
2–10 years	Influenza (annual)
3 years and 4 months	4-in-1 preschool booster (diphtheria, polio, tetanus, pertussis)
	MMR (second dose)
12–13 years	Human papillomavirus (HPV)
14 years	3-in-1 teenage booster (diphtheria, polio, tetanus)
	Meningococcal types A, C, W and Y (MenACWY)

School

- What is the child's stage in education?
- Are there any learning issues at school?
- Are there any social issues at school (including behaviour, bullying and absconding)?

Other

- Does the child have an assigned social worker?
- Has the child been abroad recently?

14.4.5 Family history

Establish if there is any family history of disease or any genetic conditions known about previously. Sometimes, an inherited condition has not yet been diagnosed so ask if any older generations had similar symptoms.

Drawing a family tree is beneficial in considering particular patterns of inheritance of potential genetic conditions. It is also a sensitive way to elicit any consanguinity.

> Consanguinity relates to parents being close blood relatives (such as siblings, cousins or aunts / uncles and nieces / nephews). The practice is more common in some cultures than others and should be approached sensitively. Consanguinity increases the risk of inherited genetic and metabolic conditions being passed on to children from that union.

14.4.6 Systems review

As with any history, a full systems review elicits symptoms otherwise missed during the consultation and allows screening for otherwise unnoticed symptoms (**Table 14.4**).

Table 14.4 *Key topics for paediatric systems review*

Feeding	Volume
	Frequency
Vomiting	Timing
	Projectile?
	Bloody / bilious?
Fever	Established by touch or thermometer?
Wet nappies	Amount per day
Stools	Consistency
	Colour
	'Redcurrant jelly'?
Rash	Triggers
	Distribution
	Blanching?
Behaviour	Irritability
	Responsiveness
Cough	Productive?
	Breathing difficulty?
Weight	Change?
Sleeping pattern	Change?
Unwell contacts	Home
	School
Localising symptoms	Ear tugging?
	Holding abdomen?
	Not using particular limb?

14.5 Neonatal examination

All newborns should receive a top-to-toe physical examination within the first 72 hours of life. This examination is standardised across the UK as part of the Newborn and Infant Physical Examination (NIPE) screening programme for early detection and diagnosis of newborn abnormalities.

14.5.1 'ID CHECK'

- Identify: introduce yourself and check the identity of the neonate and parents
- Consent gained: ask for permission to examine the infant

- Hand washing
- Exposure: the neonate should be in their nappy; always examine in a private room to allow open discussion with the parents
- Comfort maintained: ensure the infant and parents are comfortable; explain that no part of the examination will hurt their child
- Kindly proceed.

14.5.2 Endobedogram

Have a good look at the neonate:
- Does the baby look well?
- Is their skin colour normal, pale, cyanosed or jaundiced?
- Is their cry loud or weak?
- Is their posture normal?
- Are they moving all four limbs normally?

> Trauma to the brachial plexus, especially C5 and C6, occurs from shoulder dystocia during difficult childbirth. This causes a characteristic 'waiter's tip' posture where the arm hangs medially rotated and close to the body with the forearm extended and pronated (**Figure 14.3**).

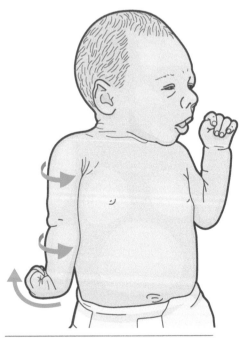

Figure 14.3 Brachial plexus trauma causing 'waiter's tip' posture.

14.5.3 Questions

Ask the parents:
- How was the pregnancy and birth? Were there any complications for mother and/or baby?
- Is there a family history of hearing, cardiac or hip problems?
- Has the infant been feeding and sleeping?
- Is the neonate passing urine and opening their bowels?

> The first bowel movement a neonate passes is of a thick, dark, tarry substance called meconium. This is entirely normal.

14.5.4 Head

Size
Measure the size of the head. Macrocephaly (a larger-than-normal head) can be normal or related to conditions such as cranial hyperostosis, megalencephaly or hydrocephalus. Microcephaly (a smaller-than-normal head) occurs as a result of brain underdevelopment.

Shape
Note the shape of the head and proximity of the cranial sutures (**Figure 14.4**). Head moulding (the periodic abnormal shaping of the head such as a flat side if the neonate sleeps on that side) is entirely normal after birth, as the cranial sutures have not yet fused. Haematomata and fluid collections occur during delivery, especially following instrumental deliveries. These usually resolve spontaneously.

Fontanelle
Gently palpate the anterior fontanelle; it should feel flat (**Figure 14.4**). A raised fontanelle indicates raised intracranial pressure whilst a sunken fontanelle indicates dehydration.

14.5.5 Skin

Inspect the skin for evidence of bruising or lacerations which may have occurred during labour, and for other abnormalities (**Table 14.5**).

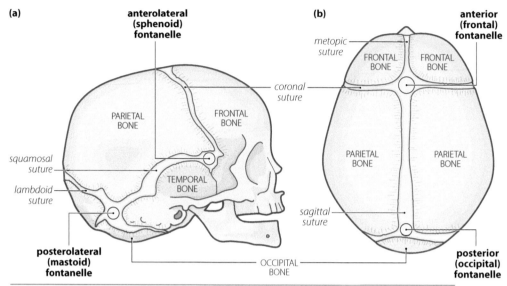

Figure 14.4 Neonatal cranial sutures and fontanelles viewed (a) from the side; (b) from the top.

Table 14.5 Common neonatal dermatological findings

Common name	Description	Pathology
Port wine stain	Purple / red mark on face	Capillary malformations
Stork bite	Purple / red mark on back of neck	
Angel's kiss / salmon patch	Pink / red patch on inner upper eyelid	
Vernix	Waxy / cheese-like substance	Intrauterine protective skin coating
Mongolian spot	Blue / black mark on lower back, buttocks or shoulders	Benign melanocytosis
Milia	White spots, usually on the face	Blocked pores
Toxic erythema of the newborn	Blotchy red spots over white / yellow papules	Benign immune system activation
Neonatal jaundice	Yellow skin and sclera	Multiple

14.5.6 Face

Inspect for dysmorphic features / syndromic appearance (**Figure 14.5**). Note any asymmetry of the facial muscles / expression, which is associated with facial nerve palsies. Check each nostril's patency. Small nostrils reduce a neonate's ability to inhale through their nose, affecting their ability to suckle.

14.5.7 Eyes

Inspect the eyes for signs of infection such as injection or discharge. Check the sclera for icterus, indicating possible liver disease. Note pupil size and shape and whether there is a difference between the two. Pupillary differences may be normal. Test for the red reflex (see Section 10.6.4). Its absence could indicate the presence of cataracts or a neuroblastoma.

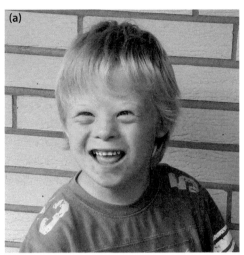

DOWN SYNDROME
round face, flattened nose, short stature, downward slanted eyes, prominent epicanthic folds

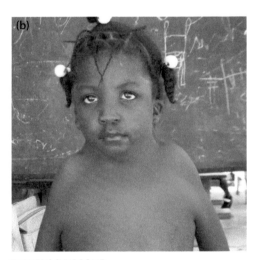

TURNER'S SYNDROME
a short, webbed neck, low-set ears and wide-set nipples are among the physical features

Figure 14.5 Stereotypical appearances of common genetic disorders: (a) Down syndrome; (b) Turner's syndrome.

14.5.8 Ears

Inspect the shape of the ears and for the presence of any skin tags. Small ears are seen in some congenital syndromes and deformed ears have an impact on a child's hearing.

14.5.9 Mouth and palate

Look inside the mouth for the presence of a cleft in the hard or soft palate. This is usually easier whilst the infant is crying. Inspect the tongue and gums for ankyloglossia. A shortened lingual frenulum reduces tongue movement and affects speech. This is more commonly known as 'tongue-tied'.

14.5.10 Neck

Note any shortening or webbing of the neck, which is associated with Turner's syndrome. Palpate for any neck swellings and along the clavicles for fractures that may occur during childbirth.

14.5.11 Upper limbs

Inspect the size and length of the arms and the number and shape of the fingers.
- Inspect the number and shape of the fingers.
- Note the number of palmar creases (two creases are normal; one crease is associated with Down syndrome).
- Palpate the brachial pulses.

14.5.12 Chest

Inspection
- Note any chest wall deformities.
- Observe chest expansion.
- Note any intercostal recession, indicating respiratory distress.

Lungs
- Auscultate both lungs for air entry and any added sounds.

Heart
- Auscultate for cardiac murmurs (see **Table 4.2** in *Chapter 4: Cardiology*).

14.5.13 Abdomen

- Note any abdominal distension and umbilical or inguinal herniae.
- Palpate for enlarged liver, spleen, kidneys and bladder. A normal liver is felt up to 2cm below the costal margin.

14.5.14 Genitalia

Are the genitalia obviously sexed or ambiguous? This indicates congenital adrenal hyperplasia.

Males

Locate the urethral opening. Hypospadias describes a condition where it is not at the tip of the penis. Palpate the presence of the testes or any abnormal lumps within the scrotum. An absent testis may be undescended. Transilluminate any lumps to diagnose a hydrocele.

Females

Exclude labial fusion (complete closure of the labia, obstructing the vaginal orifice) then inspect the clitoris and note its size. Check for any vaginal discharge.

14.5.15 Lower limbs

Inspect the size and length of the legs. Assess for any oedema or ankle deformity, indicating low albumin levels or cardiac dysfunction (particularly associated with congenital cardiac abnormalities). Inspect the number and shape of the toes then palpate the femoral pulses. Absent pulses suggests problems with arterial blood supply.

14.5.16 Hips

Barlow's test

Hold the hip joint with one hand (**Figure 14.6a**). With the other, slowly adduct the hip whilst placing gentle pressure through the knee to push posteriorly. If the hip is unstable you should feel the femoral head move outside the joint as it subluxes and dislocates (a positive Barlow's test). If this is felt, confirm it with Ortolani's test.

Ortolani's test

Only perform this test (**Figure 14.6b**) if Barlow's test is positive. Lay the baby on their back, hold the hips and knees flexed at 90°. Use your index finger to put pressure on the top of the thighs and slowly abduct the hips. If the hip is already dislocated, you will feel a 'clunk' as the femoral head relocates into the acetabulum.

14.5.17 Back and spine

Inspect the back for abnormal spinal curvature. Scoliosis describes medial curvature (side to side) and kyphosis describes anterior–posterior curvature (front to back). Hair tufts and pits over the sacrum are associated with spina bifida.

(a)

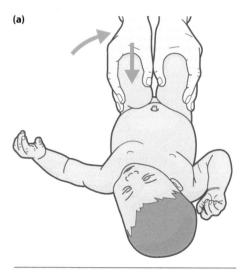

(b)

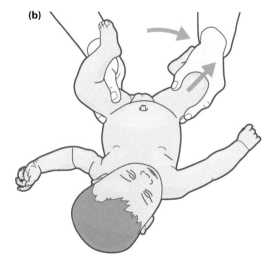

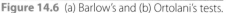

Figure 14.6 (a) Barlow's and (b) Ortolani's tests.

14.5.18 Anus

Check the patency of the anus. Meconium should be passed within the first 24 hours.

14.5.19 Reflexes

There are several reflexes that are normal within neonates that then disappear as they mature. These are residual evolutionary reflexes from primates.

Palmar grasp reflex

Stroking the infant's palm should stimulate their fingers to grip. This primitive reflex persists to around 6 months.

Sucking reflex

Inserting a clean finger to the roof of the infant's mouth should stimulate sucking. This is a good time to feel along the palate for palatal clefts.

Stepping reflex

Holding the infant up and allowing the soles of their feet to touch a firm surface should stimulate a walking movement. This reflex disappears at around 6 weeks when the legs become too heavy for the muscles. It reappears around 8–12 months once the muscles have developed.

> **The Moro reflex** describes a stereotypical neck and leg extension alongside arm jerking with upturned palms, extended thumbs and flexed fingers that occurs with a sudden noise, temperature change or rapidly dipping the infant's head. It disappears at around 2 months. It is somewhat distressing to parents to watch without prior explanation and the test is not routinely performed as part of the neonatal examination.

14.5.20 Finishing off

Thank the parents, allow them to dress their child and explain your findings. A normal neonatal examination does not generate any routine investigations. If an abnormality is found, the child should be reviewed by the appropriate specialist before confirming the diagnosis and discussing potential investigations and treatment.

14.6 Examining a child

14.6.1 'ID CHECK'

- Identify: introduce yourself and check the identity of the child and parents
- Consent gained: ask for permission to examine the child
- Hand washing
- Exposure: ask the child or their parents to uncover the relevant body area that is to be examined
- Comfort maintained: ensure both the child and parents are comfortable
  - ☐ infants are best examined lying on a couch
  - ☐ toddlers can sit on a parent's lap
  - ☐ small children can be either sitting or standing
  - ☐ for teenagers, it is important to offer a chaperone
- Kindly proceed.

14.6.2 Endobedogram

Have a good look at the child:
- Do they look well?
- Is their skin colour normal, pale, cyanosed or jaundiced?
- Are they in any discomfort?
- Is their posture normal?
- Are they localising to any part of their body, such as tugging at an ear or holding their abdomen?

14.6.3 Examination sequence

As explored above, diagnosing paediatric illness can be challenging through the difficulty in taking a history of symptoms or through the symptoms being presented relating to an illness from a different body system (such as abdominal pain from mesenteric adenitis associated with viral infections). A sensible sequential examination

Table 14.6 *Normal range for routine observations in infants and children*

Age	Heart rate (bpm)	Systolic blood pressure (mmHg)	Respiratory rate (per minute)
<1 year	110–160	70–90	30–40
1–2 years	100–150	80–95	25–35
2–5 years	95–140	80–100	25–30
5–12 years	80–120	80–110	20–25
>12 years	60–100	100–120	15–20

approach is required to ensure that the child is as comfortable as possible throughout.

Remember that as the child develops, their physiology goes through great changes; hence the normal ranges for observations change depending on the age (**Table 14.6**).

Being examined by a stranger can be confusing and frightening for a child and in turn stressful for the parents. Easy ways to reassure them are:
- ■ sitting or squatting next to the child so as to not tower over them
- ■ talking to them using words they understand (e.g. 'tummy' instead of 'abdomen')
- ■ showing them procedures such as auscultation on someone else (yourself, a parent or a teddy) before performing it on them
- ■ leaving more distressing examinations (such as otoscopy) to the end.

14.6.4 Respiratory examination

The paediatric respiratory examination follows the same sequence as for adults (see *Section 5.6*). Key elements relating to children are:

Peripheral
The peripheral respiratory examination is the same as for adults. Cyanosis is best seen under the tongue. Finger clubbing in childhood respiratory disease is most commonly associated with cystic fibrosis.

Inspection
Look for evidence of breathing difficulty (**Table 14.7**) and note any chest wall deformities.

Palpation
Normal chest expansion for a child aged 5–12 years is 3–5cm.

Percussion
Always perform lightly. Percussion is rarely useful when examining neonates, as their bodies are so small that the organs are too close together.

Auscultation
Use a paediatric stethoscope, which is much smaller than an adult stethoscope. This will allow a more detailed examination.

14.6.5 Cardiovascular examination

The paediatric cardiovascular examination also follows the same sequence as for adults (see *Section 4.6*). Key elements relating to children are:

Peripheral
Cyanosis is associated with congenital cardiac defects. Finger clubbing in childhood cardiac

Table 14.7 *Signs of paediatric respiratory distress*

Nasal flaring

Grunting

Accessory muscle use

Intercostal muscle retraction

Difficulty speaking

Poor feeding (infants)

disease is associated with congenital cardiac defects. A dysmorphic appearance suggesting a genetic disorder such as Down or Turner's syndromes is important to the cardiovascular examination as these syndromes are associated with congenital cardiac defects. Look out particularly for radio-radial and radio-femoral delays when palpating the pulses, as these are associated with aortic coarctation. Check blood pressure at the end of the consultation as this is often uncomfortable and distressing for younger children.

Inspection
A bulging over the praecordium is a sign of cardiomegaly.

Palpation
This is the same as for the adult cardiovascular examination. Note that a right ventricular tap may be felt in healthy, thin children and is not likely to be pathological.

Auscultation
As for the respiratory examination, use a paediatric stethoscope. Auscultate the praecordium as per the adult cardiovascular examination. Always listen at the back, between the shoulder blades for the continuous machinery murmur of aortic coarctation.

14.6.6 Abdominal examination

Reliable examination requires the muscles of the abdominal wall to be relaxed. If the child is crying, this may require waiting until they are more settled before proceeding.

Peripheral
Look for jaundice and pallor.

Inspection
Young children's abdomens often protrude. If you are concerned about distension, ask the parents if their child's abdomen has changed size. Localised abdominal distension is always abnormal. Upper abdominal distension could be caused by hepatomegaly, splenomegaly or pyloric stenosis. Lower abdominal distension could be caused by an obstructed bladder. Visible peristalsis is associated with pyloric stenosis and intestinal obstruction.

Palpation
Always watch the child's face for signs of discomfort when palpating the abdomen, especially if they cannot yet talk. In infants and children up to the age of 5, a normal liver is palpated up to 2cm below the costal angle and palpating the tip of the spleen is also possible.

Percussion and auscultation
Percussion for organomegaly and ascites and auscultation for bowel sounds and renal bruits is performed in the same manner as when examining adults.

Finishing off
Be sure to palpate the inguinal areas for herniae, asking the child to cough if necessary. In boys, ask about the presence of testicular lumps or any undescended testes. This may require a testicular examination with parental consent and the accompaniment of a chaperone.

14.6.7 Neurological examination

A full neurological examination is not necessary in every child. Ask the parents if they have noted any changes or abnormalities in the child's movement. Ask about any behavioural concerns of changes. Watch the child moving and playing and note if this is normal.

If concerned about a neurological problem, follow the pattern of examination as for an adult. Always be alert to meningitis in an unwell child. Kernig's sign and Brudzinski's neck sign are particularly sensitive for meningism (**Figure 14.7**).

Tone
Tone steadily increases through infancy as the child gains muscle strength and control of their limbs. A 'floppy' tone is normal in a neonate.

Power
For children who cannot follow commands, it is easier to observe movement closely and note whether it is symmetrical and appropriate for their stage of development

Reflexes
Abnormal reflexes do not always indicate abnormal neurology; an anxious child can have

(a)

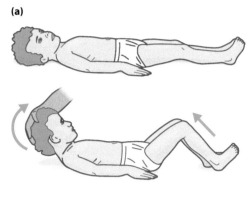

(b)

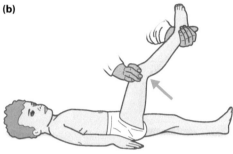

Figure 14.7 Examining for meningeal irritation: (a) Kernig's sign; (b) Brudzinski's sign.

brisk reflexes. Plantar reflexes are not reliable in infants and are not routinely tested.

Sensation

Light touch is easily assessed in patients who are able to communicate. Assessing pain, vibration and joint position sense is difficult and should only be assessed if absolutely necessary and (in the case of pain) only by a specialised clinician.

Cranial nerves

Cranial nerve examination is difficult with patients who cannot understand or follow commands. It is usually only possible for children over 4 years. For all children, observe the face for any asymmetry, hearing deficit or abnormal eye movement.

14.6.8 Musculoskeletal examination

Observe

Observe the child moving or playing and note whether there are any restrictions. Ask the parents

if they have noticed any change in their child's movement.

Look

Inspect the joints for any swelling or tenderness and note any abnormal posturing or muscle wasting of the limbs. Watch the child walk and note whether it is appropriate for their age. Look at the shape of the spine, particularly for any scoliosis.

Feel

Lightly feel over any abnormal or painful joint for warmth. Gently move it and feel for any crepitus.

Move

If able to follow simple commands, ask the child to perform a particular movement to check the range and ease of joint movement; if unable to follow a command, gently move the joints passively and note any tenderness of restriction.

14.6.9 Lymphadenopathy examination

Palpate the neck and inguinal areas for lymphadenopathy. In children, being able to palpate multiple small volume lymph nodes is normal. Cervical lymphadenopathy is common with viral upper respiratory tract infections. If lymphadenopathy is present, always ensure the abdomen has been examined for splenomegaly, which is associated with haematological malignancies.

14.6.10 Eyes, ears and throat

Examining the eyes, ears and throat is uncomfortable and may be distressing for the child, especially if they are unable to understand what is happening. If a child is unlikely to tolerate the examination, ask the parents to hold them on their lap with their head held in position (**Figure 14.8**).

Eyes

Note any abnormal eye shape or alignment. Hold a light or toy and move it around for the child to follow. Do both eyes move normally and together? Is there any nystagmus? Assess the red reflex in both eyes. This is absent if cataracts are

(a)

(b)

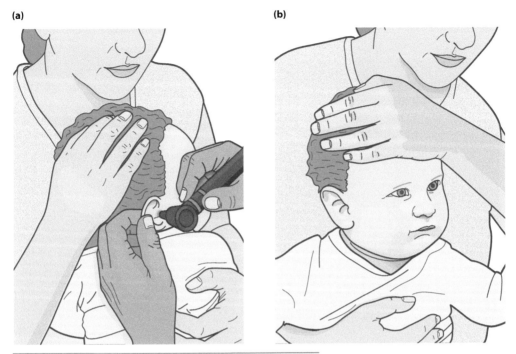

Figure 14.8 Positioning of child for (a) otoscopy; (b) fundoscopy.

present. Fundoscopy is often difficult if the child cannot keep their eye open and may be referred to a specialist if indicated.

Ears

Assess the auditory meatus for any redness or discharge indicating infection. When performing otoscopy, note any redness, dryness or wax within the auditory canal and the colour and contour of the tympanic membrane. Hearing tests are a normal part of health screening in infants. Ask the parents about the child's hearing and refer for formal audiology testing if there are any concerns.

Throat

This part of the examination is normally performed last as it usually causes infants and young children to cry, which makes any ongoing examination difficult. Ensure the child is held firmly so that their movement is limited. Ask the child to open their mouth whilst saying 'aah'. Shine a bright light at the back of the throat and note the colour of the pharynx and the size and colour of both tonsils. Is there any pus or discharge? A disposable tongue depressor may need to be used to ensure an adequate view. Fetor (bad breath) is a sign of poor oral hygiene and is particularly bad with quinsy.

14.6.11 Finishing off

Thank the child and/or their parents, allow the child to dress and explain your findings. Consider referring to a specialist if there are any concerns. Always discuss with a senior colleague before proceeding to investigations such as blood tests or radiographs.

14.7 Developmental assessment

Childhood development is categorised into four main domains:

■ Gross motor
■ Fine motor and vision
■ Hearing, speech and language
■ Social, emotional and behaviour.

The term 'developmental milestone' refers to the skill or ability expected at a certain age (**Table 14.8**). It

Table 14.8 *Age-specific developmental milestones*

Age	Gross motor	Fine motor and vision	Hearing, speech and language	Social, emotional and behavioural
6 weeks	Able to hold head level with body when lying on front	Fixes and follows with eyes	Becomes still in response to sound	Smiles
3 months	Raises head to 90° when lying on front	Able to hold an object if placed in hand	Turns towards sound	Notices own hands Laughs and squeals
6 months	No head lag when pulled up to sit Able to sit with support Able to push up on to forearms when lying on front	Able to palmar grasp objects Able to transfer objects from one hand to the other	Vocalises sounds	Able to feed self with fingers
9 months	Able to crawl Able to sit unsupported Able to pivot when seated	Able to pincer grasp objects Able to bang two objects together	Able to babble 2-syllable words like 'mama' and 'dada'	Waves bye-bye Able to play pat-a-cake Able to indicate if wants something Develops anxiety with strangers
12 months	Able to pull self up to stand Can cruise along furniture May stand briefly unsupported May unsteadily walk	Able to put a block in a cup Able to look around for things	Able to speak a few words Imitates sounds made by others speaking	Imitates activities of others Understands objects continue to exist after they're hidden (object permanence) Stranger anxiety fully established Able to point towards something wanted

Table 14.8 *Age-specific developmental milestones – continued*

Age	Gross motor	Fine motor and vision	Hearing, speech and language	Social, emotional and behavioural
18 months	Walks steadily	Able to build a tower of 2–4 blocks	Able to speak 6–12 words	Able to use a spoon
	Runs short distances	Develops preference of one hand		Plays symbolically – 'talks' into telephone
				Able to 'help' with household chores
2 years	Able to kick a ball	Able to build a tower of 6–7 blocks	Able to make 2–3-word sentences	Can remove some clothes
	Able to climb stairs with two feet per step	Able to scribble in circles	Able to identify some body parts	
			Can identify objects in pictures	
3 years	Able to stand on one foot	Able to build a tower of 9 blocks	Able to talk in short sentences that a stranger can understand	Able to use a fork
	Able to climb stairs with one foot per step	Able to copy a circle		Puts on own clothes
				May be toilet trained

is important to note that the ages stated are mean values; they are the age by which half, not all, of the population acquires a skill. It is important to reassure parents that each child develops differently.

Milestones are achieved sequentially, meaning that a child must be able to perform a task from one age range before being able to perform a task from the next. Put simply, one must be able to walk before one can run!

A child's development relies on both genetic and social factors which impact both positively and negatively. The developmental assessment aims to appreciate both where a delay in development occurs and the underlying contributing factors. A simple approach is to:

- ask screening questions
- observe the child
- note any red flag signs
- investigate for underlying problems.

14.7.1 Screening questions

Briefly discuss with the parents:

- "Do you have any specific concerns about your child's development?" Parents are the most likely to notice if their child's development or behaviour has changed or is not as expected. Often, this is as a comparison to the rate of development of other children and brings great anxiety. Reassure parents that 'normal' development is a broad term and the time course can vary for different children.
- "Were there any problems during the pregnancy or birth?" Certain maternal health issues during pregnancy and birth complications greatly affect a child's neurocognitive development (**Table 14.9**).
- "Have there been any health or social issues for the child since birth?" Similarly to pregnancy and birth, the child's physical health affects development (**Table 14.10**). When asking about social issues, be sensitive to different cultural practices and avoid accusing parents or caregivers of maltreatment.

Table 14.9 *Prenatal and perinatal events affecting neurocognitive development*

Timing	Event	Example	Consequence to foetus/infant
Antenatal	Early maternal infections	Rubella	Sensorineural deafness, blindness
		Toxoplasmosis	Neurocognitive deficit
		Cytomegalovirus	Low IQ, sensorineural deafness, psychomotor retardation
	Late maternal infections	Varicella	Encephalitis, eye pathology, limb hypoplasia
		Malaria	Stillbirth, spontaneous abortion, low birthweight
		HIV	Foetal HIV infection, side-effects of antiretrovirals
	Toxins	Alcohol	Craniofacial abnormalities, learning difficulties
		Smoking	Premature birth, brainstem immaturity, sudden infant death syndrome, stillbirth
		Radiation	Haematological malignancy
	Drugs	Cytotoxics	Foetal death, impaired nervous system development
		Anti-epileptics	Cognitive deficit, impaired neuronal development, neural tube defects
	Metabolic disorders	Diabetes	Growth abnormalities, increased risk of instrumental delivery
		Hypothyroidism	Low IQ
Perinatal	Prematurity	n/a	Neurocognitive delay
	Birth asphyxia	Cord around neck	Hypoxic brain injury
	Brain injury	Instrumental delivery	Cerebral trauma and cerebral palsy

14.7.2 Observation

Provide the child with toys and observe them:
- Are their gross motor, fine motor and visual skills appropriate for their age?
- Are they able to listen and communicate as expected?
- Do they interact with their parents, toys and other people appropriately?

14.7.3 Red flags

Some signs should raise immediate concern and require further investigation to understand the underlying cause. These include:

- developmental regression at any age
- not fixing on or following an object
- hearing loss
- low or increased muscle tone
- inability to hold an object by 5 months
- inability to sit unsupported at 12 months
- inability to walk by 18 months (male) or 2 years (female)
- no speech by 18 months.

14.7.4 Investigation

Different developmental concerns should be referred to the appropriate specialty to investigate

Table 14.10 *Childhood issues affecting neurocognitive development*

Infections	Meningitis
	Encephalitis
	Cytomegalovirus
Metabolic disorders	Hypoglycaemia
	Hyponatraemia
	Dehydration
Toxins	Heavy metals
	Solvents
Trauma	Head injury
	Other
Abuse	Understimulation
	Malnourishment
	Physical
Caregiver mental health	Depression
	Psychosis

and address any underlying problems in a manner supportive to the child and family as a whole. These specialties encompass the entire multidisciplinary team and include:

- clinical geneticists, audiologists, ophthalmologists and neurologists
- allied healthcare professionals, including physiotherapists and speech and language therapists
- psychiatrists
- social workers and health visitors.

14.8 Answers to starter questions

1. Macrocephaly (a large head) describes a head circumference that is two standard deviations above the mean according to age. The commonest pathological causes of macrocephaly include hydrocephalus (excess CSF within the ventricles) or hyperostosis (cranial bone overgrowth). However, physical size and shape is also genetic and most macrocephaly is inherited and not clinically problematic. Investigations for cranial and neurological disease can be difficult in children and involve large amounts of radiation. Before proceeding, clinicians take a clear history, look at the parents and also investigate for any neurological or developmental deficit that might indicate any underlying disease.

2. Changing a nappy, or rather investigating what is in it, provides a great amount of information as to the child's health. A reduced volume and frequency of urination is an early sign of

dehydration. Additionally, stools change with different underlying GI disease:

- Hard pellets of stool indicate constipation which may be caused by dehydration.
- Red stools could signify bleeding, such as from fissures or inflammatory bowel diseases, or be the 'redcurrant jelly' stool typical of intussusception.
- Black stools are normal as a child's first bowel motion (called meconium) but signify higher GI bleeding if occurring later in development.
- Pale stools are caused by malabsorption associated with liver and pancreatic diseases.

3. In the UK, a child between the ages of 16 and 18 years is assumed to have the emotional and intellectual capacity to decide regarding their healthcare unless there is a specific problem or deficit that is known to prevent them from doing so. For those under 16 years, if a child "achieves

sufficient understanding and intelligence to understand fully what is proposed" then they are deemed to hold 'Gillick competence' and are able to decide without requiring parental approval. Always remember that competence to make a decision is specific to a particular scenario; competence to make one decision does not equal competence to make a different decision.

4.   Children's interactions often bring concern to parents. To play, a child must recognise a new person and trust them enough to interact. Stranger mistrust is common and normal up to 1 year of age. All children have personalities and, like adults, not all get along. Communication is a key part of interaction between children. This communication can be verbal and those with hearing or speaking difficulties may struggle to play. The more complex ability of understanding social communications, i.e. being intuitive towards others, is lacking in children with autism spectrum disorders.

Chapter 15
Critically ill patients

Starter questions

1. Why don't we treat every patient in the Intensive Therapy Unit?
2. Who should we 'trauma call'?

Answers to questions are to be found in *Section 15.8*.

15.1 Introduction

Critically unwell patients have the potential to deteriorate quickly. There is often not the opportunity to take a full history before examining the patient and initiating care. A comprehensive, rapid and easy to follow standardised approach to assessment and management is used (**Figure 15.1**).
■ Primary survey – identification of life-threatening problems or injuries via 'DR ABCDE' approach (danger, response, airway, breathing, circulation, disability, exposure); this is covered in more detail in *Section 15.2*
■ Resuscitation
■ Secondary survey – focused history and head-to-toe assessment

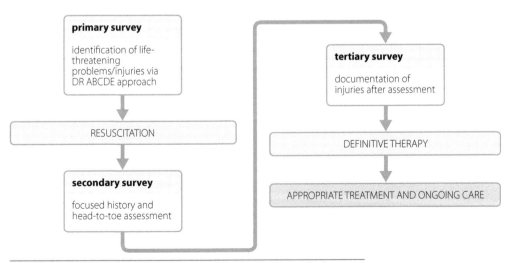

Figure 15.1 The standardised approach to assessing the critically ill patient.

- Tertiary survey – documentation of injuries after investigation
- Definitive therapy
- Appropriate ongoing care.

The theory behind this approach is that the most life-threatening problems are addressed first before moving on to the next. If a problem is encountered (such as a low BP), immediate measures are undertaken to correct this before continuing on to the next part of the assessment.

The assessment of critically unwell patients is best undertaken by a team – either the resuscitation team (for medical emergencies where no surgical intervention is needed, such as cardiac arrest or status epilepticus) or the trauma team (for traumatic / surgical emergencies such as life-threatening bleeding or road traffic accidents). Each person has a designated role in the pathway to ensure efficiency and allow multiple assessments and interventions to be undertaken simultaneously, under the guidance of a single team leader. However, all doctors are expected to be able to complete a primary survey and to provide resuscitation treatments (including basic and intermediate life support) and will often do this alone as they assess patients encountered in clinical practice.

Ideally, the assessment of unwell patients should be in a safe area where emergency equipment that might be needed is readily available, such as the resuscitation area of an emergency department. In reality, emergencies happen anywhere and at any time: by the roadside, in a GP's clinic room or even the corridor of a hospital. A good grounding of rapid, yet thorough, assessment and treatment processes helps healthcare professionals stabilise unwell patients so that they get the treatment they need, wherever they are.

Case 15.1 Fall

Presentation

Mr Jones is 84 years old. He has been 'blue-lighted' to the Emergency Department following a fall down a flight of stairs. A trauma call has been put out so that the trauma team are present when he arrives.

> **'Blue-lighting' a patient to hospital is when an ambulance transports someone at speed with the sirens and flashing blue lights on**. It is reserved for critically unwell patients who require urgent treatment on arrival.

Initial interpretation

There are two main concerns here: why did Mr Jones fall, and has he injured himself during the fall?

Falls are a common problem in the elderly with a plethora of causes:
- Motor problems: muscle weakness, reduced mobility
- Sensory impairment: visual impairment, peripheral neuropathy
- Orthostatic hypotension (including side-effects from medications)
- Cardiac disease: arrhythmia, myocardial infarction
- Respiratory disease: hypoxia, massive pulmonary embolus
- Neurological disease: stroke, epilepsy.

As an older person, Mr Jones is much more likely to sustain an injury due to frailty. He is also more likely to be on medications such as warfarin that predispose to bleeding.

Falling down a flight of stairs is a significant injury (compared to falling from bed or a chair) and immediate concern should be paid to his cervical spine, as spinal fractures risk spinal cord damage leading to permanent disability.

Primary survey

Mr Jones arrives with his cervical spine immobilised. The paramedics report he was found at the bottom of the stairs by his carers. He was last seen at 8pm the following evening. A primary survey is undertaken:

Case 15.1 *continued*

- Danger: it is safe to approach Mr Jones.
- Response: moaning and thrashing on the trolley.
- Airway: patent with no obstruction.
- Breathing: chest clear with equal expansion and normal breath sounds. His respiratory rate is 22 and oxygen saturations are 100% on maximum oxygen therapy.
- Circulation: cool skin to the elbows. His JVP is not visible but heart sounds are normal. His heart rate is 140bpm and irregular. His blood pressure is 85/44mmHg. His central capillary refill time is 4 seconds.
- Disability: Glasgow Coma Scale (GCS) is 8/15 (E2, V2, M4). His pupils are 3mm and react to light. His capillary blood glucose (CBG) is 6.3mmol/L.
- Exposure: a large bruise is noted on his right forehead and on all his limbs but there are no obvious deformities. He has a large pressure area on his left cheek and hip. His temperature is 35.3°C.

Interpretation of primary survey

Mr Jones has fallen a significant distance and has hit his head and limbs. It is unclear when he fell but given his pressure areas and hypothermia it is likely he has been on the floor for some time. He is at risk of rhabdomyolysis, the breakdown of muscle leading to high levels of circulating creatine kinase which leads to kidney damage, and should have IV fluids.

He is hypovolaemic as evidenced by his tachycardia, hypotension, prolonged capillary refill time and peripherally shut-down state. He requires urgent IV access and rehydration. Given his extensive bruising, he may have had significant bleeding, so his haemoglobin should be checked urgently.

The irregular tachycardia is atrial fibrillation with a rapid ventricular response. This could be due to underlying atrial fibrillation and missing medications that morning, his hypovolaemic state, electrolyte imbalance or sepsis. A full panel of blood tests including blood cultures are taken and sent to the laboratory.

He is drowsy and agitated. A GCS of less than 8 is an indication for sedation, intubation and artificial ventilation. This secures his airway which is at risk of becoming obstructed and also allows for faster assessment, given his thrashing movements. He requires a CT head to assess for any intracerebral cause for his drowsiness and agitation such as subdural or subarachnoid haemorrhage.

Secondary survey

Mr Jones has no medical alert bracelets and is unable to give a history. His carer has accompanied him in the ambulance and states that he has atrial fibrillation and takes warfarin. She is not aware of any other medical problems.

- Head: he has a large bruise on his right forehead but there is no underlying bogginess.
- Neck: as he is intubated and ventilated, it is not possible to assess for cervical spine tenderness.
- Chest: there are some bruises on the right side of his chest.
- Abdomen: again, there are bruises but no other injuries.
- Spine: as he is intubated and ventilated, his spine is not formally assessed.
- Pelvis: his pelvis appears stable with no deformities.
- Genitals: there is no obvious trauma to his genital region.
- Extremities: he has bruising over all four limbs. His right leg appears shorter and rotated externally when compared to the left. He has palpable pulses throughout.

Interpretation of secondary survey

Mr Jones has evidence of head injury and given this, plus the mechanism of his fall, he has a high risk for a spinal injury. He also has a fractured right neck of femur as evidenced by his shortened and externally rotated leg.

His chest and abdomen do not show obvious evidence of injury or pathology but full examination is not possible.

Case 15.1 *continued*

Investigations

An arterial blood gas after intubation shows a metabolic acidosis with normal gas exchange. His laboratory bloods show:

- haemoglobin 99g/L (normal = 130–170g/L)
- white blood cell count 14.2 × 10^9/L (normal = 4.5–11.0 × 10^9/L)
- neutrophil count 10.1 × 10^9/L (normal = 2.0–7.0 × 10^9/L)
- impaired kidney function with:
  - □ urea 14.7mmol/L (normal = 4.0–8.2mmol/L)
  - □ creatinine 158µmol/L (normal = 50–110µmol/L)
- C-reactive protein (CRP) 253mg/L (normal = <5mg/L)
- creatine kinase 21 048IU/L (normal = 20–215IU/L)
- international normalised ratio (INR) 4.8 (normal = 0.9–1.1).

A 12-lead ECG shows atrial fibrillation with a fast ventricular response but no evidence of regional ischaemia.

A FAST scan (focused assessment with sonography for trauma – see *Section 15.2.8*) is performed which reveals no pericardial or free intra-abdominal fluid.

Mr Jones undergoes a whole body 'trauma protocol' CT. This shows multiple fractured ribs and a small right-sided pleural effusion. He has no evidence of pneumothorax or consolidation. There is no cervical spine fracture. He has no pelvic fracture but has a neck of femur fracture on the right. He has a large subdural haemorrhage.

Tertiary survey

Mr Jones has multiple problems:

- Sepsis as evidenced by raised white blood cells and CRP, tachycardia, hypotension and hypothermia.
- Hypovolaemia with an acute kidney injury from sepsis, dehydration and rhabdomyolysis.
- A large traumatic subdural haemorrhage in the context of an abnormally prolonged INR.
- A right neck of femur fracture.
- Atrial fibrillation with fast ventricular response from sepsis and hypovolaemia.

Management

Mr Jones is given IV fluid resuscitation and commenced on broad-spectrum antibiotics. Warming is started with warm fluids and blankets. He is given recombinant clotting factors to rapidly correct his INR.

He is discussed with a neurosurgeon, who suggests that he be stabilised and his INR reversed before considering decompressive surgery for his subdural haemorrhage. An orthopaedic surgeon reviews, who states he can undergo surgery with a dynamic hip screw when well enough.

Given that he is invasively ventilated and requires continuous invasive monitoring, he is transferred to the intensive care unit for further management.

15.2 The primary survey

The primary survey is performed anywhere and is the initial screen for emergency problems affecting the unwell patient. It is rapid (usually taking less than 5 minutes) and follows the 'DR ABCDE' approach, whereby each body system is assessed in order of acuity (i.e. in order of which will cause most harm if a problem is not rectified first). At each letter, there are six steps: look, feel, listen, measure, intervene and reassess. In doing so, the clinician has a full appreciation of the problems, and addresses these as they are found before moving on. Ideally, the patient should be lying flat on the floor or on a trolley to be assessed.

15.2.1 Danger

- Check for hazards before approaching the patient (such as glass and debris on the ground

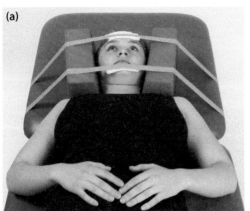
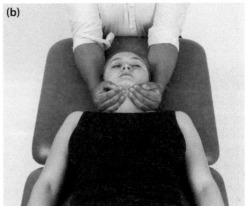

Figure 15.2 Isolation of the cervical spine using (a) collar and blocks; (b) holding.

at a road traffic accident that could cause injury). If it is unsafe, do not put yourself at risk.

■ If available, always put on personal protective equipment (gloves, plastic aprons, face masks). Without knowing the patient's medical history, you do not know whether they have a blood-borne virus (such as HIV or hepatitis) that could be contracted if you come in contact with their blood.

■ Is there any risk that the patient has sustained a cervical spine injury? These typically occur with trauma where a patient is either thrown across a distance, stops suddenly from speed or falls. If so, ensure the cervical spine is immobilised immediately by using collar and blocks (**Figure 15.2a**) or holding the head still and continuously throughout assessment (**Figure 15.2b**). For the latter, it is necessary to have a trained colleague to hold the head so that you are able to continue your assessment.

15.2.2 Response

■ Is the patient responsive? Shout their name or "Hello, can you hear me?". If they answer coherently and appropriately, their responsiveness is normal.

■ If the patient makes no response or responds with noises or movements only, this is a worrying sign that they are unwell. If unresponsive, call for help immediately, either by calling to a member of staff for support,

pulling the emergency buzzer at a hospital bedside or phoning for the emergency services if outside a hospital. If a patient is unresponsive, check for cardiopulmonary effort:

☐ if there is no suspected cervical spine injury, perform the head-tilt, chin-lift manoeuvre (**Figure 15.3**)

☐ lean side of head over the patient's mouth and 'look, feel, listen' (**Figure 15.4**):

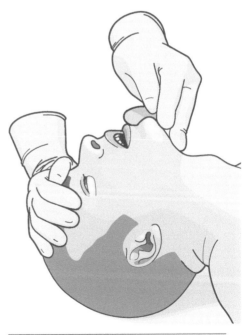

Figure 15.3 The head-tilt chin-lift manoeuvre.

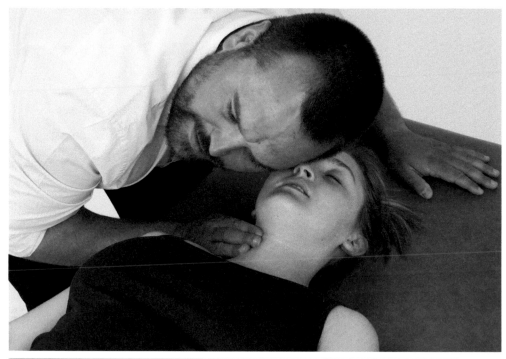

Figure 15.4 Look, feel and listen for respiratory effort and a central pulse before beginning CPR.

- – **look** for chest wall movement
- – **feel** for their carotid pulse
- – **listen** for their breathing
- ☐ if any of these are absent, begin CPR
  (**Figure 15.5**).

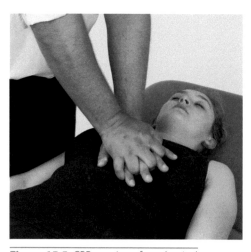

Figure 15.5 CPR consists of mechanical ventilation and chest compressions (chest compressions pictured).

15.2.3 Airway

Assessment of the airway always takes place first. Without a patent airway, air cannot enter the lungs to allow oxygen to be absorbed and transported to the tissues.

Look
- ▪ Look in the mouth. Is there blood, vomit or foreign bodies?

Listen
- ▪ Are there any sounds of airway compromise (stridor, snoring, gurgling, wheeze)?

Intervention
- ▪ Remove any obvious obstructing objects with suction or forceps. Do not put your own fingers inside a patient's mouth to remove objects as this risks pushing them down further or you being bitten. Remember dentures cause airway obstruction and should be removed.
- ▪ Perform airway interventions (**Table 15.1**).

Table 15.1 Summary of airway adjuncts, their indications, contraindications and necessary monitoring needs

Adjunct	Method	Indication	Contraindications	Monitoring
Airway manoeuvres	Head-tilt, chin-lift	Low GCS with airway obstruction	Suspected cervical spine injuries	Continue throughout if safe to do so
	Jaw thrust	Low GCS with airway obstruction	Facial or jaw injuries	Continue until airway adjunct inserted
Bag-valve mask	Tightly seals face to mask with positive pressure air from bag	Any airway concern / Used alongside airway adjuncts	Facial injuries	Does little to support airway patency
Nasopharyngeal airway	Tube insertion to pharynx via a nostril	Low GCS (<8) with no evidence of airway obstruction	Suspected basal skull, facial or nasal injuries / GCS <8	Needs upgrading to OPA if obstruction from tongue
Oropharyngeal airway (OPA, Guedel)	Tube insertion to pharynx via the mouth; pulls tongue forward	Low GCS (<8) with airway obstruction (from tongue)	Oral injuries / GCS <8	Needs upgrading to LMA/ETT if GCS <8
Laryngeal mask airway (LMA)	Tube insertion without direct vision; inflated end sits above vocal cords	Low GCS (<8) where ETT insertion not possible	Upper airway constriction (late anaphylaxis)	Needs upgrading to ETT at earliest opportunity
Endotracheal intubation (ETT)	Tube insertion under direct vision into trachea (i.e. past the vocal cords) via the mouth	Low GCS (<8) / Respiratory failure / Cardiorespiratory arrest / Agitation	Upper airway constriction (late anaphylaxis) where entry to trachea cannot be seen	Specialist anaesthetic insertion and management
Tracheostomy	Tube insertion to trachea below level of glottis via anterior neck	Any airway obstruction where ETT not possible		Specialist anaesthetic insertion and management

Agitation is common and can be severe, especially in cases of head injury. If a patient becomes unmanageable, they are at risk of not receiving the emergency treatment they need and require sedation or even a general anaesthetic and intubation to allow life-saving treatment.

Reassessment after an intervention has been made is a key non-technical skill in medicine. Once a treatment has been given, always re-examine the patient to see if there has been a response.

15.2.4 Breathing

Breathing is assessed second. Once air enters the lungs, it requires healthy and functioning lungs to allow gas transfer to and from blood. Without functioning lungs, a patient will not absorb the oxygen they require. The pattern of findings relates to the underlying process causing the patient to be unwell (**Table 15.2**).

Look
- Is the patient struggling to breathe or are they breathing comfortably?
- Are both sides of the chest moving? If so, is it equal? Sudden breathing difficulty with unequal chest wall movement is most commonly caused by a pneumothorax or flail chest (*Section 5.3.5*).

Feel
- Feel the trachea. Is it central? If it is deviated, which side has it moved to?
- Feel both sides of the chest. Does it expand equally?
- Percuss both sides of the chest. Is the note normal, dull or hyper-resonant?

Listen
- Auscultate the anterior thorax for breath sounds.
- Is there air entry on each side of the chest? If so, is it equal?
- Are there any added breath sounds (wheeze, crackles, rubs)?

Measure
- Measure respiratory rate and oxygen saturations.
- Take an arterial blood gas to assess ventilatory function.

Intervention
- If the patient has low peripheral oxygen saturations, give high flow oxygen at 15L/min via a non-rebreathe or bag-valve mask.
- Consider airway adjuncts or intubation if any concern of airway compromise or severe ventilator dysfunction.
- Consider intercostal procedures for life-threatening conditions.

Intra-thoracic bleeding, causing a haemothorax, is an important 'hidden' source of blood loss. Some patients tolerate several litres of blood loss into the thorax with little sign of respiratory compromise.

15.2.5 Circulation

Maintaining the circulation allows the patient's organs to be perfused, allowing them to continue functioning normally, or as close to normal as possible. The mainstay is assessing the patient's 'fluid status': do they have too much fluid, too little fluid or a normal amount of fluid (hyper-, hypo- and euvolaemic, respectively) and is there enough blood pressure present to perfuse the organs? The easiest organs to measure perfusion at are the brain (through responsiveness) and the kidneys (through urine output).

Hypovolaemia describes a state in which blood volume is too low to support normal cardiovascular function (i.e. with severe dehydration or heavy bleeding). It presents clinically as a low blood pressure, high heart rate and prolonged capillary refill time. The treatment is urgent volume replacement with IV fluid and blood. Those who fail to respond to treatment (with normalising blood pressure and heart rate) are in cardiovascular shock and require inotropic medications to support their blood pressure.

Table 15.2 *Emergency thoracic trauma diagnoses and their management*

Emergency condition	Description	Signs	Intervention
Tension pneumothorax	Air within pleural space causing ipsilateral lung collapse and pushing mediastinum away from affected side	Tracheal deviation **away** from affected side Absent breath sounds and reduced expansion on affected side Hyper-resonant percussion note on affected side	Needle thoracostomy Surgical chest drain insertion
Pneumothorax	Air within pleural space causing ipsilateral lung collapse and pulling mediastinum towards affected side	Tracheal deviation **towards** affected side Absent breath sounds and reduced expansion on affected side Hyper-resonant percussion note on affected side	Intercostal or surgical chest drain insertion
Massive pleural effusion ■ haemothorax: blood ■ chylothorax: lymph	Fluid within pleural space (usually blood or lymph in trauma) causing collapse of ipsilateral lung and pushing mediastinum away from affected side	Tracheal deviation away from affected side Absent breath sounds and reduced expansion of affected side Stony dull percussion note on affected side	Surgical chest drain insertion – this is usually a large bore surgical drain to prevent clogging Urgent cardiothoracic surgery
Mixed (i.e. haemopneumothorax)	Air and fluid within pleural space	Tracheal deviation Absent breath sounds and reduced expansion on affected side Stony dull percussion note over area of effusion	Surgical chest drain insertion Urgent cardiothoracic surgery

> **Patients on beta blockers or rate-limiting CCBs have a falsely normal heart rate despite being hypovolaemic.**

A patient who does not have a normal BP and/or heart rate is termed 'haemodynamically unstable'. This signifies that without treatment, they have the potential to become more unwell, or even die.

Look

- Is the patient pale or sweaty?
- Look at the JVP. Is it raised (suggesting cardiac tamponade or pericardial effusion)?

Feel

- Feel the hands and feet. A patient is 'peripherally shut down' if their extremities are cold and have a slow capillary refill time.
- Feel the carotid pulse. What is the pulse volume?

Listen

- Listen to the heart sounds. Are they muffled (suggesting a pericardial effusion)? Are there any murmurs (suggesting valvular dysfunction)?

Measure

- Measure the heart rate and blood pressure.

- Measure central and peripheral capillary refill time.
- Perform a 12-lead ECG.
- Consider continuous cardiac monitoring.

Intervention

- Gain multiple (at least two) sites of large-bore IV access. This is essential for any unwell patient.
- Send urgent blood samples for full blood count, renal function, liver function, amylase, inflammatory markers (such as CRP), blood cultures, clotting activity and blood group – these are basic screening blood tests for common causes of a patient being unwell.
- Give a fluid bolus and assess response to BP and heart rate.
- If bleeding, order urgent 'O negative' blood and blood products to give until the patient's blood group is known. Transfusion should not be delayed if a patient is unstable from bleeding.

> **O negative blood has no A, B or rhesus antigens on the red cell membranes so is suitable to be transfused to any person.** Those with O negative blood are called 'universal donors'.

15.2.6 Disability

Disability relates to the patient's neurological status rather than functional ability.

Look

- Is the patient normally responsive, drowsy, confused or agitated?

Measure

- The Glasgow Coma Scale (GCS) is a measure of neurological function relating to consciousness (**Table 15.3**). If unable to assess GCS, use the Alert, Voice, Pain, Unresponsive (AVPU) scale (**Table 15.4**). The AVPU scale is not as sensitive to subtle changes as the GCS.

> **The Glasgow Coma Scale was developed to assess consciousness in patients with head injuries.** It has since been extrapolated to assess responsiveness in all unwell patients. The initial scoring system gave a maximum score of 14 but modified scores are out of 15. The lowest score possible is 3.

- Shine a torch into each pupil to measure size and response to light.
- Ask the patient to move each hand and foot in turn to assess gross power.
- Measure the capillary blood glucose (CBG).

Intervention

- Ensure appropriate airway protection with any GCS <15 or AVPU score of P or U.
- Give rapid intravenous glucose if the CBG is <4mmol/L.

Table 15.3 *The Glasgow Coma Scale – the maximum possible score is 15 and the lowest is 3*

Score	Eyes	Voice	Movement
1	No eye opening	None	No motor response
2	Eyes opening to pain	Incomprehensible sounds	Extension to pain
3	Eyes opening to voice	Inappropriate words	Flexion to pain
4	Eyes open spontaneously	Confused speech	Withdrawal from pain
5		Normal speech	Localising to pain
6			Obeying commands

Table 15.4 The AVPU (Alert, Voice, Pain, Unresponsive) scale

	Description	Equivalent GCS
A	Alert and orientated	13–15
V	Not alert initially but responding to voice	9–12
P	Alert to pain but not to voice	4–8
U	Unresponsive to pain or voice	3

In states of reduced consciousness, skeletal muscle tone is relaxed, allowing the airway to close and the tongue to slip backwards in the pharynx, causing airway obstruction.

A GCS of ≤8, or an AVPU of P or U, is an indication to consider inserting an endotracheal tube (ETT).

15.2.7 Exposure

The aim of exposure is to assess for any 'hidden' abnormalities. If the patient is relatively well and able to assist you, ask them to lift their top to allow you to examine their abdomen. In critically unwell patients or in those who cannot assist you, remove all their clothing (this usually requires clothes to be cut off).

Whilst full exposure is essential to quickly assess for injury, be mindful of the patient's dignity. Once the assessment is complete, cover them wherever possible or examine each area in turn. Blankets or hospital gowns should be placed over patients after their clothes are removed.

Look
- Is there any obvious deformity, bleeding or bruising?
- Pay special attention to any evidence of bleeding from the back / underneath the patient as this is easily missed if not specifically checked for. This requires you to turn the

patient so only carry out this manoeuvre when it is safe to do so.
- Are there any skin changes such as a rash, pressure area or signs of IV drug use?

Feel
- Palpate the abdomen. Is it rigid, tense or tender (indicating intra-abdominal pathology)?
- Feel all four limbs. Are they warm, indicating appropriate blood supply?

Measure
- Measure the patient's temperature using a thermometer in the ear, axilla or rectum.

Intervention
- Apply physical pressure to any sites of major bleeding by holding gauze firmly against the wound.
- Replace blankets (with or without warming blankets) to preserve dignity and prevent / treat hypothermia.

15.2.8 Other

Whilst the primary survey is ongoing, other investigations and interventions also take place if felt to be necessary:
- X-ray or CT of chest, cervical spine and pelvis (especially in cases of trauma)
- Insertion of NG tube (after intubation) to allow stomach decompression
- Insertion of urinary catheter for fluid balance monitoring
- FAST (focused assessment with sonography for trauma) scan (**Figure 15.6**). This is a US scan assessing for bleeding in four common areas:
  - ☐ perihepatic space (with suspected liver injuries)
  - ☐ perisplenic space (with suspected splenic injuries)
  - ☐ pericardium (suspected cardiac tamponade and pericardial effusion)
  - ☐ pelvis (suspected intra-abdominal / aortic trauma).

An extended FAST scan also includes US scanning of the thorax to look for pleural effusions, pneumothoraces or haemothoraces.

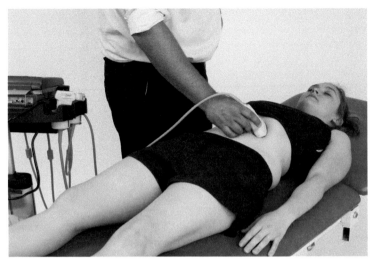

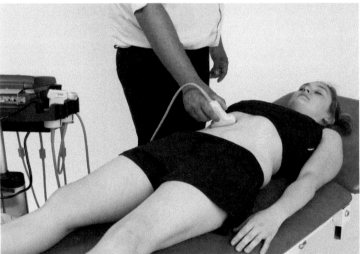

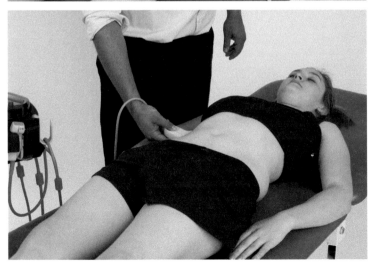

Figure 15.6 A FAST scan identifies bleeding within the peritoneal cavity or within the major organs of the abdomen.

15.3 The secondary survey

Once the primary survey has taken place and the immediately life-threatening conditions have been treated, the secondary survey follows a focused history and head-to-toe examination approach to identify any injuries in need of further investigation and management. This is less rapid than the primary survey. It is a more detailed reassessment of the patient to pick up subtler signs and to double-check that major pathologies have not been missed.

15.3.1 History

Take a focused history of important details, using family members or bystanders if present. The mnemonic 'SAMPLE' covers the key information required:
- **S**igns / symptoms
- **A**llergies
- **M**edications
- **P**ertinent past medical history
- **L**ast oral intake
- **E**vents leading to trauma or illness.

If a patient is unable to give a history, check for clues such as medical alert jewellery or cards within their belongings.

15.3.2 Head-to-toe examination

Head
- Check the scalp for injuries and deformities.
- Look around the eyes. Are there any cuts, bruises or foreign bodies?
- Check pupil size and response to light.
- Check the ears and nose for bleeding or cerebrospinal fluid leak.
- Check inside the mouth for blood, vomit or other obstructions.

Neck
- Gently palpate the cervical spine for tenderness. If present or unable to assess, assume the patient has a cervical spine injury and immobilise the neck to prevent permanent damage to the cervical spinal cord.
- Palpate for tracheal deviation.

Chest
- Inspect for chest wall injury, deformity or abnormal movement.
- Palpate for fractures and chest wall tenderness.

Abdomen
- Inspect for injuries, penetrating objects and bruising.
- Palpate the abdomen. Is there any tenderness? If so, is it localised or generalised? Is there evidence of peritonism?

Spine
- Roll the patient onto their side. If there is any suspicion of spinal injury, this should be performed as a 'log roll' (**Figure 15.7**). This technique demands a minimum of four people in order to keep the entire spine completely straight at all times. This minimises the risk of devastating spinal cord injury.
- Inspect for injury or deformity.
- Palpate each vertebra for tenderness.

Pelvis
- Palpate the pelvis for tenderness.
- Slide your hands from the small of the back to the lateral wings of the pelvis, feeling for any deformity.

Genital region
- Inspect for incontinence, bleeding or any injuries.

> **Priapism is the presence of a sustained erection in males.** It is a sign of spinal injury.

Extremities
- Inspect each limb for deformity or injury, noting the level of any traumatic amputation.
- Palpate the radial and posterior tibial pulses (or lowest palpable pulse if amputations have occurred).
- Examine power and sensation in the hands and feet (*Section 9.6*).

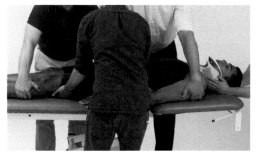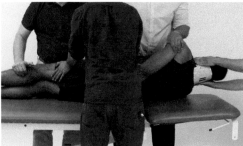

Figure 15.7 All trauma patients must be 'log-rolled' on turning by a team of healthcare workers, in order to protect the spinal cord.

15.4 Common investigations

The choice of investigations utilised for critically unwell patients depends on their needs. If the patient is unstable, resuscitative efforts should continue until the patient is stable enough to safely undergo the investigation, particularly in situations where the patient needs to be moved between rooms (e.g. CT scanning) or potentially be moved to a different hospital (such as to an angiography centre).

15.4.1 Blood tests

Blood tests give a rapid and time-specific reflection of the patient's physiology (**Table 15.5**).

15.4.2 X-ray

X-rays are usually performed in the emergency room without the need to move the patient. Bony X-rays require the patient to be transferred onto a trolley.

- Chest radiographs assess for and confirm pneumothorax, pleural effusions or rib fractures.
- Spinal radiographs assess for fractures. If unable to fully image each vertebra, a CT scan should be performed before declaring the spine safe to move.
- Bony radiographs confirm location and type of fracture.

15.4.3 Ultrasound

Ultrasound is performed at the bedside and does not require the patient to be moved.

- FAST scan quickly identifies any major injuries requiring urgent intervention.
- Ultrasound is used to guide safe insertion of intercostal devices during drainage.

15.4.4 Computed tomography

CT is performed by a dedicated scanner and requires the patient to be moved into a specially designed room. It gives three-dimensional, cross-sectional images of the head, neck, thorax, abdomen, aorta and pelvis. These diagnose organ trauma and identify evidence of bleeding. The addition of IV contrast allows identification of the source of bleeding and characterisation of whether bleeding is arterial or venous.

15.4.5 Angiography

Angiography is performed within a specially designed room, and only in hospitals with a specialist able to perform it. It utilises X-ray scanning together with IV contrast to give real-time images of blood vessels that are bleeding. Catheters are then passed into these vessels and objects inserted to block the vessel to stem bleeding – a process called embolisation.

Table 15.5 *Common blood tests used to investigate unwell patients*

Blood test	Aspect of blood test	Relevance
Full blood count (FBC)	Haemoglobin (Hb)	Anaemia associated with blood loss or bone marrow failure
	White blood cell count (WBC)	Infection
	Platelets (Plt)	Consumption (platelet usage in response to massive/multiple bleeding) or bone marrow failure
Renal function (U&E)	Sodium and potassium (Na & K)	Electrolyte disturbances
	Urea and creatinine (Ur and Cr)	Dehydration, GI bleeding and AKI
Liver function (LFT)	n/a	Hepatic or biliary function
Amylase	n/a	Pancreatitis
Clotting screen	n/a	Clotting disorders leading to bleeding; hepatic function
Cross-match	n/a	Identification of blood group for transfusion
Blood gas sampling	pH, carbon dioxide, bicarbonate, base excess and lactate (CO_2, HCO_3, BE & Lac)	Acid–base balance
	pH, carbon dioxide and oxygen (CO_2 & O_2)	Respiratory function

15.5 Tertiary survey

The tertiary survey encompasses full documentation of all examination and imaging and laboratory findings in the order of the primary and secondary surveys. The purpose is to make a problems list that is arranged in order of most severe (and thus in need of the most urgent management) to least severe. From this a comprehensive summary and management plan is made using all the information gathered.

Always consider a patient's welfare when summarising their problems. If the patient's illness or injury might have been caused by abuse or neglect (including by the patient to themself), this must be highlighted and addressed. In the UK, patient deaths from abuse or neglect must be referred to the coroner.

15.6 Definitive management

After completing the primary and secondary surveys and stabilising the patient, the next step of management needs addressing:

■ Does the patient require surgery or any other intervention? Is this an emergency or can it wait?

- Does the patient require ventilatory support?
- Does the patient require medications such as antibiotics, beta blockers or fluids?

- Does the patient require transfer to another centre? If so, do they need intubation and ventilation to allow safe transfer?

15.7 Appropriate ongoing care

Once emergency management has taken place, the patient needs to be cared for in the most appropriate setting. Where this happens within the hospital depends on their clinical requirements and is referred to as their level of care (**Table 15.6**).

For some people, certain interventions may never be successful or if successful, result in an unacceptable quality of life afterwards. Some patients do not want certain treatments. The 'treatment escalation plan' refers to a limit that is decided on what amount of treatment is appropriate. It influences the maximum level of treatment a patient receives and whether CPR should be started if their heart stops beating.

Table 15.6 *Descriptions of level of care*

Level of care	Definition	Examples
0	Needs admission to normal ward care	Intravenous medications
		Vital sign observations at a maximum of every 4 hours
1	Heightened observation in a normal ward	Oxygen therapy
		Intravenous fluids
		Parenteral nutrition
		Vital sign observations at a minimum of every 4 hours
2	High dependency care in a designated area (High Dependency Unit, HDU)	Basic cardiovascular, renal or respiratory support (inotropes, or haemofiltration or non-invasive ventilation)
		Invasive monitoring
		Vital sign observations at a minimum of every hour
3	Intensive care	Multiple organ support
		Invasive monitoring
		Continuous vital sign monitoring

15.8 Answers to starter questions

1. There are many factors influencing the most appropriate intensity of treatment. First, as the level of therapy received increases, cost and staffing levels increase. Treating every patient on intensive care would not be a sustainable option. Secondly, intensive therapy involves invasive monitoring (i.e. intravascular BP monitoring, regular blood tests, etc.). These are not without risks and side-effects which should be avoided if not necessary. Thirdly, intensive therapies such as inotropic medications or invasive ventilation are not appropriate for some patients; they are either futile and will not affect the overall outcome, they could make the patient worse, or the patient may not want them. Overriding all of these decisions is patient choice. If a patient with the capacity to decide does not want invasive or intensive therapy then this cannot be forced upon them against their wishes.

2. A 'trauma call' is an alert that mobilises a team of nurses, doctors, surgeons, anaesthetists, radiologists, radiographers and porters to a patient at risk of critical illness following major injury. The level of injury required to prompt a 'trauma call' is relatively high and includes those with evidence or risk of head or spinal injury, penetrating thoracic or abdominal wounds, amputations or major haemorrhage. For head and spinal injuries, the cut-off for a significant and non-significant injury is difficult to define and has many variables. For example, a young person with strong bones is less likely to suffer a spinal injury when falling from standing than an older person with severe osteoporosis. Put these scenarios in context and remember to always keep the differential open, however unlikely the risk of trauma is seen to be.

Chapter 16
Special circumstances

Starter questions

1. How do you assess a patient who speaks no English?
2. How do you assess a patient who cannot speak? Or cannot hear?
3. In what circumstances might a doctor treat a patient before taking a history and performing an examination?
4. What does 'acopia' mean?
5. Why do most terminally unwell patients die in hospital?

Answers to questions are to be found in *Section 16.2*.

16.1 Introduction

There are some instances where the usual format of history, examination, investigations is not possible or not appropriate. If a history is not available, for example, the doctor must rely upon their ability to detect signs on examination to direct their investigations and diagnosis. Sometimes the doctor must become a detective in order to discover the medical issues affecting patients, and liaise with people from the wider multidisciplinary team.

Doctors never work in isolation; there are numerous allied healthcare professionals who provide invaluable assistance in complex clinical cases. Understanding the nature of each person's expertise is an important part of the doctor's responsibilities. The cases below illustrate how a collaborative approach to unusual clinical circumstances provides holistic, patient-centred healthcare.

Case 16.1 An agitated patient

Presentation

A 47-year-old patient is brought into the ED by the police, who found him acting strangely in the street. He is extremely agitated. He is shouting obscenities and paranoid ideas about being attacked by some unknown force. He accuses the police escort of stealing his thoughts with magic. He is physically lashing out, and requires four members of staff to restrain him from hurting himself or others.

Initial interpretation

The patient has an acute confusional state. Causes of this are divided into organic (conditions pertaining to altered or abnormal physiology, e.g. delirium), or psychiatric, such as acute psychosis. Organic causes should be sought and ruled out before an acute psychiatric condition is diagnosed, because organic causes are usually reversible if treated.

History and examination

The ED staff first attempt de-escalation. They move the patient to a quiet area with no people he might perceive as threatening, such as security guards. They speak to him in a calm manner, with no confrontational or aggressive body language.

> **Safety of healthcare workers is paramount when dealing with patients with aggressively disturbed behaviour.** De-escalation must not be attempted if there is a real chance of the doctor or nurse being harmed by the patient. If the patient presents a danger to themselves, other patients or hospital staff, then rapid tranquillisation is the safest treatment course.

Despite these measures, he remains extremely agitated and combative. He is screaming accusations that the doctors and police are trying to kill him. He refuses to believe that he is in a hospital despite repeated explanations, perceiving himself to be in a prison.

Further interpretation

The patient is exhibiting signs of acute behavioural disturbance (ABD). ABD is associated with abnormal behaviour and hyper-adrenergic autonomic response. Common features include:

- extremely aggressive behaviour
- acute psychosis
- apparent insensitivity to pain
- excessive sweating
- tachycardia and tachypnoea
- hyperthermia
- decreased response to chemical sedation
- excessive or 'superhuman' strength.

ABD is a medical emergency, as the patient is at risk of developing sudden haemodynamic collapse or even cardiac arrest. Improper restraint techniques contribute to patient injury or even asphyxia, and over-treatment with sedatives causes neurological and respiratory depression.

Immediate intervention

The ED consultant decides to treat him with rapid tranquillisation with benzodiazepines. She administers an intramuscular dose of lorazepam. The patient no longer presents a physical danger to himself or the hospital staff. They are able to nurse him in a hospital bed, and perform blood tests and a CT brain scan to rule out an organic cause of his behaviour. A urinary toxicology screen is negative for drugs of abuse. The nursing staff find a phone number for the patient's brother in his possessions, and he is able to confirm that the patient's name is Ashley, and that he has a diagnosis of schizophrenia. His family have been searching for him for 24 hours.

Differential diagnosis

Determining whether an episode of ABD is organic or psychiatric in nature is challenging. It should not be assumed that just because a patient has a pre-existing psychiatric diagnosis, the episode is psychiatric in origin.

Organic causes of an acute confusional state are the '4 Is': **I**nfection, **I**ntoxication (and withdrawal), brain **I**njury and **I**ctus (seizures).

Case 16.1 *continued*

Infection

In older people, infection of any body system may cause an acute delirium, as older people have less 'cognitive reserve', i.e. they have less resistance to physiological insult. This is because the brain undergoes certain age-related changes, such as small vessel ischaemia and generalised involutional changes. People of any age develop acute confusion in the presence of a CNS infection, such as viral encephalitis.

Intoxication

Recreational drugs are associated with abnormal cognition and behaviour. Drugs taken for their calming or tranquillising effects ('downers') include heroin / other opiates, benzodiazepines such as diazepam, cannabis and GHB. These cause a hypoactive, or stuporous state. Drugs taken for their stimulant properties ('uppers'), including Ecstasy, cocaine and amphetamines, can cause a hyperactive confusional state, as exhibited by this patient.

Withdrawal

Acute cessation of tranquillising drugs after a period of chronic use causes an agitated confusional state which is very similar to acute psychosis. This is seen in sudden withdrawal of alcohol, benzodiazepines and opiates.

Brain injury

In addition to CNS infection, acute concussion or any other process that alters the brain structure can lead to acute confusion. This includes intracranial haemorrhage, a brain tumour or hydrocephalus (accumulation of CSF in the brain's ventricles).

Ictus

'Ictus' means 'seizure', and the post-ictal phase is the minutes and hours following a seizure. Patients in the post-ictal phase often exhibit very abnormal behaviour and confusion, which is hypoactive or hyperactive in nature.

16.1.1 De-escalation

De-escalation is interacting with agitated patients to avoid conflict and restore a sense of calm, using verbal and non-verbal communication (**Figure 16.1**). It is an important method of averting violence, particular in clinical areas where tensions run high, such as the ED and acute psychiatric units.

Unlike chemical sedation or physical restraint, de-escalation does not have injurious side-effects, so it is the first tactic used with aggressive or angry patients. Effective de-escalation techniques include:

- speaking in a calm, level voice, even if the patient is shouting
- using non-threatening body language such as an open posture and non-confrontational eye contact
- moving into a quiet area
- using active listening skills, such as head nodding, sympathetic smiles, saying 'mm-hmm'
- acknowledging that the patient is upset and empathising
- apologising if they have a grievance about their healthcare
- ensuring there are no people present that could be perceived as threatening or aggressive, such as security officers.

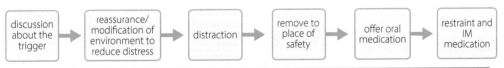

Figure 16.1 Management of agitation. Patients require close monitoring and continued discussion and reassurance.

Case 16.2 Suspicious bruising

Presentation

Mrs Hall is a 96-year-old patient who has been transferred to hospital from her care home with a UTI. Mrs Hall has severe Alzheimer's disease, and is bed-bound and non-communicative. Whilst examining Mrs Hall, her doctor notices excessive bruising to her upper arms and legs. Some of the bruises have the appearance of handprints.

Initial interpretation

Excessive bruising can be due to clotting disorders. Congenital clotting disorders (e.g. haemophilia), acquired disorders (e.g. idiopathic thrombocytopenic purpura or leukaemia), and iatrogenic problems (e.g. excessive anticoagulant medication) are all associated with bruising in the context of trivial or non-existent trauma. Absence of clotting disorders points to either sustained or repeated trauma, which demands further investigation.

History and examination

Close examination of Mrs Hall does not reveal any clinically evident bone fractures, and a phone call to the nursing home confirms that Mrs Hall does not walk and has not suffered any recent falls which might explain the bruising. Whilst she is unable to communicate, she seems to grimace in pain when the bruises are palpated.

Mrs Hall's doctor discusses the case with her consultant, who is similarly concerned about the bruises. They discuss the case with the ward sister, who decides to raise a safeguarding alert.

Further interpretation

It is difficult to assess pain and restricted movement with a patient who is unable to communicate. X-rays of any bruised or seemingly painful area will show any covert broken bones. Whilst communication with the care home is important, there needs to be a more comprehensive enquiry into how Mrs Hall sustained these injuries.

Immediate intervention

As a result of the safeguarding alert, a thorough investigation takes place at Mrs Hall's care home. It transpires that some of the healthcare assistants have been transferring Mrs Hall from her bed to the commode by gripping her arms and legs and lifting her. This is against NHS policy, which instructs carers to use a mechanical hoist to transfer dependent patients, in order to avoid injury.

The responsible carers are suspended during the investigation. They are eventually permitted to return to the care home, on the condition that they attend additional training in moving and handling, and caring for vulnerable patients.

16.1.2 Vulnerable adults

A vulnerable adult is one who is unable to independently take care of themselves and protect themselves from harm, neglect, exploitation or abuse. An adult is considered vulnerable if they:
- have an intellectual disability
- have a mental health disorder that limits their ability to function, such as schizophrenia
- are elderly and frail, with limited ability to carry out basic activities of daily living
- have dementia, or any chronic cognitive disability, e.g. brain injury

- are homeless
- abuse drugs or alcohol
- have a long-term health disorder that requires the assistance of daily carers.

Vulnerable adults are at particular risk of abuse, of which there are several forms (**Table 16.1**).

16.1.3 Safeguarding alerts

Safeguarding is about keeping vulnerable individuals safe from harm. Any medical professional can raise a safeguarding alert if they have concerns or suspicions that a vulnerable adult is being abused. An alert is raised by

Table 16.1 *Types of abuse, from which vulnerable adults require safeguarding*

Type of abuse	Features	Possible warning signs
Financial	Theft from patient Misuse or unauthorised use of funds and saving, arranging financial affairs without permission Coercing patient to give money or goods	Patient no longer has treasured possessions Patient no longer able to pay bills Patient has given bank card or details to another person
Physical	Assault Slapping, hitting, punching, twisting Physical restraints Administration of harmful or inappropriate medications	Unexplained bruising, fractures or other injuries Patient has reluctance to see a certain person, or exhibits fear in regard to certain person
Sexual	Non-consensual activity with a person for sexual gratification Indecent exposure to patient	Patient has reluctance to see a certain person, or exhibits fear in regard to certain person STI in vulnerable populations, e.g. children, frail patients Patient becomes withdrawn or shows personality changes
Psychological	Bullying Humiliation Taunting Verbal abuse Controlling or restrictive behaviour toward patient	Patient becomes emotionally labile, fearful or withdrawn Depression or anxiety Weight loss / poor nutrition
Neglect	Abuse by omission – withholding treatment or medications, obstructing access to healthcare Deliberately failing to meet nutritional needs Ignoring medical advice	Patient is unkempt Weight loss / poor nutrition Chronic illnesses showing no response to treatment Constant presence of dominant / controlling friend or relative during consultation

completing a form and sending it to the safeguarding officer for the hospital, Trust or GP surgery. This alert instigates a multi-agency investigation of the patient's circumstances. Whilst a safeguarding investigation is being carried out, the patient must remain in a place of safety, which is usually a hospital bed. Investigation of a safeguarding alert is usually completed within a few days.

Case 16.3 A frail patient

Presentation

Mr Roberts is 80 years old. At 2am, Mr Roberts attempts to get out of bed to go to the toilet, but falls over his walking frame. He is unable to get up off the floor due to leg weakness. He is unable to call for help, as his only telephone is downstairs. He is discovered by his daughter when she visits him 12 hours later, still lying on the floor. He has been incontinent of urine and is in significant pain and distress. She calls an ambulance, which brings Mr Roberts into the local hospital.

Initial interpretation

Falls in elderly patients are common. There is no key element of Mr Roberts' history thus far that explains why he fell. Patients who lie on a hard surface for more than two hours are at risk of developing pressure areas, breakdown of skeletal muscle (rhabdomyolysis), dehydration and hypothermia, so a more comprehensive assessment of Mr Roberts is required.

History and examination

The acute medicine team assess Mr Roberts in the ED. They perform an X-ray of his pelvis to ensure that he has not fractured his hip. They perform blood tests to rule out an infection, and an ECG to rule out arrhythmias which could have contributed to his fall. As they find no acute medical pathology, they refer Mr Roberts to a geriatrician who specialises in frailty.

The doctor takes a comprehensive history from Mr Roberts, and learns that he has been falling with increasing frequency over the last few months, but has not mentioned it to anyone

for fear of 'being put in a home'. He finds cooking quite exhausting, and often skips meals. Mr Roberts explains that his legs sometimes give way, and whilst he is usually able to pull himself back to standing position, this time he simply didn't have the strength. Dr Ravi notes that Mr Roberts is very thin, with little muscle mass. He performs a lying / standing BP, which reveals a postural drop of 30mmHg.

Further interpretation

This orthostatic hypotension contributes to Mr Roberts' falls by making him experience light-headedness and poor balance whilst in the standing position. His low body mass and undernourished state had led to a state of sarcopenia: decreased muscle mass. This contributes to Mr Roberts' perception of his legs giving way following prolonged standing, and his inability to raise himself from the floor following a fall.

Immediate intervention

Mr Roberts' doctor decides to stop his antihypertensive medication, which is exacerbating his postural hypotension. Mr Roberts is assessed by the occupational therapists and physiotherapists, who carry out a home visit with Mr Roberts. They feel that he would be safe to return home with a package of care: twice-daily carers to visit him to ensure that he is able to eat a proper meal, help him get washed and dressed safely, and ensure that he is safe from falls. They give him a pendant alarm to wear around his neck, to press if he does fall again and is unable to get up.

16.1.4 Frailty

Frailty is a health state of the ageing body, signifying its gradual loss of the inbuilt reserves that protect one from ill health. An illness event that would cause only minor problems for a younger patient, such as an infection or an MSK

injury, has severe effects on a frail patient. Some of the physical manifestations of frailty are:
- progressive unintentional weight loss
- decreased exercise tolerance and general fatigue
- minimal physical activity

- decreased strength and reduced muscle mass (sarcopenia).

Frail people are at greater risk of:
- falls
- fractures, especially neck of femur fractures
- delirium
- infections
- depression and social isolation.

Management

When a patient is identified as frail, the multidisciplinary team (MDT) takes a holistic approach to maximising the patient's quality of life and maintaining their good health (**Table 16.2**). Whilst the MDT is common to all aspects of modern medical care, the team plays a particularly crucial role in geriatric medicine. This is because much of the care of older patients focuses on maintaining independence and mobility, which often requires adaptations to their living environment, and preventing illness and harm, such as falls.

Table 16.2 *Members of the MDT (in addition to 'doctor' and 'nurse')*

Member	Role
Healthcare assistant	Cares for the daily needs of the patient, including toileting, eating and drinking, and performs basic nursing duties, such as measuring vital signs
Physiotherapist	Cares for patients with regard to mobility, movement and maintaining independence
Occupational therapist	Assesses and adapts the patient's home environment and daily activities to maximise quality of life and health status
Speech and language therapist	Works with patients who have problems with swallowing or communication to maintain adequate and safe nutrition, and helps them engage in the world around them
Social worker	Responsible for patients' needs in regard to welfare support, social care needs and living environments
Dietitian	Ensures that patients are obtaining the optimal nutrition for their health needs
Pharmacist	Regulates the medications patients receive, ensures they don't come to inadvertent harm from medication errors, educates patients about their prescriptions to improve compliance and dispenses medications safely
Physician associate	These professionals from a medical science background perform many of the tasks of the physician and work as part of the general medicine team
Other	
Clinical psychologist	Helps patients with the psychological demands of ill health, such as major surgery / transplantation
Independent mental capacity advocate (IMCA)	Practitioners who act as advocates for patients who do not have the mental capacity or ability to make informed decisions about their healthcare

Case 16.4   End of life care

Presentation

Diana is a 59-year-old female with metastatic breast cancer. She presents to hospital with pneumonia, having completed her most recent cycle of chemotherapy. She has severe bone pain from her bone metastases, and experiences nausea and constipation due to her opiate medication. Her breathing has deteriorated to the point where she requires oxygen to breathe comfortably.

Initial interpretation

It is important to establish Diana's priorities at this point. Her pneumonia is a potentially reversible cause of her current health condition, and antibiotics may well improve her condition enough to re-engage with her cancer treatment. Her diagnosis of advanced cancer and her immunosuppressive treatment with chemotherapy mean that Diana will find it much more difficult to overcome a bout of pneumonia than other patients.

History and examination

Her nurse, Anna, spends some time with Diana, and discovers that Diana does not feel up to another round of chemotherapy. She wants to enjoy the remaining time she has left, spending it with her family.

David, a palliative care nurse, sits with Diana and her husband. Diana explains that she is desperate for her pain and nausea to improve, so that she can sit up in bed, have visitors, and enjoy some food and a cup of tea now and then. She understands that she has a terminal diagnosis, and that any further treatment would be for the purpose of extending her life by months, at best. Diana would like to stop chemotherapy and expresses the desire to die at home rather than the hospital, surrounded by her family and a familiar environment. Her husband supports this decision, but is worried that he will not know how to look after her properly at home without help.

Further interpretation

Diana is in the final stages of her life. She has made an informed and balanced decision about her preferred end of life care. These decisions are very difficult for patients. Relatives also find them very upsetting. Palliative care teams help gather information for the patient, and communicate with patients how they are supported throughout the process. For example, community palliative care teams could visit Diana regularly at home and assist her husband with giving medication and help Diana with her basic needs, such as washing and toileting.

Immediate intervention

Unfortunately, Diana's need for oxygen does not improve, and she becomes increasingly frail. It becomes apparent that transferring her home for end of life care will not be feasible, as she requires regular nursing, constant adjustment of her pain medications, and oxygen therapy. Diana decides that she would prefer to transfer to her local hospice, where her medical, psychological and emotional needs will be met.

At the hospice, the palliative care team give Diana a constant infusion of opiates and anti-sickness medication, which vastly improves her symptoms. She is able to sit up in bed and enjoy visits from her grandchildren. As her status deteriorates, the hospice team give her small doses of midazolam (a benzodiazepine) to treat her agitation and anxiety. She eventually passes away peacefully with her family at her bedside, exactly as she hoped.

16.1.5   Palliative care

Palliative care is the branch of medicine dedicated to treating patients with life-limiting disease, and with chronic health conditions that cause severe disability. Rather than focus on curative treatment, palliation focuses on symptom management and maximising the quality of life within the context of an incurable disease.

The transition from usual medical care to palliation is problematic, as many patients feel that by agreeing to palliative care, they are being 'doomed' to die and that all hope is lost. Careful communication helps the patient understand that palliation is a different approach to treatment, not a sign of surrender.

Palliative care doctors look after patients with many conditions, such as cancer, chronic organ failure and progressive neurodegenerative diseases, but there are several symptoms that are common to most palliative care patients (**Table 16.3**).

Table 16.3 *Common symptoms experienced by patients at the end of life, that are addressed by palliative care*

Symptom	Potential causes	Treatment options
Pain	MSK pain due to prolonged immobility	Appropriate analgesia
	Large tumours causing mass effect	Debulking surgery Localised radiotherapy Opiate analgesia
	Metastatic cancer, e.g. to bones causing bony pain	Opiate analgesia
	Neuropathic pain due to neurological disorders	Appropriate analgesia
Breathlessness	Respiratory disease, e.g. lung cancer, end-stage COPD, end-stage fibrosis	Oxygen Fan (blowing air onto the face can relieve symptoms of breathlessness)
	End-stage heart failure	Diuretics
	Gradual multi-organ failure as patient approaches death	Low dose morphine relieves feelings of breathlessness
Nausea	Medication, such as opiates	Anti-emetics
	Obstruction of GI tract due to tumour (usually associated with vomiting)	Palliative stenting
	Loss of appetite due to severe organ failure	Anti-emetics Nil by mouth
Constipation	Medication, such as opiates	Laxative
	Obstruction of GI tract due to tumour	Laxatives, stenting if appropriate
	Immobility	Fluid hydration
Agitation	Fear of prognosis or loss of function / independence	Reassurance
	'Terminal agitation' is associated with fluctuating delirium and personality changes, and is seen at the very final stages of dying	Anxiolytics (benzodiazepines)
Secretions	Poor cough, leading to accumulation of airway secretions and a sensation of drowning	Regular airway suction
		Anti-secretory medication, e.g. hyoscine

Case 16.5 Perioperative medicine

Presentation

Mr Mohammed is an 88-year-old man who lives with his family. He has a past medical history of AF, heart failure and asthma. His chronic breathlessness makes walking a difficult process, and one morning he trips and falls, sustaining a fracture of his left femoral neck. He is quickly transferred to hospital for urgent orthopaedic intervention.

Initial interpretation

A fractured neck of femur is a common emergency in older adults. Mr Mohammed requires urgent surgery to repair the break. This is major surgery, usually involving a general anaesthetic, and Mr Mohammed's age and co-morbidities place him at a higher risk of perioperative complications.

History and examination

Two days after his surgery, doctors review Mr Mohammed once more on the orthopaedic ward. The surgeons are worried that Mr Mohammed is not making good progress with the physiotherapists, and seems more short of breath

than usual. On examination Mr Mohammed is hypoxic with saturations of 90% on room air, a resting tachycardia of 120bpm, a respiratory rate of 28 breaths per minute, and a blood pressure of 140/92mmHg. On auscultation of the chest there are bilateral crackles, and there is pitting oedema of the lower limbs and sacrum. The JVP is elevated.

Further interpretation

Mr Mohammed has unfortunately developed decompensated heart failure following his surgery. Potential causes include aggressive IV fluid therapy, omission of usual diuretic therapy due to vomiting or drowsiness, or acute cardiac problems, such as arrhythmia or ACS. It is not clear whether his fast AF is a consequence or a precipitant of his acute cardiac failure.

Immediate intervention

Mr Mohammed receives intravenous diuretics (furosemide) to improve his peripheral and pulmonary oedema, and oxygen to improve his hypoxia. He is given a beta blocker and higher dose of oral digoxin to reduce his heart rate to a normal level (<100bpm).

16.1.6 Perioperative medicine

Orthogeriatricians are specialists who see older patients undergoing emergency orthopaedic surgery, and perioperative medicine has emerged as a new subspecialty within medicine in recent years. Whilst surgeons bring their technical expertise to the operating theatre, there is evidence that medical complications of surgery are best treated by physicians.

One role of the perioperative physician is to make a careful assessment of the patient prior to

surgery and to improve their medical condition as best they can. This includes:

- treating acute organ failure, such as acute heart failure
- optimising chronic organ problems, such as CKD
- treating infection
- ensuring the patient is adequately hydrated.

Perioperative physicians review patients after surgery, and monitor them for any of the common medical complications of surgery (**Table 16.4**).

Table 16.4 *Common postoperative medical problems*

Complication	Symptoms	Signs	Cause	Management plan
Pulmonary embolism	Breathlessness Pleuritic chest pain	Hypoxia Tachycardia	Hypercoagulable postoperative state	Anticoagulation Oxygen
Heart failure	Breathlessness	Peripheral oedema Raised JVP Crackles on chest	Excessive IV fluids Perioperative MI Arrhythmia	Diuretics Oxygen
Arrhythmia	Palpitations Syncope	Tachy- or bradycardia Hypotension if severe	Perioperative MI Electrolyte abnormality	Correct cause Control rate
Delirium	Fluctuation, confusion and mental clouding	Disorientation Hypoactive or hyperactive behaviour	Physiological stress of surgery Infection Hypoxia Uncontrolled pain Postoperative constipation Excessive analgesia	Correct cause
Loss of function	Inability to perform usual tasks of daily living Poor mobility Decreased confidence following illness and surgery		Decreased confidence following illness and surgery Pain Physically limited e.g. by plaster cast	MDT approach to supporting patient in their own environment

Case 16.6 Patients with learning disability

Presentation

A doctor in a GP practice is due to see Kevin, who is a 32-year-old man with learning difficulties. He is attending for an asthma review. The doctor is aware that Kevin has previously seen his GP colleague, and it was a very difficult consultation. Kevin became quite frustrated and angry, and walked out of the GP surgery before finishing the consultation. The doctor has decided to ask Kevin's support worker Dave to come to the consultation.

Initial interpretation

Triadic communication (involving three people rather than two) is a useful tool when treating these patients, much as is used with a child patient and their parent. The presence of a familiar and non-threatening person helps negate feelings of fear and mistrust. This sort of consultation takes much longer than usual, and longer time slots must be allotted for them.

History and examination

When Kevin first comes in he seems sullen and withdrawn. The doctor asks his permission to speak about his asthma in front of Dave, and Kevin agrees. Dave knows Kevin very well, and explains to Dr Sharma that Kevin sometimes struggles to express himself clearly, which makes him angry and stressed. He is also quite frightened of doctors and nurses, and has a fear that they are going to 'give him an injection'. The doctor is sympathetic, and promises Kevin that there will be no injections today.

Further interpretation

It is important that patients with an intellectual disability are treated with dignity and afforded the usual autonomy and confidentiality that any other patient is given. Interactions must be slow and comprehensible, so it is important to allow extra time for these consultations; being rushed or hurried is often a frightening experience. Any physical examination should be introduced, explained and, if possible, demonstrated before being performed on the patient.

Immediate intervention

Whilst Dave often helps Kevin answer questions by prompting and encouraging him, the doctor is careful to speak directly to Kevin himself. He keeps his body language and tone calm and non-threatening. He shows him how to perform a peak flow measurement, first by demonstrating it with Dave. He asks him questions about his inhalers, and asks Kevin to show him how he uses his inhaler. He congratulates him on his technique and shows him a spacer device, explaining that it helps get the inhaler medicine into his lungs. Kevin doesn't like it, but allows Dave to keep it to discuss it with him at a later date.

16.1.7 Disabilities, difficulties and disorders

There are multiple terms used to describe patients with learning difficulties and learning disorders. The term 'learning disability' indicates an intellectual impairment that usually limits the patient's ability to cope independently and maintain their own safety. The term 'learning difficulties' (sometimes termed 'learning disorder') describes an obstacle to learning, that requires dedicated attention on the part of the teacher and the learner. Learning disabilities are lifelong and start in childhood. They are associated with other disorders such as Down syndrome, or are idiopathic.

Triadic consultations are the mainstay of paediatrics, where much of the child's history comes from a parent, and instructions from the doctor often require the parent's encouragement before the shy child complies.

They are also used when working with an

interpreter – an increasingly common occurrence in modern medicine. When working with an interpreter, remember:

- Speak directly to the patient. The doctor and interpreter should not converse with each other and refer to the patient in the third person, as this makes the patient feel very excluded and inhibited.
- Use short sentences. Interpreters are not merely translating word for word, they are adjusting phrases to better align with the cultural norms of the patient. Asking them to translate large blocks of information at a time is unfair, and will lead to communication errors.
- Be sensitive to the interpreter's impressions. They will be able to better detect and interpret the patient's non-verbal communication. They usually notice when the patient seems confused or uncertain.

Case 16.7 Patients with no history

Presentation

An elderly woman is brought into the ED. She was found wandering the streets, confused and disoriented, by a member of the public. She states that her name is Vera Morgan, but is unable to recall her address or any other personal information. She is fearful and distressed. The first person to see Mrs Morgan is Ana Maria, a nurse in the ED. She brings Mrs Morgan a cup of tea and tries to soothe her whilst recording her baseline observations. She records a normal blood pressure, heart rate, respiratory rate and temperature.

Initial interpretation

It is not certain from initial assessment whether Mrs Morgan has an acute delirium, or if her behaviour is part of a chronic dementia. Whilst a clear history is not possible, a basic examination seems reassuring. No matter what the true diagnosis is, Mrs Morgan is obviously in need of reassurance and comfort.

History and examination

Ana Maria discusses the case with the ED doctor, and they try to find out who Mrs Morgan is, and what has happened to her. First, the doctor checks the hospital records to see whether anyone by the name Vera Morgan has been admitted to the hospital before. He finds two entries: one was a 46-year-old woman, and one was a 79-year-old woman. Investigation of the second entry reveals that a 79-year-old woman called Vera Morgan attended the outpatient phlebotomy department for some blood tests 4 years ago. Fortunately the electronic notes list the patient's GP, and a quick phone call to the surgery reveals that Mrs Morgan is a patient with vascular dementia who lives alone, and has previously managed to live safely at home with regular visits from her family. Her next of kin is her son.

Further interpretation

Traditionally, assessment of patients like Mrs Morgan has been challenging. The advent of electronic health records has changed this markedly. It allows doctors to instantly review documentation from hospital admissions and outpatient clinics, and access blood results and imaging from many years ago. This is a very useful tool, allowing you to fully appraise yourself of any patient's care to date.

Immediate intervention

Ana Maria calls Mrs Morgan's son Philip, who was due to visit his mother today. He explains that she has become prone to wandering out of the house during recent days, and that her confusion is much worse than usual. The doctor tests Mrs Morgan's urine and finds evidence of a UTI, which he treats with a course of oral antibiotics.

The hospital team carries out an MDT assessment, and after 3 days Mrs Morgan is able to return home with plans for a carer to visit her three times per day to ensure her safety.

Case 16.7 *continued*

Differential diagnosis

There are different causes of dementia, but these causes are not usually distinguishable from the history and examination (**Table 16.5**). Patients with dementia are vulnerable adults. Their diminished cognitive reserve makes them readily susceptible to delirium (i.e. they are frail). Delirium manifests as an acute deterioration in their mental status, worse than their normal cognitive baseline. A full list of precipitants of delirium is explored in *Section 12.3.7*.

When meeting a patient for the first time, it is difficult to know whether a patient has dementia or delirium. A collateral history is the only way of differentiating between the two.

> **When a patient can't give a history, the collateral history is paramount.** This is a history 'by proxy', given by someone who knows the patient well. A collateral history can be obtained from another healthcare professional, such as the patient's GP or caregiver, or from a family member or close friend. Computerised records and review of previous blood and imaging results also provide insights into the patient's history.

Table 16.5 *Subtypes of dementia*

Name	Pathology	Features	Treatment options
Alzheimer's disease	Atrophy of cerebrum, with development of amyloid plaques and neurofibrillary tangles	Begins as short-term memory problems, and progresses to degeneration of self-care, speech and higher cognitive function	Acetylcholinesterase inhibitors (e.g. donepezil) and NMDA receptor antagonists (e.g. memantine) slow progression of disease and ameliorate symptoms but strong evidence is lacking
Vascular dementia	Chronic ischaemic changes and multi-infarcts in the brain	History of stroke Stepwise decline in cognitive function	Optimise vascular risk factors, e.g. aspirin, statin
Frontotemporal dementia	Frontotemporal lobar degeneration	Personality changes and loss of inhibition Problems with language comprehension and expression	Mainly supportive SSRI antidepressants may help with blunting of emotion or severe apathy
Dementia with Lewy bodies	Cerebral accumulation of Lewy body (proteinous material)	Hallucinations, occasionally psychosis Parkinsonism	Parkinsonian features – dopamine therapy Antipsychotics if appropriate

Case 16.8 Multiple co-morbidities

Presentation

Mrs Phipps is a 73-year-old patient who has come to the geriatric outpatient clinic. She was discharged from hospital 6 weeks ago following a 4-day inpatient stay for pneumonia. She has type 2 diabetes, hypertension, previous breast cancer, osteoarthritis, kyphosis due to degenerative spine disease, and mild heart failure. She has previously had a coronary artery bypass graft (CABG) for severe coronary disease, and suffered a small stroke several years ago, which has left her with a mild left-sided weakness. She is an ex-smoker of 25 years, and has a 40 pack year history. Her GP is concerned about her decreasing exercise tolerance, which Mrs Phipps blames on breathlessness and pain in her knees.

Initial interpretation

Mrs Phipps has many potential causes of her symptoms. The pain in her knees is likely due to osteoarthritis. She may have undetected heart failure, and her breathlessness is a manifestation of pulmonary oedema. Her spine kyphosis is causing restriction to her lung function. She has either non-resolving pneumonia, or a recurrence of infection. Her smoking history raises the possibility of COPD. We should consider a 'silent' MI during her recent hospital admission: pneumonia is a big physiological stressor that impairs coronary perfusion, and patients with diabetes do not always experience chest pain during an MI.

History and examination

Susan, the doctor working in the geriatric clinic, establishes that Mrs Phipps has experienced breathlessness on exertion for many years, but has always managed to carry on with her normal life. Recently, the breathlessness has become oppressive and debilitating, and she is now struggling to walk to her local shops, which are only 100 metres from her home.

The clinical examination reveals normal O_2 saturations on air at rest, but a slight expiratory wheeze in the upper lung zones. There is mild pitting oedema to the level of the ankles, and Mrs Phipps' chest X-ray is clear. Susan performs lung function testing (spirometry) which shows an obstructive lung defect. There are no effusions in the knee joints, and an X-ray reveals arthritic changes. Mrs Phipps' blood tests show mild CKD.

Further interpretation

An obstructive lung defect indicates small airways disease. By contrast, lung restriction due to kyphosis would produce a restrictive spirometry result. The absence of significant ankle oedema, orthopnoea and PND makes CCF unlikely. This information, together with the wheeze and the smoking history, confirms Susan's suspicion of undiagnosed COPD.

Her CKD is probably due to both diabetes and hypertension. Susan must take a drug history to ensure that Mrs Phipps is not taking any nephrotoxic medications, or drugs that require a lower dose in CKD.

Immediate intervention

Susan prescribes Mrs Phipps inhalers to help her breathlessness. She requests an echocardiogram to evaluate Mrs Phipps' heart function – this will reveal if the mild ankle oedema is due to right heart failure secondary to untreated chronic lung disease (cor pulmonale). She changes Mrs Phipps' antihypertensive amlodipine (a CCB that causes ankle oedema as a common side-effect) to ramipril (an ACE inhibitor), with a plan to recheck her kidney function in one week.

She asks Mrs Phipps to stop taking ibuprofen for her knee pain, as NSAIDs worsen kidney disease. Instead, she prescribes regular paracetamol and a weak opiate.

Case 16.8 *continued*

Differential diagnosis

As patients are living longer, it is increasingly common for older patients to have a long list of co-morbidities, which interact in many ways. These interactions mean that it is rare for these patients to present with merely one problem. One of the inevitable effects of multi-morbidity is polypharmacy – prescription of several medications. Patients dislike swallowing multiple pills every day, and often get mixed up about which pill to take at what time. Patients are less likely to be compliant with polypharmacy, which leads to worsening of chronic health issues. The problem is compounded when patients see different specialists for their various conditions, as each specialist prescribes in isolation. It takes a generalist such as a GP or a geriatrician to rationalise a medication list in order to reduce the amount of drugs to an absolute minimum to keep the patient healthy.

> **Multi-morbidity is not solely a burden of the elderly.** Patients with psychiatric illness often have multi-morbidity, due to self-neglect, engaging in harmful behaviours such as smoking, excessive alcohol or using recreational drugs, and side-effects from powerful psychotropic medications (see *Table 12.10*). It is estimated that individual homeless patients have between six and eight medical conditions, which are often untreated due to a lack of health-seeking behaviour and difficulty in accessing healthcare services. This is reflected in their very poor life expectancy: usually late forties to early fifties.

16.2 Answers to starter questions

1. A common scenario in healthcare is a patient who speaks little or no English. Many patients bring friends or family members to their consultations to act as interpreters. This is not best practice, as there are inherent biases and conflicts of interests. Interpreters (available to all medical centres in the UK) should be booked in advance for any interaction with a language barrier. There are also telephone services for healthcare professionals that instantly connect clinicians to interpreters of any language.

2. Patients with profound deafness often lip-read to some degree but it is better to book a professional sign language interpreter for these consultations. Alternatively, using simple pen and paper is often sufficient to communicate, and many hospitals and clinics have small whiteboards and pens for this purpose.

    Patients who have had a laryngectomy often use a digital voice device, which is a small microphone pressed against the neck as they mime speech.

    Patients in severe pain, such as those suffering trauma or kidney stones, often can't give a coherent history or participate in a clinical examination until they receive analgesia, such as morphine.

3. Recent advances in sepsis recognition and management have led to protocols that facilitate rapid administration of life-saving treatments, including antibiotics and IV fluids. These treatments are given by a triaging nurse or a paramedic before the patient sees a doctor, leading to improved sepsis survival rates.

4. 'Acopia' is a common shorthand seen in medical notes to denote 'inability to cope'. It is rather a derogatory term which should be avoided. It does not capture the complex interaction between patient and environment which results in a patient's difficulty in keeping themselves safe and healthy, and instead implies a failure on the part of the patient.

5. Most people would prefer to die at home, yet the overwhelming majority die in hospital. The UK healthcare system has traditionally struggled to support terminally unwell patients in their own home if they require intensive nursing, regular medication, feeding and oxygen. Community palliative care programmes have made great inroads in improving this.

    If a patient has a terminal diagnosis, such as metastatic cancer, discussions about end of life care should take place early to determine the patient's preferences.

Appendix
Figure acknowledgements

Clinical photographs are © Sam Scott-Hunter, except where indicated below.

Figure 2.3 James Pollitt

Figure 3.5 Adapted from image at https://www.toraks.org.tr/halk/News.aspx?detail=2793

Figure 4.6 James Pollitt

Figure 4.8 Reproduced from www.footiq.com

Figure 4.9 Licensed under: Public domain
Available at: http://commons.wikimedia.org/wiki/File:Splinter_hemorrhage.jpg

Figure 4.10 Reproduced under a Creative Commons Attribution-Share Alike 4.0 International Licence
Available at: https://flic.kr/p/e8SkaN

Figure 4.11 Reproduced under a Creative Commons Attribution 2.0 Generic Licence. © 2008 Zech and
Hoeg, licensee BioMed Central Ltd.
Available at: https://commons.wikimedia.org/wiki/File:Four_representative_slides_of_corneal_arcus.jpg

Figure 4.12 Reproduced under a Creative Commons Attribution 3.0 Germany licence.
Author: Klaus D. Peter, Gummersbach, Germany

Figure 4.15 Reproduced from Morris, P., Warriner, D. and Morton, A. (2015) *Eureka: Cardiovascular
Medicine*. JP Medical Publishers.

Figure 5.7 From the authors' collection

Figure 5.11 James Pollitt

Figure 6.5 Licensed under: Public domain
CDC/Dr Thomas F. Sellers/Emory University

Figure 6.7 Reproduced from https://healthool.com/palmar-erythema

Figure 6.8 Licensed under: Public domain
Author: Londonsista

Figure 6.10 From the authors' collection

Figure 8.6 Licensed under: Public domain
Author: Lily Chu, National Naval Medical Center, Bethesda, MD.
Available at https://upload.wikimedia.org/wikipedia/commons/3/30/Paget_Disease_of_the_Nipple.jpg

Figure 8.11 Reproduced under a Creative Commons Attribution-Share Alike 3.0 Unported Licence.
Available at https://commons.wikimedia.org/wiki/File:Melasmablemish.jpg. User: Elord.

Figure 9.10 Reproduced from Collins, D., Goodfellow, J.A., Silva, A.H. *et al.* (2018) *Eureka: Neurology &
Neurosurgery*. JP Medical Publishers.

Figure 10.8 Reproduced under a Creative Commons Attribution-Share Alike 3.0 Unported Licence. Available at https://commons.wikimedia.org/wiki/File:Snellen_chart.svg

Figure 11.3 Reproduced from Dogra, A. and Arora, A.K. (2014) Nail psoriasis: the journey so far. *Indian Journal of Dermatology*, **59(4):** 319–333. www.e-ijd.org

Figure 12.3 Reproduced from Fenton, F., Lodge, K-M. and Henderson, J. (2016) *Eureka: Psychiatry*. JP Medical Publishers.

Figure 12.5 Reproduced from Fenton, F., Lodge, K-M. and Henderson, J. (2016) *Eureka: Psychiatry*. JP Medical Publishers.

Figure 13.7 James Pollitt

Figure 13.8 James Pollitt

Figure 13.9 Reproduced from Fox, T., Brooke, A. and Vaidya, B. (2015) *Eureka: Endocrinology*. JP Medical Publishers.

Figure 13.10 Reproduced from Fox, T., Brooke, A. and Vaidya, B. (2015) *Eureka: Endocrinology*. JP Medical Publishers.

Figure 13.12 Reproduced from Fox, T., Brooke, A. and Vaidya, B. (2015) *Eureka: Endocrinology*. JP Medical Publishers.

Figure 14.2 Main picture reproduced under a Creative Commons Attribution 3.0 Unported Licence. Attribution: Biswarup Ganguly. Available at https://commons.wikimedia.org/wiki/File:Vicki_Pandit_-_Howrah_2014-04-06_9845.JPG. Parts (a)–(d) reproduced from https://healthlifemag.com

Figure 14.5a Reproduced under a Creative Commons Attribution-Share Alike 3.0 Unported Licence. Available at https://commons.wikimedia.org/wiki/File:Boy_with_Down_Syndrome.JPG. Author: Vanellus Foto.

Figure 14.5b Reproduced from www.reddit.com/r/WTF/comments/19w7xe/turners_syndrome/

Index

Abdominal distension, 153, 198–9
Abdominal pain, 137–9, 165–6, 359
Abdominal scars, 151, 176
Abducens nerve, 251, 253, 262, 267
Abuse, 399
Acanthosis nigricans, 53, 152, 201
Accessory nerve, 252, 253, 263, 269
Accommodation, 264
Achalasia, 130, 131, 141
Acromegaly, 47, 330, 344, 345, 351
Active listening, 8
Acute behavioural disturbance, 396
Acute coronary syndrome (ACS), 68, 71
Acute kidney injury, 163
Addison's disease, 333, 337
Adrenal gland, 331–3
Adrenal insufficiency, *see* Hypocortisolism
Affect, 322–3
Agitation, 384, 396–7, 403
Airway, 382–3
    adjuncts, 383
Alcohol, 14, 81, 147, 171, 204, 232, 261, 286, 320
    in pregnancy, 211
    withdrawal, 311, 315
Aldosterone, 330, 332, 333
Alopecia, 288
Alveoli, 103
Amenorrhoea, 195
Anaemia
    iron deficiency, 28, 131, 141–2, 144, 150, 151,
        158, 201, 206
    B12 deficiency, 42, 51, 142, 228, 325
    folate deficiency, 42, 142, 326
Anal fissure, 133, 144
Anaphylaxis, 357

Angina
    definition, 68
    unstable, 68
Angiotensin, 333
Anisocoria, 270
Ankle brachial pressure index (ABPI), 96
Ankyloglossia, 365
Ankylosing spondylitis, 281, 289, 299
Anorexia nervosa, *see* Eating disorders
Antepartum haemorrhage, 203–4
Anterior drawer test, 297
Antidiuretic hormone (ADH), 330
Anxiety, 312–14
Aorta, 64
    dissection, 69
Aortic regurgitation, 86
Aortic stenosis, 87, 355
Apex beat, 86, 91, 118, 122
Appendicitis, 359
Archetypes, 20, 22
Arrhythmia, 69, 71–2, 74, 405
Arterioles, 65–6
Arthralgia, 282, 359
Ascites, 149, 153, 156, 199
Aspiration pneumonia, 259
Asthma, 107, 108, 109, 114, 120, 357
Asterixis, *see* Flap
Ataxia, 231, 245
Atherosclerosis, 66
Atrial fibrillation, 71–2, 73, 85, 90
Atrial flutter, 71–2, 73, 85
Atrial septal defect, 355
Atrioventricular node, 67
Attire, 4–6
Auscultation, 57, 59

Autoimmune hepatitis, *see* Hepatitis
Autonomic nervous system, 215
Avascular necrosis, 360
AVPU scale, 386, 387

Babinski's sign, *see* Plantar response
Bad news, *see* Breaking bad news
Baker's cyst, 291
Balance, *see* Coordination
Barlow's test, 366
Barrett's oesophagus, 131
Bell's palsy, 259, 273
Bipolar affective disorder (BAD), 309
Bitemporal hemianopia, 257
Bladder, 164
Blindness, *see* Visual impairment
Blood pressure, 68
    measurement, 38–40
Body hair, 56
Bone, 277–8, 282
Bone marrow, 277
Bone remodelling, 278
Bouchard's nodes, 288
Boutonnière deformity, 287, 288
Bowel habit, 139–40
Brachial plexus trauma, 363
Bradycardia, *see* Heart rate
Bradypnoea, *see* Respiratory rate
Brain, 215–17
Brainstem, 217, 252
Breaking bad news, 15–17
Breast, 183–4
    cyst, 189
    examination, 191–3
    masses, 188, 193
    pain, 190
    scars, 191
Breath sounds, 119, 123
Breathlessness, 77, 106–8, 403
Bronchiectasis, 107, 108, 109
Brudzinski's sign, 369, 370
Bruising, 149, 151, 398
Bruits, 87, 93, 349
Buerger's test, 95
Bulimia nervosa, *see* Eating disorders
Butterfly rash, 289

Cancer
    breast, 189–90
    colorectal, 133, 142, 144
    endometrial, 196, 199, 210
    lung, 107, 108, 109, 110, 126
    oesophageal, 143
    ovarian, 198, 210
    renal, 168
    stomach, 143
Capacity, 306, 375–6
Capillary refill time, 83, 94, 116, 384, 385, 386
Caput medusa, 151
Cardiotocography, 210
Care package, 400
Carotid pulse
    palpation, 44
Carpal tunnel syndrome, 283
Cartilage, 278–9
Cataract, 256
Catecholamines, 333
Cellulitis, 75–7
Central nervous system (CNS), 215, 216, 303
Central retinal artery occlusion, 257, 271
Central retinal vein occlusion, 257, 271
Cerebellum, 226, 260
    dysfunction, 245
Cerebrospinal fluid, 247
Cerebrum, 217
Cervical smear, 209, 210
Cervical spine injury, 381, 389
Cervical spine isolation, 381
Cervix, 184, 202
    ectropion, 196
    polyp, 196
Chaperone, 6, 11, 37, 60, 158, 176, 192
Charcot's arthropathy, 350
Chest expansion, 118, 122
    hyperexpansion, 117
Chest pain, 68–70, 72
Chickenpox, 358
Chondrocalcinosis, *see* Pseudogout
Chorea, 237
Chronic fatigue syndrome, 284
Chronic kidney disease (CKD), 89, 163–7, 179, 261, 409
Chronic liver disease, 135–6, 149, 158
Chronic obstructive pulmonary disease (COPD), 107, 108, 109, 114, 120, 126

Chvostek's sign, 345
Ciliary muscles, 251
Claudication, 78–9
Clubbing, 41–2, 116, 150
Coagulopathy, 135, 398
Coarctation of the aorta, 85–6
Coeliac disease, 130
Cognitive behavioural therapy (CBT), 305–6
Cognitive bias, 25
Cognitive disorders, 223, 227
Cognitive function, 220, 223, 246, 324
Colic, 137, 138
    renal, 166
Colitis, 131, 133
Collapse, 73
Collateral history, 408
Collateral ligaments, 297, 298
Colour vision, 266
Communication skills, 3, 6–8, 11, 355–6
    cultural awareness, 8
    difficulties, 9–10
    jargon, 11, 14
    non-verbal, 7–8
Computed tomography (CT), 125, 157, 178, 247,
    272, 298, 325, 390
Confidentiality, 15, 30
Confusion, 314, 407
Congenital hip dysplasia, 359
Conjunctiva, 46, 84, 117, 173, 270
Conn's syndrome, 333
Consanguinity, 362
Consent, 36, 356
Constipation, 140, 341, 359, 403
Consultation room, 6
Contraception, 200
Coordination, 266–7, 244, 245, 260
Cor pulmonale, 112, 120, 126
Cornea, 256
Corneal arcus, 84, 91
Corneal reflex, 267
Coronary heart disease (CHD), 61, 64, 68, 69, 75,
    82, 87, 97, 337
Cortisol, 330, 331–3
Cough, 20, 69, 74, 109, 268, 356, 357
Crackles, 88, 119
Crepitations, see Crackles
Crohn's disease, see Inflammatory bowel disease
Croup, 356, 357

Cushing's disease, 47, 251, 331, 338
Cushing's syndrome, 331
Cyanosis, 42, 83, 88, 116
Cyclothymia, 310
Cystoscopy, 178

Data protection, 15, 30
Deafness, see Hearing impairment
Deep vein thrombosis (DVT), 75, 94
De-escalation, 397
Delirium, 314–15, 405, 407
    causes, 316
Delusions, 311, 312
Dementia, 315, 407, 408
Demyelination, 256
Depression, 307, 324
    postnatal, 307
Deprivation of Liberty Safeguards (DoLS), 306
Dermatitis herpetiformis, 151
Dermatomes, 220, 221, 227, 244
Dermatomyositis, 281, 286, 289
Developmental milestones, 372–3, 374, 375
Dexamethasone suppression test, 351
Diabetes insipidus, 340
Diabetes mellitus, 97, 210, 339, 351
    complications, 266, 271, 337, 338
    type 1, 336
    type 2, 337, 338
Diabetic ketoacidosis (DKA), 345, 346, 358
Diabetic retinopathy, 266, 271
Diarrhoea, 139–40, 158
Differential diagnosis, 3, 29
Digestion, 129, 131–2, 135, 136
Digital rectal examination (DRE), 156
Diplopia, 226, 256, 347
Disorganised thinking, 311
Diverticulosis, 140
Dizziness, 47
Do Not Attempt Cardiopulmonary Resuscitation
    (DNACPR), 34
Down syndrome, 365, 369, 406
Dual process theory, 20–1, 23
Duodenum, 132
Dupuytren's contracture, 150, 172, 287–8, 294
Dysarthria, 51
Dysdiadochokinesis, 245
Dysmenorrhoea, 183, 197

Dyspareunia, 197
Dyspepsia, *see* Heartburn
Dysphagia, 130, 140, 141, 259
Dysphasia, 51
Dysphonia, 51
Dyspnoea, 108, 116
Dyspraxia, 223
Dysthymia, 307
Dystonia, 237
Dysuria, 159–60, 166

Ear, 49
Eating disorders, 314
Echocardiography, 95–6, 125
Electrocardiogram (ECG), 95–6
Electroencephalogram (EEG), 247, 235
Employment, 13, 114, 171, 286
End of life care, 402, 410
Endocarditis, 83, 97
Endometriosis, 197, 203
Endoscopy, 157–8
Epiglottitis, 357
Epilepsy, 316, 232, 247, 248, 316
Epistaxis, 48
Erectile dysfunction, 168
Errors
    clinical, 26, 31
cognitive, 22, 24
Erythema nodosum, 53, 139, 151, 289
Euvolaemia, 56
Exophthalmos, 270, 346, 348
Extrapyramidal system, 233–4
Eye
    anatomy, 255
    movements, 267

Facial movements, 267
Facial nerve, 251–2, 253, 259, 262, 267
Falls, 400–1
Fasciculations, 223
FAST scan, 387–8, 390
Fatigue, 284
    endocrine causes, 334, 337–8
    gastrointestinal causes, 141–2, 158
Femoral stretch test, 295–6
Fibroids, 199, 206

Fibromyalgia, 282
Flight of ideas, 324
Fluid overload, 56, 81, 87, 92, 121, 164, 169, 170, 173
Fluid status, 56
Flap
    hepatic, 150
    respiratory, 116
Foetal lie, 207, 208, 209
Fontanelle, 363, 364
Foot drop, 231
Frailty, 400–1
Frontal lobe, 217
Functional status, 13, 82, 115, 232, 261, 287, 405, 410
Fundoscopy, 226, 271, 350, 371

Gag reflex, 268
Gait, 231, 244, 246, 290, 291, 292
Galactorrhoea, 190, 203
Gall bladder, 134–5
GALS, 290–4
Gangrene, 88
Gas transfer, 105
Gastric outlet obstruction, 130
Gastritis, 130, 143
    autoimmune, 130, 142
Gastroenteritis, 138, 140, 359
Gastrointestinal bleeding, 142–4
Gastro-oesophageal reflux disease (GORD), 130, 136–7, 143
Gastroparesis, 130
Generalised anxiety disorder, 313
Genital examination, 176–7
Giant cell arteritis, 257, 261
Gilbert's disease, 146
Glasgow-Blatchford score, 143
Glasgow Coma Scale (GCS), 386, 387
Glaucoma, 256, 272
Glomerulonephritis, 163
Glossopharyngeal nerve, 263, 268–9
Goitre, 334, 348
Gonadotrophins, 330, 331
Gonads, 335–6
Gottron's papules, 286, 289
Gout, 281, 283
Granuloma annulare, 344

Graves' disease, 334
Group therapy, 306
Growth hormone (GH), 330, 331
Guillain–Barré syndrome, 228
Gynaecomastia, 149, 152

Haemarthrosis, 283
Haematemesis, 143
Haematuria, 168
Haemoglobinopathy, 360
Haemoptysis, 110
Haemorrhoids, 133, 144
Haemothorax, 384
Hair loss, 55
Hallucinations, 310–11
Hand washing, 36–7
Hashimoto's thyroiditis, 334
Head injury, 389
Headache, 229, 231
Head-tilt chin-lift, 381, 383
Hearing impairment, 9–10, 47, 258–9, 267–8,
    410
Heart
    anatomy, 64
    cardiac cycle, 67
    cardiac output, 68
    innervation, 67–8
    stroke volume, 68
Heart attack, see Acute coronary syndrome
Heart failure, 69, 73, 78, 87, 97, 108, 404, 405
Heart rate
    autonomic control, 67–8
bradycardia, 73, 85
    measurement, 38, 42
    tachycardia, 73, 85
Heart sounds, 91–2
Heartburn, 136–7
Heaves, 86, 118–19, 122
Heberden's nodes, 287, 288
Helicobacter pylori, 137, 143
Hemiparesis, 224–5
Hepatic encephalopathy, 135, 150–1
Hepatitis
    autoimmune, 146
    viral, 146
Hepatomegaly, 145, 153, 289
Hernia, 145

Heuristics, 21–3
Hirsutism, 195, 197, 201, 203, 344
Homonymous hemianopia, 257
Hormone replacement therapy (HRT), 187, 190
Horner's syndrome, 117, 121, 270
Human factors, 24, 25–6
Human immunodeficiency virus (HIV), 179
Hypercalcaemia, 340
Hypercholesterolaemia, 82
Hypercortisolism, 331, 338, 340, 351
Hyperemesis gravidarum, 204
Hyperosmolar hyperglycaemic state (HHS), 345,
    346
Hyperprolactinaemia, 203
Hypertension, 88–9
    complications, 39
    pregnancy-induced, 205
Hypertensive retinopathy, 89, 271
Hyperthyroidism, 47, 334, 338, 345
Hypervolaemia, see Fluid overload
Hypocalcaemia, 345
Hypocortisolism, 333, 337, 338, 339, 345, 351
Hypoglossal nerve, 253, 263, 269
Hypoglycaemia, 345, 346
Hypogonadism, 341
Hypomania, 310
Hypospadias, 366
Hypotension, 39
Hypothalamic–pituitary–adrenocortical axis, 332
Hypothalamic–pituitary–gonadal axis, 336
Hypothalamic–pituitary–ovarian axis, 186, 197
Hypothalamic–pituitary–thyroid axis, 334
Hypothalamus, 329
Hypothetico-deductive reasoning, 20
Hypothyroidism, 47, 334–5, 337, 338, 348
Hypovolaemia, 56, 86, 88, 344, 345, 384–5
Hysteroscopy, 209

Ileum, 132
Illness script, 20
Illusions, 324
Immunisations, 361
Infertility, see Subfertility
Inflammatory bowel disease (IBD), 133, 138, 139,
    140, 144, 145–6
Insight, 317, 325–6
Inspection, 58

Insulin, 342, 343, 351
Intermenstrual bleeding, 195–6
Interpreters, 407, 410
Interstitial lung disease, 108, 109, 114
Intoxication, 397
Intrauterine growth restriction (IUGR), 207
Iris, 270
Irregular periods, 195, 197
Irritable bowel syndrome (IBS), 138
Ishihara plates, 266

Janeway lesions, 42, 82, 97
Jaundice, 147–9, 151
    neonatal, 364
Jaw jerk, 267
Jejunum, 132
Joint aspiration, 298
Joint effusion, 283, 297
Joint pain, *see* Arthralgia
Joint swelling, 283
Joints, 278–9
Jugular venous pressure (JVP), 43–4, 117, 120, 173, 385
    measurement, 43
    physiology, 43
    waveform, 44

Kayser–Fleischer rings, 152
Kernig's sign, 369, 370
Kidney
    examination, 155–6, 176
    function, 160–4
Knight's move thinking, 324
Koilonychia, 42, 150
Korsakoff's syndrome, 232
Kussmaul's respiration, 358
Kyphoscoliosis, 117
Kyphosis, 117, 289, 294, 299, 366

Labyrinthitis, 258, 260
Lactation, 183
Language, 217, 223, 246
Learning difficulties, 9, 406–7
Learning disability, 406–7
Left ventricular hypertrophy, 89

Leg length, 296
Leg swelling, 75–7, 112
Leukaemia, 360
Leukonychia, 42, 150, 173
Libido, 309, 341
Lid lag, 348
Ligaments, 279
Limb ischaemia, 88
    signs, 94
Liver, 134, 135
    examination, 155
'Log roll' manoeuvre, 389, 390
Lower urinary tract symptoms (LUTS), 166–7
Lumbar puncture (LP), 247, 325
Lung fibrosis, 107, 108, 120, 289, 299
Lungs
    anatomy, 102
    physiology, 105–6, 125
Lymphadenopathy, 46, 117, 175, 177, 190, 348, 359, 370

Macrocephaly, 363, 375
Macrosomia, 206
Macular degeneration, 266, 271
Magnetic resonance imaging (MRI), 247, 272, 298, 325, 350
Malabsorption, 131, 139
Malar flush, 91
Mallory–Weiss tear, 143
Malnutrition, 158
Mammography, 209
Management plans, 32–3
Mania, 307–10, 312, 324
    drug-induced, 310
Mastitis, 190, 191
Meconium, 363
Median nerve, 222, 239
Medicolegal records, 15
Melaena, 144
Memory, 246
Meningitis, 358–9
Menopause, 186–7
Menorrhagia, 183, 194, 210, 341
Menstrual cycle, 185–7
Mental Capacity Act, 306
Mental Health Act, 306
Mental state examination (MSE), 320–6

Metabolic acidosis, 358
Metacognition, 26
Microcephaly, 363
Microsomia, 206
Migraine, 229
    hemiplegic, 215
Milia, 364
Mini-mental state examination (MMSE), 324
Mistakes, *see* Errors
Mitral regurgitation, 86, 87
Mitral stenosis, 87
Mongolian spot, 364
Mononeuropathy, 226, 256
Mood, 307–10, 322
Morning sickness, 204
Moro reflex, 367
Motor neurone disease, 235
Multidisciplinary team (MDT), 235, 401, 407
Multimorbidity, 409–10
Multiple sclerosis (MS), 235, 261
Murmurs, 86–7, 92–3
Muscle fibres, 279
Muscles, 279
Myalgia, 282
Myalgic encephalomyelitis (ME), *see* Chronic
        fatigue syndrome
Myocardial infarction (MI), *see* Acute coronary
        syndrome
Myocytes, 279

Nail changes, 41–2
    cardiovascular disease, 82–3
    gastrointestinal disease, 150, 154
    genitourinary disease, 173, 176
    musculoskeletal disease, 286, 288
    respiratory disease, 116
    thyroid disease, 347
Nail pitting, 286
Nausea, 140, 142
Neck masses, 45–6
Necrobiosis lipoidica diabeticorum, 53, 344
Neglect, 399
Neonates, 355
Nephritic syndrome, 163
Nephron, 160–2
Nephrotic syndrome, 163
Nerve conduction studies, 247

Nerve entrapment, 282–3, 288
Nerve root, 220, 222, 227, 238, 239, 240
Neurofibromatosis, 233, 234, 259
Neurons, 303
Neurotransmitters, 303–4
Nipple
    discharge, 190
    inversion, 192
Non-accidental injury, 360
Non-alcoholic fatty liver disease (NAFLD), 134, 158
Non-epileptic attack disorder (NEAD), 74, 228, 230
Nystagmus, 245, 267

Obesity, 134, 146, 153, 197, 203, 211
Obsessive–compulsive disorder (OCD), 313
Occipital lobe, 217
Oculomotor, 251, 252, 262, 267
Oedema, 75–6, 153, 173, 176, 409
Oesophagus, 129
Olfactory nerve, 251, 253, 262, 263
Oligohydramnios, 206–7
Oligomenorrhoea, 195, 341
Onycholysis, 42, 286
Ophthalmoplegia, 346–7, 348
Ophthalmoscopy, *see* Fundoscopy
Optic atrophy, 271
Optic chiasm, 254
Optic nerve, 251, 253, 254, 262, 263–6
Optic tract, 254, 257
Oral glucose tolerance test (OGTT), 351
Oropharynx, 50–1
Orthopnoea, 78
Orthostatic hypotension, 400
Ortolani's test, 366
Osler's nodes, 42, 82, 84, 97
Ossification, 277–8
Osteoarthritis, 281, 283, 287, 288
Osteoblasts, 278
Osteoclasts, 278
Osteomyelitis, 359
Otoscopy, 48, 50, 371
Ovary, 184–5, 186

Paget's disease of the breast, 192
Pain, 78, 403, 410
Palliative care, 402–3

Pallor, 151, 201
Palmar crease, 365
Palmar erythema, 42, 149, 150, 206, 347
Palmar grasp reflex, 367
Palpation, 57, 58
Palpitations, 70, 341
    associated symptoms, 72
    causes, 70, 73
    history, 71–2
Pancreas, 134, 336–7
Pancreatitis, 138–9, 140
Papilloedema, 271
Paraparesis, 225–6
Parasympathetic nervous system, 68, 251
Parathyroid gland, 335
Parathyroid hormone (PTH), 330, 340
Parietal lobe, 217
Parkinsonism, 232, 234, 235, 236, 317
Patellar tap, 292, 293, 294, 297
Patent ductus arteriosus, 355
Peau d'orange, 191
Pelvic examination, 202
Pelvic inflammatory disease (PID), 203
Pelvic pain, 197–8, 203
Pelvic prolapse, 197–8
Penis, 165
Per rectum (PR) examination, see Digital rectal
        examination
Percussion, 57, 58–9
Paroxysmal nocturnal dyspnoea (PND), 78
Pectus carinatum, 117–18
Pectus excavatum, 117–18
Peptic ulcer disease (PUD), 137, 143, 144
Perception, 324
Percussion, 58–9, 123
Pericarditis, 68–9, 385
Perioperative medicine, 404–5
Peripheral nervous system (PNS), 215, 216,
        219–20
Peripheral neuropathy, 227, 228, 350
Peripheral pulses, 51–2, 66, 95
Peripheral vascular disease (PVD), 69, 88, 94–5
Personality disorders, 314, 315
Perthes' disease, 360
Pets, 115
Phaeochromocytoma, 333, 345
Phalen's test, 295
Phobias, 313–14

Pituitary gland, 186, 330
    anatomy, 331
    apoplexy, 330
Placenta praevia, 204
Placental abruption, 204
Plantar fasciitis, 282
Plantar response, 243
Pleurae, 104
Pleural effusion, 107, 108, 111, 120, 385
Pleural rub, 119
Pleuritis, 69, 110
Pneumonia, 107, 108, 110, 120, 357
Pneumothorax, 69, 107, 108, 110–11, 120, 385
Polycystic kidney disease, 174
Polycystic ovarian syndrome (PCOS), 197, 203, 341
Polydipsia, 339
    psychogenic, 341
Polyhydramnios, 206–7
Polymyalgia rheumatica, 281
Polymyositis, 281, 289
Polyuria, 339, 341, 346
Popliteal cyst, 77
Port wine stain, 364
Postcoital bleeding, 195
Posterior drawer test, 297
Postmenopausal bleeding, 196
Post-traumatic stress disorder (PTSD), 313
Postural drop, see Orthostatic hypotension
Poverty of thought, 324
Pre-eclampsia, 205
Pregnancy, 186, 187, 188
    examination, 207–9
    physiological changes, 188, 204, 206
Presbyacusis, 258
Pressure of thought, 324
Pretibial myxoedema, 348
Priapism, 389
Primary biliary cholangitis, 146
Primary sclerosing cholangitis, 146
Primary survey, 377–8, 380–8
Prolactin, 331, 341
Proprioception, 227, 231, 244
Prostate, 164, 175
Pseudogout, 281, 283
Psoriasis, 288, 289
Psoriatic arthritis, 281, 286, 288
Psychodynamic psychotherapy, 305
Psychology, 305–6

Psychomotor agitation, 308, 322
Psychomotor retardation, 308
Psychosis, 310–12, 316
    causes, 312
Ptosis, 267, 270
Pulmonary embolus, 110, 112, 405
Pulmonary stenosis, 355
Pulse
    character, 86, 90, 91, 173
    volume, 86
Pupil, 253, 256, 270
Pupillary reflex, 264
Pyelonephritis, 137–8, 359
Pyloric stenosis, 369
Pyoderma gangrenosum, 53, 151

Questioning style, 6–7

Radial nerve, 222, 226, 239
Radio-femoral delay, 52, 85, 91, 92
Radio-radial delay, 85, 91, 92
Ramsay Hunt syndrome, 259
Rapport, 10, 11, 322, 406
Rash, 54, 55, 358–9
Reactive arthritis, 281
Recreational drugs, 310, 320
Red flags, 27, 28, 374
Reflective practice, 26
Reflexes, 235, 236, 238, 243, 346
Regurgitation, 141
Relative afferent pupillary defect, 264
Renal calculi, 359
Renal replacement therapy, 164, 173, 176, 179
Renin–angiotensin–aldosterone system, 333
Respiratory buffering, 108
Respiratory distress, 368
Respiratory failure, 106, 126
Respiratory rate
    bradypnoea, 85
    measurement, 40
    tachypnoea, 85
Retina, 253–4, 257, 266
Rheumatoid arthritis, 281, 286, 287, 288, 289, 299
Rheumatoid nodules, 286, 289
Rinne's test, 267, 269
Risk, 25

Risk assessment
    cardiovascular, 82
    psychiatric, 320

Safeguarding alert, 298–9
Sarcopenia, 400
Schizophrenia, 311, 312, 321, 324
    negative symptoms, 312, 313
Schober's test, 295, 296
Sciatic nerve, 222, 240
Sciatic stretch test, 295
Sclera, 270
Scleritis, 286, 288
Scleroderma, 152, 281, 288
Scoliosis, 117, 294, 366
Scotoma, 257
Scrubs, 6
Secondary survey, 377–8, 389
Seizures, 228–30, 231, 397
Selective serotonin reuptake inhibitors (SSRIs), 304
Self-harm, 309, 314, 320
Self-neglect, 321
Sensation, 227, 243–4
Sensitivity, 31
Septic arthritis, 281, 283, 360
Serum osmolality, 350
Sexually transmitted infections (STIs), 169, 179, 198
Short bowel syndrome, 130
Sicca, 130
Sickle cell disease, 172
Sinoatrial node, 67
Sjögren's syndrome, 130, 281, 288
Skin
    examination, 55
    history, 53
Smell, 258
Smoking, 13–14, 81, 109, 113, 126, 147, 171, 204, 232, 261, 286, 320
Smooth muscle, 279
Snellen chart, 264–5
Space-occupying lesion, 255
Spasticity, 233, 238
Specificity, 31
Speech, 51, 217, 245, 259, 322
Spider naevi, 149, 152
Spina bifida, 366

Spinal cord, 217, 220
    anatomy, 218
Spinal nerves, 220, 222
Spirometry, 409
Spleen, 135
    examination, 155
Splenomegaly, 145, 153, 289
Splinter haemorrhages, 42, 286, 288
Sputum, 109–10, 125
Steatorrhoea, 140
Stepping reflex, 367
Steroids, 285
Stomach epithelium, 131
Stork bite, 364
Stridor, 112, 356, 382
Stroke, 224–5, 235, 248, 259, 261
Stye, 270
Subarachnoid haemorrhage, 228
Subfertility, 203, 341
Sucking reflex, 367
Suicidality, 309, 320
Summarising, 29–30
Swallowing, 51
Swan neck deformity, 287, 288
Symphyseal fundal height (SFH), 206–7, 208
Synapses, 303–4
Syncope, 72, 73
Systemic lupus erythematosus (SLE), 286, 288, 289

Tachycardia, see Heart rate
Tachypnoea, see Respiratory rate
Tactile vocal fremitus, 118, 119, 122
Taste, 258
Telangiectasia, 152
Temporal arteritis, see Giant cell arteritis
Temporal lobe, 217
Tendon, 282
Tendonitis, 282
Tertiary survey, 377–8, 391
Testes, 165
    pain, 169, 170
    undescended, 366
Thirst, 339–41, 346
Thrills, 87, 91
Thought blocking, 346
Thought disorder, 324
Thyroid acropachy, 347

Thyroid examination, 347–9
Thyroid gland, 333–5
Thyroid-stimulating hormone (TSH), 331
Tinel's test, 295
Tone, 223, 233–4, 238
Tonometry, 272
Tourette's syndrome, 237
Trachea
    anatomy, 102
    deviation, 118, 122
Tracheitis, 356–7
Transient ischaemic attack (TIA), 248
Treatment escalation planning, 33–4, 392
Tremor, 116, 234, 245, 345, 347
Trendelenburg's test, 297
Triadic communication, 406
Trichotillomania, 322
Trigeminal nerve, 251, 253, 262, 267
Trochlear nerve, 251, 253, 262, 267
Trousseau's sign, 345
Tuberculosis (TB), 113, 126
Tuberous sclerosis, 233
Turner's syndrome, 365, 369

Ulcerative colitis (UC), see Inflammatory bowel
    disease
Ulcers
    genital, 174
    limb, 78–9, 88, 344, 350
    mouth, 152, 288
    peptic, 130
Ulnar nerve, 222, 226, 239
Ultrasound, 390
    foetal, 210
    joint, 298
    transvaginal, 209, 210
Unequal pulses, 85–6
Ureters, 164
Urethra, 164
Urethral discharge, 169
Urinalysis, 178
Urinary tract infection (UTI), 359
Urine output, 40–1
Urticaria, 358
Uterine tubes, 185
Uterus, 184, 186
Uvular deviation, 268

Vagina, 184
Vaginal discharge, 198
Vagus nerve, 252, 253, 263, 268–9
Valves, 92
Varices, 143
Vasculitis, 358
Vasovagal syncope, 74
Veins, 66
Ventilation, 104–6
Ventricular septal defect (VSD), 355
Ventricular tachycardia, 73, 85
Vestibulocochlear nerve, 252, 253, 262, 267–8
Visual acuity, 264–5
Visual fields, 263, 265
Visual impairment, 9, 256–8, 260
Visual neglect, 265–6
Visual pathways, 254
Vitiligo, 289
Vocal cords, 259
Vocal resonance, 119, 120

Vomiting, 140, 142, 362
Vulnerable adult, 398
Vulva, 184, 201

Walking aids, 287
Weakness, 223–6, 235, 238, 284, 345–6
    fatiguable, 226
Weber's test, 267, 269
Weight
    change, 338–9
    loss, 144–5
Wheeze, 112, 119
White coat, 6
    hypertension, 89

Xanthelasma, 91, 151
Xanthomata, 84, 90
X-ray, 124–5, 157, 390